Fragments for a History of the Human Body   Part One

Fragments for a
History of the Human Body

Part One

Edited by Michel Feher

with Ramona Naddaff and Nadia Tazi

Editors: Jonathan Crary, Michel Feher, Hal Foster, Sanford Kwinter

Special Editor of this Issue: Michel Feher

Associate Editors of this Issue: Ramona Naddaff, Nadia Tazi

Managing Editor: Ramona Naddaff

Designer: Bruce Mau

Translation Editor: Siri Hustvedt

Translations: Anna Cancogni, Lydia Davis, Roger Friedman, Janet Lloyd, Ughetta Lubin, Ralph Manheim, Sarah Matthews, Ian Patterson, Alyson Waters.

Editorial Assistance: Judith Aminoff, Ted Byfield, Reynolds Childress, Barbara Czarnecki, Deborah Drier, Meighan Gale, Freya Godard, Astrid Hustvedt, Mike Taylor, Nancy Worman.

Production: Steven Bock, John Calvelli, Alison Hahn, Anita Matusevics, Damian McShane, Susan Meggs-Becker, Greg Van Alstyne, Dorothy Vreeker.

Picture Research: CLAM! (Christine de Coninck, Anne Mensior) and Marie-Hélène Agueros.

Special thanks to: Archie, Ron Date, Mark Elvin, Mickey Fear, Madeleine Feher, Albert Fuss, Marvin Green, Judith Gurewich, Krista Hinds, Jonathan Joaquin, Barbara Kerr, Gus Kiley, Kerri Kwinter, Rick Lambert, G.E.R. Lloyd, Janet Lloyd, Sandra Naddaff, Lisa Naftolin, Mary Picone, John Scinocco, Alice Sindzingre, Mike Tibre.

Typesetting by Canadian Composition.

Film Preparation by P.B.C. Lithoprep.

Printed in Canada by Provincial Graphics.

Distributed by The MIT Press, Cambridge, Massachusetts and London, England.

We gratefully acknowledge translation assistance provided for this volume by the French Ministry of Culture and Communication.

© 1989 Urzone, Inc.
ZONE 611 Broadway Suite 838
New York, NY 10012
All rights reserved.

First printing February, 1989
Second printing April, 1990

ISSN: 0887-0411
ISBN: 0-942299-25-6 (cloth)
ISBN: 0-942299-23-X (paper)

Library of Congress Catalog Card Number: 88-051439

ZONE 3

Contents

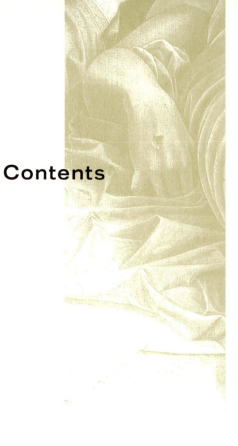

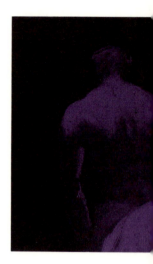

Introduction

Michel Feher

The history recorded by the following collection of essays is the history of that area where life and thought intersect. This intersection is complex, often turbulent, for the vital processes cannot fuel figures of thought without causing them to renew themselves, while concepts that attempt to reflect the living being cannot do so without constantly altering its direction. The human body affected by such interchanges is therefore transformed in response to their modalities, that is, in response to the different strategies adopted by life and thought in order to carry out their respective plans — through, and despite, one another. The changes undergone by the body — sometimes acting as an obstacle to the intelligence and sometimes as its springboard, sometimes expressing the entire universe and sometimes disappearing completely as an autonomous entity — are therefore quite real. They proceed, as Marcel Mauss put it, from body techniques which mingle physical capacities and mental mechanisms to form a body adapted to circumstances: the body of a charismatic citizen or of a visionary monk, a mirror image of the world or a reflection of the spirit.

Regarded in this light, the history of the human body is not so much the history of its representations as of its modes of construction. For the history of its representations always refers to a real body considered to be "without history" — whether this be the organism observed by the natural sciences, the body proper as perceived by phenomenology, or the instinctual, repressed body on which psychoanalysis is based — whereas the history of its modes of construction can, since it avoids the overly massive oppositions of science and ideology or of authenticity and alienation, turn the body into a thoroughly historicized and completely problematic issue. Even though the problems inherent in this issue cannot be solved once and for all, an understanding of them remains crucial if we are to acquire what Michel Foucault has called "a thickened perception of the present," or, in this case, of the body we construct for ourselves. By comparing earlier and foreign constructions with those through which we perceive our bodies today, and even more importantly by studying transformations that affect body techniques and the new problems they contain, we can define more precisely the current boundaries of an ethics of the body. This ethics goes beyond a mere determination of which values will best protect us against an epidemic fed by our carnal desires, or against the growing confusion between man and machine, or against the dissociation of procreation and sexuality. For we must first ask ourselves who or what we take the body to be when we perceive it as an immune system threatened on all sides, even by its own functions; when we seek to discover in ourselves the particular, saving deficiency that distinguishes us from machines without throwing us back to an animal state; or when the uterus no longer appears to be the unequivocal, silent locus that perpetuates the species. At the intersection of the confusions of our lives and the uneasy peregrinations of our thoughts, these questions, among many others, outline a picture of a contemporary body. Nevertheless, only by adopting a historical and pragmatic perspective can we both appreciate what is really new in its appearance and also spot certain marks of age that hint at transformations yet to come.

As the notion of fragment implies, the essays that make up these three volumes do not pretend either to form a complete survey or to define a compact portion of the history of the human body. The fact that so many problems are addressed only indicates the extent of the field to be explored and marks several axes along which current research is moving, so that the consistency of these fragments lies in a cross section in which the connections among different disciplines – history, anthropology, philosophy, etc. – are highlighted rather than in a general overview or a strictly delimited schema.

Deciding on an order for these articles was not an easy task: for one thing, the price paid for collecting "living" material was that some studies could not be finished in time for publication and others changed focus along the way. But what presented a greater problem was the fact that most of these texts are interrelated in more ways than one – through similarity of subject or methodology, historical continuity, geographical proximity – so that any one sequence disrupted some other that might have been just as pertinent. However, in the end we were forced to choose and opted for identifying three main approaches and devoting one volume to each.

The first approach, which may be regarded as a vertical axis, begins at the "top" and measures the distance and proximity between divinity and the human body. These measurements, however, are not taken in order to investigate the presence or absence of anthropomorphism in the conception of divinity. The question to be asked here then is not: given the human body, how does a warrior of ancient Greece or a Christian mystic of the late Middle Ages, a Spanish Kabbalist or a Daoist master, imagine his or her gods? But rather the opposite: what kind of body do these same Greeks, Christians, Jews or Chinese endow themselves with – or attempt to acquire – given the power they attribute to the divine? A practical question, since it amounts to asking oneself what exercises to do in order to resemble a god physically or to commune sensually with him. Should one strive to maintain one's vigor – one's "form" – and achieve a graceful mastery of one's gestures; or should one, on the contrary, expose the flesh to suffering, bruise it and inflict it with the most atrocious privations? Or perhaps it is the human couple that comes closest to resembling the god that created them through a judicious use of their power to procreate.

And conversely, we will examine what it is about the human constitution that prevents man from participating in divine perfection: it may be the lusts of the flesh that carve out a canal from the genitals to the soul in which the devil is swallowed up; or perhaps after each meal, man's digestive system draws him into a world of corruption and decay.

This last question invites us to follow the vertical axis to its "bottom," that is, to the threshold between not only human and animal but also between the living organism and the mechanical contrivances purported to be inanimate which imitate or simulate it. Here again, though what we are looking at are monstrous doubles of the human body, the point is not so much to show how they parallel a supposedly known organism, as to discover how their monstrousness affects the human body by contaminating it.

To put it another way, the problem is not so much to list images of animals or automatons as so many deforming combinations or copies that more or less conform to a human standard, but rather to make use of these same images — werewolf or marionette, chimera or robot, as well as a few hungry ghosts — in order to see what deformities we attribute to our own bodies, deformities which — unhappily or perhaps happily — pull us in the direction of animals and automatons.

The second axis of this exploration is transversal, in the sense that it concentrates on psychosomatic relations, how the "inside" relates to the "outside." Its initial question involves what the Western world calls the human soul: life principle, vector of intelligence, candidate for salvation or damnation. Invisible, even immaterial for some, it can nevertheless be contained within a man's body, express itself in his face and make itself known through his gestures. Thus, by observing the features and postures of an individual, one can catch his soul in the act and discover his true nature by interpreting what it demands of his body or what his body reveals without his knowing it. Yet if one applies a pragmatic point of view to this hermeneutics, one no longer tries to find out which soul or which conception of the soul is revealed by the body's attitudes but which regions of the body are mobilized and which types of discipline are imposed on it in order to produce the soul of a hero, a saint or a perfect courtier. Conversely, one may wonder what particular lack of discipline in gestures or features not only signifies depravity or ignominy but actually creates it — so that a feeling such as racial hatred becomes more the result of a specific cultural construction than of a universal fear of the "other."

After exploring the conformation of the soul we go on to the second fundamental articulation of "inside" and "outside," the modulation of the emotions and of the erotic in particular. Once again, the point is not so much to start with a supposedly universal emotion and examine the different ways it is expressed, as it is to insist on the singularity of the emotions immanent in the ceremonies that produce them. Not that the transports of love are artificial; but they do not exist outside a certain setting, that is, a stylization of movements and poses, each of which includes its own particular intensifications and deviations. They are comprised within a history of erotic modes, or more generally of emotional structures. Thus, several specific rituals are examined — from the *asag* in courtly love to the *geerewol* among the Wodaabe of Niger — as well as certain long-term processes of transformation — the art and the meaning of dress and undress as depicted in Western art, for example, or the adventures of both heart and body in China during the past 150 years.

Beyond the vagaries of desire and the exigencies of the soul, the body is further agitated by sensations and afflictions issuing from its "depths," that is, from a dark and mysterious interior, capable of infecting the mind and affecting the individual's relations with the outside world. At the limits of anatomy and of psychism, cenesthesia has never ceased to be a subject of intense speculation, from the mixture and balancing of the humors to the networks of nerves, including all the correspondences between microcosm and macrocosm. Indeed, the affects which make up our relationship to the inside of the body testify to the conformity or lack of conformity between a certain image of the soul and a certain map of the organism. Pleasure, suffering — physical and mental — and, even more, death itself constitute a series of inevitable nodes in the intersection of life and thought.

Yet one must take care not to endow these events with an absolute transcendence, whether in the form of the "meaninglessness" of pain and death, which would render all efforts at thinking futile, or in the form of a message, a cry from the body or from life, more real than any speech. Rather, illness and death appear as the nerve sites of both life's ritualization and life's problematization, in particular where the linking of psychic and somatic are concerned. Here, an examination of attitudes and concepts developed by Japanese healers, Indian Brahmans and Church Fathers allows us to refine the overly hasty and overly neat distinction made between Western dualism and Eastern monism or holism.

Finally, the last approach, taken in the third volume of this exploration, plays on the classical distinction between organ and function. The goal here is not, however, to separate organicism and functionalism — if indeed that debate is still alive — but to analyze the uses of certain organs and bodily substances as metaphors for or models of the functioning of human society, on the one hand, and, on the other, to describe several remarkable characteristics attributed to certain bodies because of the status of the individuals they incarnate, that is, the position they occupy in a certain conception of the social body, or even of the organization of the universe. To put it another way, the organ tends either to imply the function or, on the contrary, to challenge it, while the function makes the body of the person filling that function the organ of a larger body.

Where the organs are concerned, the reason for resorting to a metaphor or to an organic model is essentially to naturalize a political institution, a social hierarchy or a moral principle: it is, one might say, the ideological aspect of things. This is the case when the sovereignty of the Pope or of royalty seeks legitimacy in the fact that a State needs a "head," or that a society needs a "heart." This is the case when the necessity for man's domination of woman is ascribed to the superiority of sperm, with its formative power, over the merely nourishing qualities of female milk and blood. This is the case when what happens to female sexuality within marriage is attributed to a maturation process that shifts orgasm from the clitoris to the vagina. Yet it is less interesting to examine ideology as a whole — especially because such a notion implies the existence of a true, non-ideological nature — than it is to point out the practical differences and often unforeseeable theoretical consequences involved in various redundant modes of naturalization or various uses of the same organ. For different types of political or social domination are involved when it is the heart rather than the head imposing its supremacy; or when a rotten tooth, symbol of vice, is pulled in public rather than in private; or when sperm, milk and blood are seen as different in nature or merely in quality. What is more, the application of organic models to politics actually has the reciprocal effect of producing political or at least agonistic metaphors for organic life: rivalries between head, heart and liver within the organism, or even more strikingly, between male and female seeds within the embryo.

Where the function is concerned, we examine the fate of bodies that are assigned a pivotal position in perpetuating life or maintaining the social order: abused bodies such as the Roman Empire's slaves or Victorian prostitutes; bodies that are sacrificed in order to preserve the energy of the cosmos, as in Aztec rituals, or to foster economic growth in the West when there is a gap between profit and health; and finally, the bodies of royalty, whose fate is often scarcely more enviable, as in the case of the bodies of central African kings, which functioned as a sort of barometer of the world's fertility and consequently became potential sacrifices for the slightest fault. As in the case, too, of the Roman emperor, who was deified upon his death so as more effectively to prevent his taking himself for a god during his lifetime. As in the case, lastly, of the monarch by divine right as Pascal saw him, whose worldly splendor was merely a vain appearance intended to hide his true greatness, a great-

ness modelled on the passion of Christ on the Cross – which returns us to the relation between "top" and "bottom." This tortuous, fragmented and open-ended progress of essays ends, therefore, with a catalogue – itself necessarily still "in progress" –
of works devoted to the history of the human body.

Translated by Lydia Davis.

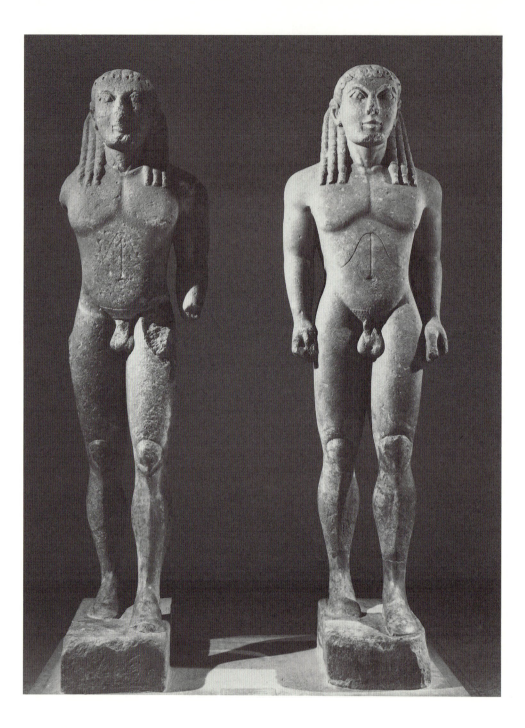

Kouroi of Cleobis and Biton, 6th century B.C. As a reward for the deeds they had just performed, Cleobis and Biton's mother, a priestess of Hera, asked that her sons may have that which is best for man. In answer to this prayer, Hera granted the two brothers, who were sleeping in the temple, never to wake up and to die at the height of their youth, in the splendor of their virile beauty — like gods — as we see them here (Delphi Museum).

Dim Body, Dazzling Body

Jean-Pierre Vernant

The body of the gods. How does this expression pose a problem for us? Can gods who have bodies — anthropomorphic gods like those of the ancient Greeks — really be considered gods? Six centuries before Christ, Xenophanes already protested the possibility of such a thing, denouncing the foolishness of mortals who believe they can measure the divine by the yardstick of their own nature: "Men believe that, like themselves, the gods have clothing, language and a body."[1] An identical body for gods and men? "The Ethiopians claim that their gods are flat-nosed and black-skinned; the Thracians, that they are blue-eyed and have red hair."[2] Why not an animal's body, then, Xenophanes ironically asks: "If oxen, horses and lions had hands with which to draw and make works like men, horses would represent the gods in the likeness of a horse, oxen in that of an ox, and each one would make for them a body like the one he himself possessed."[3]

These remarks made by the Greek poet-philosopher are conveyed to us by Clement of Alexandria in his *Stromata*, written in the second century A.D. Clement wishes to show that through the light of reason the wisest of the ancients were able to recognize the vanity of idolatry and mock the gods of Homer — those puppets invented by man in his own image, with all his faults, vices, passions and weaknesses.

That in his polemic against "false gods" a Church Father should make use of criticisms voiced by a pagan philosopher who takes a distance from the collective beliefs of a religion in which divinity occasionally appears in a too human light, is fair play. But it is certainly not the surest and most suitable way to approach the problem of the body of the gods in ancient Greece. To do this, one must put oneself in the very framework of polytheism and adopt its perspective.

Would the Greeks, in representing the gods to themselves, really have attributed

19

to them the form of corporeal existence that is proper to all perishable creatures here on earth? To pose the question in these terms would be to admit, from the outset, that for human beings "the body" is a given, a fact, one that is immediately evident, a "reality" inscribed in nature and, as such, beyond question. In the case of the Greeks, the difficulty arises only from their apparently having projected the notion of a body onto beings who, insofar as they are divine, are situated outside the body's legitimate sphere of application, since they are, by definition, supernatural and belong to the other world, the beyond.

But one can also approach the problem from the opposite angle and direct one's inquiry to the body itself, no longer posited as a fact of nature, a constant and universal reality, but as an entirely problematic notion, a historical category, steeped in imagination (to use Le Goff's expression), and one which must, in every case, be deciphered within a particular culture by defining the functions it assumes and the forms it takes on within that culture. Therefore, the real question can be formulated as: what was the body for the Greeks? Today the concept of the body gives us the illusion of self-evidence for essentially two reasons: first, because of the definitive opposition between soul and body, spiritual and material, that has established itself in our Western tradition. And consequently and correspondingly, because the body, reduced entirely to matter, depends on positivistic study; in other words, it has acquired the status of a scientific object defined in anatomical and physiological terms.

The Greeks contributed to this "objectification" of the body in two ways. First of all, within the religious context of the sectarian cults — whose teaching was later taken up and transposed by Plato into the field of philosophy — they elaborated a new notion of the soul, an immortal soul which man must isolate and purify in order to separate it from a body whose role has now become nothing more than that of a receptacle or tomb. Then, through medical practice and medical literature, the Greeks investigated the body, observing, describing, theorizing about its visible aspects, its parts, the internal organs that compose it, their function and the diverse humors that circulate in it and direct its health or illness.

But the affirmation of the presence of a noncorporeal element within us which is related to the divine and which is "our selves," like the naturalistic approach to the body, marks more than just a turning point in Greek culture: it marks a kind of rupture.

In this respect, despite Clement, Xenophanes is a good witness to that which, in reference to the most ancient Greek philosophers, one might perhaps call the pre-Socratic body. Although he lampoons the heterogeneous and restless troop of Homeric gods in order to propose a more rigorous and refined conception of divinity, a conception that evokes the spherical One of Parmenides (who some believe was his student),[4] nevertheless, Xenophanes does not radically dissociate divine nature from corporeal reality. Just as he does not postulate the existence of a unique god when he writes, "One god, the greatest among gods and men," he also does not affirm that the gods do not have bodies. Xenophanes merely claims that the body of a god is not like that of a mortal. It is dissimilar for precisely the same reason that a god's thought (*noēma*) – with which he is abundantly endowed – is dissimilar to a man's thought.[5] Dissimilarity of body and dissimilarity of thought are jointly proclaimed in the unity of a formula in which gods' bodies and thoughts are fused by virtue of their common difference to human beings.[6] Like everybody and anybody, a god sees, hears, understands. But for all that, he does not require specialized organs like our eyes and ears. A god is "wholly" seeing, hearing, understanding.[7] He moves without effort or fatigue; without having to budge, without even changing his place, he shakes everything up.[8] In order to traverse the gulf separating god and man, Xenophanes is not led to oppose the corporeal to the noncorporeal, to an immateriality, a pure Spirit; for him, it is enough to acknowledge the contrast between the constant and the changing, the immutable and the mutable, the perfection of that which remains eternally accomplished in the plenitude of itself, and the incompleteness and imperfection of that which is divided, dispersed, partial, transitory, perishable.

The fact is that in the archaic period Greek "corporeity" still does not acknowledge a body/soul distinction, nor does it establish a radical break between the natural and the supernatural. Man's corporeality also includes organic realities, vital forces, psychic activities, divine inspirations or influxes. The same word can refer to these various domains. On the other hand, there is no term that designates the body as an organic unity which supports the individual in the multiplicity of his vital and mental functions. The word *sōma*, translated as body, originally designated a corpse, that is to say, what remains of an individual after his incarnated life and physical vitality have left him, reducing him to a pure inert figure, an effigy. He becomes an object of exhibition and lamentation for others, before he disappears, burned or buried, into invisibility. The term *demas*, used in the accusative, designates not the body but an individual's stature, his size, his build made up of assembled pieces (the verb *demō* signifies the erecting of a construction through superimposed rows, as in a brick wall). It is often used in connection with *eidos* and *phuē*: the visible aspect, the carriage, the imposing appearance of what has grown well. Nor is *chrōs* the body; rather, it is the external envelope, the skin, the surface where there is contact between oneself and an other; it also means flesh-tint, complexion.

To the extent that man is alive, inhabited by force and energy, traversed by drives that move and stir him, his body is plural. The Greek vocabulary of the corporeal is characterized by multiplicity, even when it is a matter of expressing it in its totality. The Greeks use the word *guia*: the bodily members in their suppleness, their articulated mobility, or *melea*, the limbs as bearers of force.

They also use the word *kara*, the head, with a metonymic value: a part for the whole. Even in this case, the head is not equivalent to the body; it is a way of saying "a man himself," as an individual. In death, men are called "heads," but they are heads hooded in night, enveloped in darkness, faceless. Among the living, heads have a countenance, a face, a *prosōpon*; they are there, present before your eyes just as you are present to their eyes. The head, the face is what one sees first in a being, what is revealed of him on the surface; it is what identifies him and makes him recognizable when he is present to the gaze of others.

When one wishes to speak of the body in terms of its vitality, its life force, its emotions, as well as its ability to reflect and know, a host of terms is available: *stēthos, ētor, kardia, phrēn, prapides, thumos, menos, nous*. The values of these words are closely related. They designate, without always distinguishing among them very precisely, bodily parts or organs (heart, lungs, diaphragm, chest, guts); breaths, vapors or liquid juices; feelings, drives, desires; and thoughts, concrete operations of the intellect such as comprehension, recognition, naming and understanding.[9] This intertwining of the physical and the psychological within a self-consciousness that involves itself in the parts of the body is summarized in James Redfield's striking remark that for the Homeric heroes, "the interior I is none other than the organic I."[10]

This vocabulary of, if not the body, then at least the various dimensions or aspects of the corporeal, constitutes in its entirety the code that allowed a Greek to express and think about his relation to himself, his presence to himself, which, depending on the circumstances, was greater or smaller, more or less unified or dispersed. But it connotes equally his relations to others, to whom he is bound by all forms of bodily appearance: face, size, bearing, voice, gestures — what Mauss calls "body techniques" — not to mention all that is related to the olfactory and tactile senses. This vocabulary also encompasses the relation to the divine or supernatural, whose presence within oneself, in and through one's own body, like the outer manifestations in the case of a god's apparitions or epiphanies, expresses itself in the same symbolic register.

To pose the problem of the body of the gods is thus not to ask how the Greeks could have outfitted their gods with human bodies. It is rather an investigation of how this symbolic system functions, how the corporeal code permits one to think of the relation between man and god under the double figures of the same and the other, of the near and far, of contact and separation, while marking between the poles of the human and the divine that which associates them through a play of similitudes, mutual advances, overlapping areas, and dissociates them through the effects of contrast, opposition, incompatibility and mutual exclusion.

From this symbolic system that codifies the relation to oneself, to others and to the divine, I would like to draw attention to certain elements that are pertinent to our subject. Roughly, the problem consists of deciphering all the signs that mark the human body with the seal of limitation, deficiency, incompleteness, and that make it a sub-body. This sub-body cannot be understood except in reference to what it presupposes: corporeal plenitude, a super-body, the body of the gods. We will therefore examine the paradox of the sublimated body, of a divine super-body. By pushing to an extreme all the qualities and bodily values that are present in an always diminished, derivative, faltering and precarious form in man, one is led to endow the divinities with a set of traits which, even in their epiphanic manifestations here below, in their presence among mortals, locates them in an inaccessible beyond and causes them to transgress the corporeal code by means of which they are represented in their relation to humans.

Man and his body are embedded in the course of nature, of *phusis*, which causes all that is born here below to rise, mature, and disappear according to the rhythm of the days, seasons, years and the life span proper to each species.[11] Therefore, man and his body bear the mark of a congenital infirmity; like a stigma, the seal of the impermanent and fleeting is branded on them. In order to exist they must, like plants and other creatures living on the earth, pass through the successive phases of growth and decline: after childhood and youth, the body matures and expands in the strength of manhood, and then, when old age comes, it changes, weakens, becomes ugly and dilapidated, until it is engulfed forever in the night of death.

It is this inconstant body, vulnerable to the vicissitudes of time flowing without return, that makes human beings the creatures whom the Greeks, in order to be contrasted with "those who exist eternally"[12] — the gods endowed with the perpetuity of their full presence — have baptized with the term "the ephemeral ones," beings whose lives unfold in the quotidian, the day to day, in the narrow limits of a changing and unstable "now" whose continuity and future is always uncertain.

The human body is ephemeral. This does not merely signify that, no matter how beautiful, how strong, how perfect it may appear to be, it is destined for decrepitude and death; but, in a more essential way, it means that since nothing in it is immutable, the vital energies it deploys and the psychological and physical forces it puts into play can remain in a state of plenitude for only a brief moment. They are exhausted as soon as they become active. Like a fire that consumes itself as it burns and which must continuously be fed in order to keep it from going out, the human body functions in alternating phases of expenditure and recuperation. It does not function along a continuous line or at a constant level of intensity, but in cycles punctuated by more or less complete or lasting eclipses, pauses or fade-outs. Sleep follows waking as its necessary counterpart; every effort brings on lassitude and demands time for rest. When in any particular activity the body is put to task or strained, it must restore the inner loss, the decrease in energy that hunger soon signals and which finds only provisional remedy in the satiety of a meal. If, in order to survive, man must endlessly sit down to a meal and eat in order to abate the depletion of his forces, it is because those forces weaken with use. The more intensely arduous an activity, the more serious and difficult it is to overcome the consequent weakness.

In this way, death does not only stand out in the lives of men as the end that unremittingly limits the horizon of their existence: it is there every day, every moment, ensconced in life itself, like the hidden face of a condition of existence

24

in which the two opposing positive and negative poles — being and its privation — are again inextricably intertwined: no birth without death, no waking without sleep, no lucidity without unconsciousness, no tension without relaxation. The other side of a luminous youthful body is an ugly faded one. The body is the agent and instrument of actions, powers and forces which can only deploy themselves at the price of a loss of energy, a failure, a powerlessness caused by a congenital weakness. *Thanatos*, Death, might borrow the mask of his twin brother *Hupnos*, Sleep, or assume the appearance of some of his sinister associates — *Ponos, Limos, Gēras* — who incarnate the human ills of fatigue, hunger and old age. (Through their mother *Nux*, the Dark Night, they are all children of the same lineage, and like Death himself, they are the issue of *Chaos*, the original Chasm, the dark, primordial Abyss that existed before anything had form, solidity and foundation.)[13] But it is always Death, in person or by delegation, who sits within the intimacy of the human body, like a witness to its fragility. Tied to all the nocturnal powers of confusion, to a return to the indistinct and unformed, Death, associated with the tribe of his kin — Sleep, Fatigue, Hunger, Old Age — denounces the failure, the incompleteness of a body of which neither its visible aspect — contours, radiance, external beauty — nor its inner forces of desire, feeling, thoughts and plans are ever perfectly pure. They are never radically separated from that part of darkness and nonbeing which the world inherited from its "chaotic" origin and which remains, even in the cosmos organized and now presided over by Zeus, a stranger to the luminous domain of the divine, to its constant, inexhaustible vitality.

Thus, for the Greeks of the archaic period, man's misfortune is not that a divine and immortal soul finds itself imprisoned in the envelope of a material and perishable body, but that his body is not fully one. It does not possess, completely and definitively, that set of powers, qualities and active virtues which bring to an individual being's existence a constant, radiant, enduring life in a pure, totally alive state, a life that is imperishable because it is free from any seed of corruption and divorced from what could, from within or without, darken, wither and annihilate it.

Although they belong to the same universe as men, the gods are of a different race: they are the *athanatoi*, the nonmortals, the *ambrotoi*, the ones who do not perish.

The designation is paradoxical because, in order to make a comparison with human beings, it defines those beings whose bodies and lives possess complete positivity — without lack or defect — through negation, absence. The paradox is instructive because it implies that in order to think of the divine life and body, the required reference or point of departure for the Greeks is this defective body — this mortal life which they themselves experienced each day. To be sure, the mortal body is their point of departure so that they might better disengage themselves from it, break free from it and, through a series of deviations and successive denials, constitute a kind of purified body, an ideal body incarnating divine efficiencies and sacred values which will forever appear as the source, the foundation, the model of that which is only its poor reflection, its feeble, deformed, paltry image on this earth: those phantoms of the body and life that are at a mortal's disposal in the course of his brief existence.

In the human body, blood is life. But when it gushes out of a wound,[14] flows over the ground, mixes with earth and dust,[15] coagulates and becomes putrid, then blood means death. Because the gods are alive, there is undoubtedly blood in their bodies. Yet, even when it trickles from an open wound, this divine blood cannot tip the scales toward the side of death. A blood that flows, but that does not mean the loss of life; a blood that does not hemorrhage, that is always intact, incorruptible; in short, an "immortal blood," *ambroton haima* — is it still blood? Since the gods bleed, one must admit that their bodies have blood in them, but it must be immediately added that this is so only on the condition that this blood is not really blood, since death, the other side of life, is not present in it. Letting blood that is not blood, the gods simultaneously appear to have "immortal blood" and to be "bloodless."

The same wavering, the same oscillation occurs with respect to meals. The gods dine just as men do. Men are mortal because their bodies, inhabited by a hunger that is endlessly reborn, cannot survive without eating. Men's vitality and blood are nourished by a sustenance that, whether it is meat, bread or wine, can be defined as "ephemeral food"[16] because it is itself marked by death, decomposition, decay. Meat is the dead flesh of an animal slaughtered during sacrifice and offered to the gods. Its life has departed, leaving the field open to the internal forces of corruption in those parts of the animal reserved for man (i.e., all that is edible). Bread represents human nourishment par excellence: it is the symbol of civilized life; men are "bread eaters," and for the Greeks, "to eat bread," "to live off the fruit of the plowed earth" is another way of saying "to be mortal." If the Ethiopians, who live at the edge of the world in that islet of the golden age which it is their privilege to inhabit, are of all humanity the closest to the gods by virtue of their striking physical beauty, the fragrance they exude and their exceptional longevity, it is because their diet knows no cereals, and they consider wheat to be a kind of manure.[17] And even wine, that confounding and ambiguous drink, is worked on by fermentation, so that it too is the result of corruption.

According to the Homeric formula, to enjoy imperishable life, to possess immortal blood (or not to have blood at all) implies "not to eat bread, not to drink wine." To be true to Hesiod, one must add that this also means not to touch the flesh of the sacrificial victim, to keep for oneself only the aroma of the herbs burned on the altar, the emanations of the charred bones that rise in smoke toward heaven. The gods are always observing a fast.

Under these conditions, why do the gods sit down to a meal? The first answer: they assemble as guests for the pleasure of it, for the splendor of the celebration and the radiant joy of the banquet. They do not gather in order to appease their appetites, to satisfy their stomachs or to fill up that belly, the *gastēr*, the cause of man's misfortune that dooms him to death.[18] The second answer: just as there is ephemeral nourishment, so there is a food and drink of immortality. Whoever eats and drinks or succeeds in procuring such repast for himself becomes a god, if he is not one already. But, jealous of their privilege, the gods are careful to keep exclusively for themselves this nourishment that is "ambrosian" like their own bodies. Thus, after the table is set at the summit of Mount Olympus, the gods are, at the same time, those who, nourished by nectar and ambrosia, eat the dishes of immortality and those whose immortal bodies know no hunger and have no need at all to eat.

These paradoxes are not really perverse. Beneath their contradictory appearance, the propositions they enunciate are really saying the same thing: whatever positive forces such as vitality, energy, power, luster, the human body may harbor, the gods possess these forces in a pure and unlimited state. In order to conceive of the divine body in its plenitude and its permanence, it is thus necessary to subtract from the human body all those traits that bind it to its mortal nature and betray its transitory, precarious and unfulfilled character.

It is also necessary to correct the commonly held view that the anthropomorphism of the Greek gods means they were conceived in the image of the human body. It is rather the reverse: in all its active aspects, in all the components of its physical and psychological dynamism, the human body reflects the divine model as the inexhaustible source of a vital energy when, for an instant, the brilliance of divinity happens to fall upon a mortal creature, illuminating him, as in a fleeting reflection, with a little of that splendor that always clothes the body of a god.

Splendor of the gods. That is what shows through in all the *dunameis*, the powers, that the body manifests when it is as it should be: radiating youth, vigor and beauty, "similar to a god, like unto the Immortals." Let us look, with the *Homeric Hymns*, at the Ionians on the island of Delos, as they engage in dance, song, wrestling, and in the Games to please Apollo: "An unexpected arrival would think them immortal and forever free from old age for he would see, in all, their grace."[20] Grace, *charis*, makes the body shine with a joyful luster that is like the emanation of life itself, like the charm that continually wells from it. First of all, then, there is *charis*, and with it there is stature, breadth, presence, speed of leg, strength of arm, freshness of complexion, and a relaxation, suppleness and agility of the limbs. And all of these are no longer perceived through someone else's eyes but are grasped by everyone within himself, in his *stēthos, thumos, phrenes, nous*, fortitude, enthusiasm for combat, the warrior's frenzy, and the momentum of anger, fear, desire, self-mastery, prudent intellection and subtle guile — these are some of the powers for which the body is the depository, powers that can be read upon it like marks that attest to what a man is and what he is worth.

The Greek body of Antiquity did not appear as a group morphology of fitted organs in the manner of an anatomical drawing, nor in the form of physical particularities proper to each one of us, as in a portrait. Rather, it appears in the manner of a coat of arms and presents through emblematic traits the multiple "values" — concerning his life, beauty and power — with which an individual is endowed, values which he bears and which proclaim his *timē*, his dignity and rank. To designate nobility of soul, the generosity of the hearts of the best men, the *aristoi*, the Greeks used the phrase *kalos kagathos*, underlining the indissolubility of physical beauty and moral superiority. The latter can be evaluated only through a comparison with the former. Through a combination of its qualities, powers and "vital" values, which in their reference to a divine model always bear a sacred dimension, and which each individual has in varying amounts, the body takes on the form of a sort of heraldic painting upon which each person's social and personal status is inscribed and deci-pherable: the admiration, fear, longing and respect he inspires, the esteem in which he is held, the honors to which he is entitled — in short, his value, his price, his place on a scale of "perfection" that rises as high as the gods encamped upon its summit, and whose lower rungs, at various levels, human beings share.

Two orders of remark will complete this sketch. The first concerns the body's fron-tiers. The human body is, of course, strictly delimited. It is circumscribed like the figure of a distinct being, separate, with its inside and outside: its skin marks the surface of contact, while its mouth, anus and genitals are the orifices that assure communication with the outside. Nevertheless, it is not shut up on itself, closed, isolated or cut off from the outside, like an empire within an empire. On the con-trary, it is fundamentally permeable to the forces that animate it, accessible to the intrusion of the vital powers that make it act. When a man feels joy, irritation or pity, when he suffers, is bold or feels any emotion, he is inhabited by drives that he senses within himself, in his "organic consciousness," but which, breathed into him by a god, run through and across him like a visitor coming from the outside. By touching the Aiantes with his staff, Poseidon "fills them both with a powerful pas-sion [*meneos krateroio*]; he makes their limbs agile, first the legs, then, rising, the arms."[21] *Menos*, vital ardor, *alkē*, fortitude, *kratos*, the power of domination, *phobos*, fear, *erōs*, the impetus of desire and *lussa*, the warrior's frenzy, are all localized in the body, tied to this body which they invest; but as "powers" they exceed and surpass every individual carnal envelope. They can abandon it just as they invaded it. In the same way, when a man's spirit is blinded or enlightened, it is most often because, in the intimacy of his *noos* or his *phrenes*, a god intervenes to inspire the aberration of error, *atē*, or a wise resolve.

The powers which, in penetrating the body, act upon the inner scene in order to move and animate it, find on its outside, in what a man wears or handles — clothing, cover, adornments, weapons, tools — extensions that permit them to enlarge their field of action and to reinforce their effects. Let us take an example. The ardor of *menos* burns in the warrior's breast; it shines in his eyes. Sometimes, in exceptional cases when it becomes incandescent, as with Achilles, it bursts into flames above his head. But it also manifests itself in the dazzling brilliance of the bronze worn by the warrior. Rising skyward, the gleam of weapons that incites panic in the enemy's ranks is like an exhalation of the fire that burns in the warrior's body. The hero's accoutrements, the prestigious arms that allude to his career, his exploits and his personal value, are a direct extension of his body. They adhere to him, form an alliance with him, are integrated into his unusual figure like every other trait of his bodily armory.[22]

What military panoplies are to the body of a warrior, rouge, ointment, jewelry, iridescent fabrics and bust-ribbons are to a woman's body. The grace and seductiveness, the power to attract that are part of these adornments, emanate from them like magical charms whose effect on others is no different than that exercised by the charms of the feminine body itself.

When the gods create Pandora, so that she, this "marvel to behold," will become the deep, inextricable trap where men will be caught, they create in the same gesture a virgin's body and the vestmental trappings that will make this body "operative": dress, veil, belt, necklaces, tiara....[23] This provision of Pandora's clothing is integrated into her anatomy to compose the bodily physiognomy of a creature one cannot behold without admiring and loving because in the femininity of her appearance she is as beautiful as an immortal goddess. The lion's skin that Hercules wears on his shoulders, Ajax's bow, Peleus's javelin in Achilles' hand, the scepter of the Atreides carried by Agamemnon, and, among the gods, the aegis on Athena's breast, the dogskin cap worn by Hades, the thunder brandished by Zeus, the caduceus that Hermes waves — all these precious objects are efficacious symbols of powers held, functions exercised. Serving as a support or link to the inner energies with which a person is endowed, they belong to his "appurtenances," like his arms or his legs, and, together with the other parts of his body, they define his bodily configuration.

It is necessary to go one step further. Physical appearance itself, with all that it entails and that seems to our eyes congenitally determined — size, stature, bearing, complexion, the brightness of the eyes, the liveliness and elegance of movements, in brief, a person's beauty — can be, on occasion, "poured" from the outside onto the body in order to modify, revivify and embellish one's appearance. These "salves" of youth, grace, power and radiance which the gods sometimes give their protégés by suddenly "clothing" them in supernatural beauty, and which operate at a more modest level in the activities of grooming, bathing, and applying oils, function to transfigure the body through cleaning and purifying, ridding it of everything that makes it blemished or dirty, of anything that pollutes, disfigures, defiles or soils it.[24] Suddenly made unrecognizable as if he had exchanged his sordid old rags for sumptuous apparel, the individual, newly clothed in strength and grace, appears radiant in the bloom of youthful vitality.

Thus, when Nausicaa discovers Odysseus on the beach where he has been deposited by the tide, his naked body swollen from the sea, Odysseus is fearful, terrible to look on (*smerdaleos*).[25] The hero washes himself, rubs himself with oil and puts on new clothes. Athena makes him "taller and more massive, with his hair curling down over his forehead." When Nausicaa sees him again, "he is radiant with charm and beauty."[26] The same scenario, the same metamorphosis takes place in Odysseus's meeting with Telemachus. Odysseus is in the courtyard, like an old beggar with a withered body, bald and bleary-eyed.[27] Athena, touching him with her golden wand, "gives him back his handsome bearing and his youth"; his skin becomes ruddy, his cheeks fill out, his beard grows back blue-tinged on his chin. When Telemachus sees him like this, he is afraid, and turns his eyes away for fear of looking on a god. "Stranger, how you have changed," he confides to Odysseus. "A moment ago I saw you in other clothes and with a completely different skin [*chros*]. Are you perhaps some god, a lord of the heavens?"[28]

To this sudden beautification of the body through the exaltation of its positive qualities and the effacing of what taints and darkens it, may be contrasted mourning rituals and the brutalities leveled against the enemy's corpse, procedures that pollute the body, make it dirty, and commit outrage upon it. Here it is a matter of destroying all the values the body incarnates, all the vital, aesthetic, social and religious qualities it once bore, to make it ugly and to dishonor it by sending it, deprived of form and vitality, to the dark world of the formless.

Therefore, for a Greek of this period to conceive of the category of the body is less a matter of precisely determining its general morphology or the particular form nature gives to one individual or another than it is a matter of situating the body between the opposite poles of luminosity and darkness, beauty and ugliness, value and foulness. And it must be situated all the more rigorously, because when it does not have a definitively fixed position, it tends to oscillate between extremes, moving from one pole to the other. Not that in such a case a person would actually change bodies. Frightful or splendid, Odysseus always has the same body. But corporeal identity lends itself to these sudden mutations and changes in appearance. The young, strong body that becomes old and weak with age, that moves in action from enthusiasm to dejection, can also, without ceasing to be itself, rise or descend in that hierarchy of life's values which it reflects and to which it bears witness, from the darkness and ugliness of disgrace all the way to the brilliant beauty of glory.

This leads us to the second order of our remarks. Epic characters are often represented as being perfectly sure of their powers in the hour of combat. They overflow with confidence and enthusiasm or, as we would say today, they are in great shape, all keyed up. They express this feeling of corporeal plenitude and strength by saying that their *menos* is *atromon*,[29] unshakeable, that, similar in its inflexible ardor "to blazing iron [*aithōni sidērōi*],"[30] it remains *empedon*,[31] unalterable, sure within them. *Héroisme oblige!* In reality, like everything human, like strength, suppleness or speed, the ardor of *menos* is subject to vicissitudes: it relaxes, waivers, weakens and disappears with death. In Hades, the dead form the troops of the *armenēna karēna*, the heads that are without *menos*.[32] With age, the physical and psychic qualities make a complete man, leave the body, delivering the old man up to nostalgia for his lost strength, his extinguished ardor: "Why isn't your strength intact [*biē empedos*],"[33] Agamemnon says to Nestor who is overwhelmed by the weight of years; and the old man, in a litany, exhales his regret at no longer being what he was: "My strength today is no longer the same as that which once inhabited my supple limbs. Oh! If only I were young now, if only my strength were still intact [*biē empedos*]."[34] And again: "No, my limbs no longer have the same sureness [*empeda guia*], neither do my feet, nor my arms — no longer do you see them shoot out rapidly to the right and the left of my shoulders. Oh! If only I were young again, if only my strength were intact [*biē empedos*]."[35]

The nature of the bronze sky is, in fact, *empedos*, unshakeable above our heads like the gods who live there. No hero can change the fact that everything in the human body is consumed and destroyed and decays. This exhaustion of vital forces which must fade with time is translated by the root *phthi* in the verbs *phthinō, phthiō, phthinuthō*. Therefore, in order to make himself *empedos*, the hero cannot count on the body or on anything connected with it. Whatever his strength, passion or valor may have been, he, too, when the day comes, will become one of those heads emptied of *menos*. His corpse, his *sōma*, would rot as carrion if the funeral ritual, in consuming his flesh on the pyre, did not previously expedite it into invisibility, its skin intact, and smooth as in the case of the young warrior fallen as a hero on the field of battle, the bloom of his virile beauty still upon him.

When his body disappears, vanishes, what remains here below of the hero? Two things. First of all the *sēma*, or *mnēma*, the stele, the funeral memorial erected on his tomb, which will remind the generations of men to come of his name, his renown, his exploits. As the *Iliad* puts it, "once set up on the tomb of a man or a woman, the stele is immutable [*menei empedon*]."[36] It is a permanent witness to the identity of a being who, together with his body, finds his end in definitive absence — and even, it would seem, somewhat more than a witness. In the sixth century, when the stele began to bear a figurative representation of the deceased, or when a funeral statue — a *kouros*, a *korē* — was erected on the tomb, this *mnēma* appeared as a kind of corporeal substitute that expressed in an immutable form the values of beauty and life that the person incarnated during his brief existence. Second, parallel to the funeral monument, there is the song of praise that faithfully remembers high deeds of the past. Endlessly conserved and revivified in the oral tradition, the poetic word, in celebrating the exploits of the warriors of yesteryear, snatches them from the anonymity of death, from the darkness of Hades where the common man disappears. Their constant remembrance in the course of epic recitation makes these vanished ones "shining heroes" whose figures, always present to the spirit of the living, radiate a splendor that nothing can dim, the splendor of *kleos aphthiton*, "imperishable glory."[37]

The mortal body must return and lose itself in the nature to which it belongs, a nature that only made the body appear in order to swallow it up again. The permanence of immortal beauty, the stability of undying glory: in its institutions, culture alone has the power to construct these by conferring upon ephemeral creatures the status of the "beautiful dead," the illustrious dead.[38] If the gods are immortal and imperishable, it is because, unlike men, their corporeality possesses, by nature and even in the very heart of nature, that constant beauty and glory which the social imagination strives to invent for mortals when they no longer have a body to display their beauty or an existence that can win them glory. Living always in strength and beauty, the gods have a super-body: a body made entirely and forever of beauty and glory.

Without claiming to be able to answer it, there is one last question one cannot avoid posing. What is a super-body? How does the splendor of a divine body manifest itself?

First of all, it is manifested by what one might call its superlative effects: the magnification or multiplication of all values which appear by comparison on the human body as diminished, paltry and laughable. The gods are much larger and "a hundred times stronger" than men. When they confront one another in hand-to-hand combat on the battlefield of Troy in order to settle their differences, the entire world trembles, shaken to its foundations: in the depths of his subterranean dwelling, Hades jumps from his throne and is alarmed. Will the earth break open, revealing the ghastly dwelling place of death and corruption hidden in its bowels?[39] When Apollo advances in front of the Trojans, he causes, with a simple playful kick of his foot, the collapse of the embankment that the Achaians have built to protect their ships. Then, effortlessly, he pulls down their wall: "As a child by the seashore makes childish playthings out of the sand and then wrecks them with a kick or a punch to amuse himself, in the same way, Phoebus, you destroy what cost the Argives so much pain and toil."[40] To Calypso, who takes pride in being equal in the beauty of her body and appearance (*demas, eidos*) to the human wife whom Odysseus longs to see again, the hero answers that, in fact, next to the goddess, as perfect as Penelope may be, she would seem "inferior in appearance and size [*eidos, megethos*] by comparison, because she is only human and you are free from death and old age [*athanatos, agērōs*]."[41]

But the difference between the body of the gods and that of men is not essentially on the order of "more" as opposed to "less." The way the gods manifest themselves to mortals when they decide to personally intervene in their affairs varies greatly. It depends on whether the god concerned is a Power, like Hades, whose status requires that he must always remain hidden and invisible to human eyes; or whether, like Pan and the nymphs, he is given to appearing in broad daylight, or during the night in a dream, like Asclepius; or whether it is a god who, like Hermes, normally enjoys human company and commerce; or, finally, whether, like Dionysus, he is one who appears by surprise, just as it pleases him, so that his presence be recognized as an imperious and baffling epiphany. Furthermore, the nature of our documents adds to this diversity: divine apparitions do not follow an analogous scenario, nor do they obey the same model in an epic narrative, a religious hymn or a scene of a tragedy.

Nevertheless, one might venture a typological schema of the forms assumed by the gods when they make corporeal appearances. The gamut of possibilities runs from complete incognito to the god's revelation in full majesty. There are two kinds of incognito: the first is for the god to hide himself by clothing his body in a fog, enveloping it in a mist so that it becomes (or remains) invisible. Master of the situation, he acts with all the more power and efficiency as the spectators, blind to his presence, neither see nor understand what is happening right under their noses. When Aphrodite wishes to save Paris from Menelaus's impending blow, she makes him vanish from the closed space where the two men are pitted against each other and deposits him in Helen's room. Everyone, both Greek and Trojan, is deceived. Paris is already resting next to his beloved while the Greek warriors are still searching the ranks of the enemy to see where the devil that Trojan could have hidden himself.[42]

Therefore, the gods have a body that they can at will make (or keep) totally invisible to mortal eyes — and it does not cease to be a body. The visibility that defines the nature of the human body (inasmuch as it necessarily has a form, *eidos*) is flesh-colored (*chroïe*), and it has a covering of skin (*chros*) that takes on a completely different meaning for the gods. In order to manifest his presence, the divinity chooses to make himself visible in the form of *a* body, rather than *his* body. From a divine perspective, the opposition visible/invisible is no longer entirely pertinent. Even in the framework of an epiphany, the god's body may appear to be perfectly visible and recognizable to one of the spectators while remaining, at the same time and in the same place, completely hidden to the eyes of others. Before the assembled Greek army, Achilles ponders in his heart whether to draw the sword and strike Agamemnon. Immediately, Athena dashes down from the heights of heaven. She stops short behind the son of Peleus and puts her hand on his blond hair, "visible to him alone; no one else sees her. The hero turns around and immediately recognizes Pallas Athena."[43]

The second type of incognito appearance is when a god gives his body a strictly human appearance. However, this frequently used trick has its limits. As well-camouflaged as a god may be in the skin of a mortal, there is something "off," something in the otherness of the divine presence that remains strange and disconcerting even when the god is in disguise. Rising from the sea, Poseidon gives himself the stature and the voice of Calchas, the diviner. He approaches the two Aiantes, exhorts them, and with his remarks he gives them confidence and an ardor that wells up in their breasts. His mission accomplished, he turns and departs. But the son of Oileus is not deceived. It is a god who has come to us in the guise of Calchas, he confides to his companion: "No, that is not Calchas the seer. Without difficulty, I recognized from behind, while he was going away, the trace of his feet and his legs. The gods are recognizable."[44] One detects a god by his trace, just as a hunter recognizes the marks of the game he pursues. In spite of his disguise, the imprint left by the god as he walks on the ground undoubtedly reveals the disorienting, paradoxical and prodigious character of a body that is "other," because, in the very effort to look as though nothing were wrong, it reveals itself to be both the heaviest and the lightest of bodies. When Athena climbs into her chariot, it creaks and buckles under her weight. But when she leaps from one place to another, the same goddess does not even touch the ground. Poseidon left the two Aiantes in the human appearance of Calchas, imitating his gait, but his step was like that of "a quick-winged falcon pursuing a bird across the plain."[45] The divine body, in all the concentrated mass of its being, weighs as much as the marble or bronze statue located in the gods' temple: yet, it is aerial, ethereal, impalpable and as weightless as a ray of light.

So that they will not be recognized when they mingle with the crowd of fighters, the gods take the precaution of throwing a mist over the warriors' eyes to prevent them from distinguishing the divine from the human. In order to support Diomedes, Athena is not content to inspire him with a passion three times greater than his usual ardor, to make his legs, then his arms and his whole body supple from top to bottom: she takes away the mist that covered his eyes so he can distinguish whether a god or a man is before him, and thus will not run the risk of hand-to-hand combat with immortal divinities.

36

The bandage of darkness that covers their eyes and causes them to confuse mortals and immortals not only gives men a disadvantage because it hides the divine presence from them, it also protects them. To see a god face-to-face, as he is authentically in his uncovered body, is far more than human strength can bear. For the experience of seeing Artemis bathe in the nude, Actaeon pays with his life; for seeing Athena, Tiresias pays with his sight. After having slept with an immortal, Aphrodite, but without fully knowing that he has been with a goddess (*ou saphra eidōs*),[46] the mortal Anchises is understandably frightened when upon waking he sees the deity. Her head touches the roof of the room; her body is dressed in all its best finery; her cheeks are "radiant with immortal beauty [*kallos ambroton*]."[47] It is enough to see Aphrodite's "neck and her lovely eyes." He turns his gaze away in terror, hides his face under the covers, and begs for mercy:[48] may the goddess spare him, may he not be made "*amenēnos*," forever deprived of *menos*, the fire of his vital ardor, for having approached too brilliant a flame. Metaneira also feels her knees weaken and is speechless, prostrate and terror-stricken when Demeter, shedding the guise of an old woman, reveals herself in all her majesty to Metaneira: tall and noble of stature, radiant with beauty, exhaling a lovely perfume, "the immortal body of the goddess gave out a light that spread far; her blonde hair fell over her shoulders and the stronghold was illuminated as if by a bolt of lightning."[49]

The body of the gods shines with such an intense brilliance that no human eye can bear it. Its splendor is blinding. Its radiance robs it of visibility through an excess of light the way darkness causes invisibility through a lack of light. Between the shadows of death where they finally must lose themselves and the pure luminosity of the divine which remains inaccessible to them, men live in a middle world, divided between day and night. Their perishable bodies stand out clearly in the light of the sun. Their mortal eyes are made to recognize that which, through the combination of light and shadow, presents a precise form with its own shape, color and solidity. The paradox of the divine body is that in order to appear to mortals, it must cease to be itself; it must clothe itself in a mist, disguise itself as a mortal, take the form of a bird, a star, a rainbow. Or, if the god chooses to be seen in all his majesty, only the tiniest bit of the splendor of the god's size, stature, beauty and radiance can be allowed to filter through, and this is already enough to strike the spectator with *thambos*, stupefaction, to plunge him into a state of reverential fear. But to show themselves openly, as they truly are — *enargeis* — is a terrible favor the gods accord no one.[50] Heracles himself, who very much wanted to see Zeus, was unable to look at the god's face. Zeus "who did not want to be seen by him," hid his face behind an animal skin.[51]

More than any other part of the body, the face, like a mirror, reveals what an individual is and what he stands for. When a human being disappears in death, he loses his face at the same instant that he loses his life. The dead, their heads covered with darkness, drowned in shadow, are "faceless" as they are "without *menos*."

For a god to show his face openly would be to give himself up: the face-to-face encounter implies a relationship of parity between partners who look one another in the eyes. Looking away, lowering one's eyes to the ground, covering one's head: mortals have no other way to acknowledge their unworthiness and avoid the risk of confronting the unequaled, unbearable splendor of the divine countenance.

A body invisible in its radiance, a face that cannot be seen directly: the apparition, rather than revealing the being of a god, hides it behind the multiple disguises of a "seeming to be" that is adapted to feeble human vision. If a god's body can take on so many forms, it is because not one of them can encompass within itself the Power that surpasses each of them and would impoverish itself if it were to be identified with any one of the figures that lends it its appearance. It is not important that Athena, in her struggle with Odysseus against the suitors, initially approaches him in the guise of a very young boy taking his herd to pasture,[52] only to take on a little later the appearance of a tall and beautiful woman.[53] As boy or girl, Athena's visible body fails equally to express what the goddess is authentically. It fails to designate that invisible body made of undying energy, power and vitality, and, in the case of Athena, a sovereign mastery of the art of cunning intelligence, ingenious stratagems, skillful know-how, shrewd lies. These are capacities that all belong to her, that constitute her attributes and define her power among the gods, just as they are Odysseus's lot and glory among mankind. Confronted with a goddess who likes to "take all manner of shapes,"[54] the only authentic criteria the hero, however cunning he may be, has by which he can ascertain whether it is Athena in person who is really facing him, is to admit that in the game of cunning, in craftiness, in deceptive discourse, he is not her match and that he must take a back seat to one who, in divine Olympus, is intelligence incarnate.[55]

One of the functions of the human body is that it precisely positions every individual, assigning him one and only one location in space. A god's body escapes this limitation no less than it does that of form. The gods are here and there at the same time. They are on earth where they show themselves by exercising their actions, and in the heavens where they reside. When Poseidon goes to the Ethiopians to feast with them in the land of the rising and setting sun, he travels, in the same movement, to the two opposite extremities of the earth.[56] Certainly, each god is attached to a particular domain of action depending on his type of power: the underworld for Hades, the ocean depths for Poseidon, cultivated land for Demeter, woods, forests and peripheral wilderness for Artemis. Thus, the gods do not enjoy absolute ubiquity anymore than any one of them possesses omniscience or omnipotence. But by travelling at a speed as fast as thought, the constraints imposed by the externality of the divisions of space are child's play to them, just as, through the independence they enjoy from natural cycles and their successive phases, they do not know the externality of the divisions of time as they relate to one another. In a single impulse, the gods' corporeal vitality extends across past, present and future, in the same way that its energy is deployed to the ends of the Universe.

Thus, if the nature of the gods seems to belie rather than to exalt the traits that define the corporeal in human existence, why speak of the body of the gods? First of all, because the Greeks of the archaic period, in order to conceive of a being of whatever kind, had no alternative but to express that being within the framework of the body's vocabulary, even though it meant skewing this code through procedures of distortion and denial, contradicting it at the very moment they used it. We have observed that the gods have blood that is not blood; that they eat the food of immortality while continuing to fast; and that sometimes they even sleep without closing their eyes or letting their vigilance fall completely asleep.[57] Should we not add: they have a body that is not a body?

We may indeed, as long as we specify that in the traditional religious system the step that would finalize the rupture between the divine and the corporeal is never taken – the step that at the same time would sever the continuity between gods and human beings established by the presence of the same vital values, the same qualities of force, radiance and beauty whose reflection is worn by the bodies of both mortals and immortals.

Moreover, all the activities of the cult presuppose the incorporation of the divine: how could mankind institute regular exchange with the gods in which homages and benefits balance out, unless the Immortals appear in this world in a visible and specific form, in a particular place and at a particular time?

But another reason, one that relates to the very nature of polytheism, must also be taken into consideration. For the Greeks, the divine world is organized into a society of the beyond, with its hierarchies of rank, its scale of grades and functions, its distribution of competencies and specialized abilities. Thus, it gathers together a multiplicity of particular divine figures, each one has its place, its role, its privileges, its signs of honor, its particular mode of action, a domain of intervention reserved for it alone: in short, each one has an individual identity.

Individual identity has two aspects: a name and a body. The proper name is that particular social mark attributed to a subject in order to consecrate its uniqueness within the species to which it belongs. Generally, things and animals do not have proper names. All human beings – as human beings – have one, because each person, even the most unknown, has a form of individual existence. As Alcinous reminds Odysseus when he invites him to say who he is: "There has never been a man without a name; whether he is noble or a peasant, everyone receives one at the time of his birth."[58] Similarly, it is the body that gives a subject his identity, by distinguishing him from all of his peers through his appearance, his physiognomy, his clothing and his insignia. Like men, the gods have proper names. Like men, too, they have bodies – that is to say, a set of specific characteristics which make them recognizable by differentiating them from the other supernatural Powers with whom they are associated.

A divine world that is multiple and therefore divided within itself by the plurality of beings composing it. Gods, each one of whom has his own name and individual body, partake of a limited and particular form of existence: this conception has not failed to arouse questions, reservations or rejection in certain marginal religious currents and sects, as well as among philosophers. These hesitations, which have expressed themselves in widely divergent ways, proceed from a single conviction: the presence of evil, misfortune and negativity in the world results from the process of individuation to which it has been subjected and which has given rise to beings who are separate, isolated, individual. Perfection, plenitude and eternity are the exclusive attributes of totally unified Being. Every fragmentation of the One, every dispersion of Being, every distinction among parts signifies death's entrance on the stage, together with a multiplicity of individual existences and the finitude that necessarily delimits each of them. To rid themselves of death, to fulfill themselves in the permanence of their perfection, the gods of Olympus would therefore have to renounce their individual bodies, dissolve themselves in the unity of a great cosmic god or be absorbed into the person of the orphic Dionysus — the god who is divided up and later reunified by Apollo. Dionysus is the guarantor of the return to primordial indistinctness and the reconquest of a divine unity that must be found again after having been lost.[59]

Hesiod's orthodox *Theogony* gives the corporeal nature of the gods its theological foundation by categorically rejecting this perspective: it places the complete, perfect and immutable not in the confusion of an original unity, in the obscure indistinctness of chaos, but rather in its opposite, in the differentiated order of a cosmos whose parts and constitutive elements have bit by bit become separate, delimited and located. Here, the divine Powers that were at first included in vague cosmic forces took on in the third generation definitive form as celestial gods living in a constant ethereal light, with their particular personalities and figures, their functions articulated each in relation to the others, their powers balanced and adjusted under the unshakeable authority of Zeus. If the gods possess plenitude, perfection, immutability, it is because at the end of the process that led to the emergence of a stable, organized and harmonious cosmos, each divine person's individuality is clearly fixed.

The divine being is one who, endowed with an existence that, like human existence, is individual, nevertheless knows neither death nor what is associated with it, because in its very particularity it has the value of a general, atemporal essence, of a universal, inexhaustible power. Aphrodite is *one* beauty: she is that particular goddess whose appearance makes her recognizable among all the others. When Aphrodite, Athena and Hera stand before Paris, it is by comparing and contrasting the bodies of the three goddesses, by registering their differences, that Helen's future seducer can divine the powers and privileges that belong to each one, privileges that

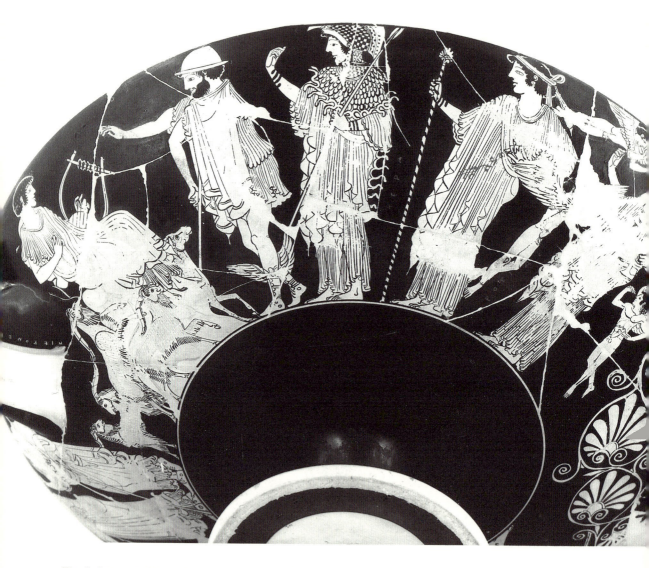

The Judgement of Paris. Each goddess displays the power that she will give to Paris if chosen. Hera incarnates royal power; Athena, military prowess; Aphrodite, erotic seduction (Berlin, Staatliche Museum).

42

will not fail to be granted him by the one whose favor he will win with his vote. If he chooses Aphrodite, if he hands her the palm, it is because she, the most beautiful one, is also Beauty itself, that Beauty by which every individual in the world, whether animal, human or divine, is made beautiful and desirable. In its splendor, the goddess's body is the very power of Eros to the extent that Eros is a universal force. Nor is Zeus any more only a king, the king of gods: he is royalty itself. A monarch who does not derive his power from Zeus does not exist, nor is there a king who does not exercise his functions through him and who does not receive from him, by delegation, the honors and glory reserved for the supreme master. The power of sovereignty finds its anchor in Zeus in the particular figure wherein it is fixed and incarnate.

The splendor, glory and radiant brilliance of a permanent, cosmic, indestructible royalty, which no person can ever overturn, have a form and a body, even if the former escapes the limitations of form and the latter is beyond a body.

In many ways, the divine super-body evokes and touches upon the non-body. It points to it; it never merges with it. If it were to swing to one side, to turn itself into the absence of body, the denial of body, it would upset the very equilibrium of Greek polytheism in its constant, necessary tension between the darkness in which the visible human body is steeped and the radiant light with which the gods' invisible body shines.

NOTES

1. Xenophanes, frag. 14, in Clement of Alexandria *Stromata* 5.109.2 = fr. 170 in *The Presocratic Philosophers*, eds. G.S. Kirk and J.E. Raven (Cambridge: Cambridge University Press, 1957) (hereafter cited as KR).

2. Xenophanes, frag. 16: *Stromata* 7.22.1 = 171 KR.

3. Xenophanes, frag. 15: *Stromata* 5.109.1 = 172 KR.

4. Aristotle, *Metaphysics* A5.986b21 = 177 KR; Diogenes Laertius 28A1 in *Die Fragmente der Vorsokratiker*, comp. H. Diels, ed. W. Kranz (Berlin, 1954) (hereafter cited as DK).

5. Xenophanes, frag. 23: *Stromata* 5.109.1 = 173 KR.

6. *Outi demas thnetoisin homoiios oude noēma*: "like mortals neither in the body nor in thought."

7. Sextus, frag. 24 = 175 KR: "Wholly [*oulos*] he sees, wholly he understands, wholly he hears."

8. Simplicius, frags. 25, 26 = 171 KR. The text specifies that, without becoming tired, without difficulty and without moving, the god makes everything shake through the "desire of his intellection [*noou phreni*]." The association of the terms *nous* and *phrēn* is reminiscent of the Homeric expression *noein phresi*, to have a thought, or a project, in one's *phrenes* (*Iliad* 9.600 and 22.235). What are the *phrenes*? A part of the body: the lungs or the membrane of the heart, and an interior place of thought, since it is through the *phrenes* that one knows; but also a site of feeling or of passion — in effect the *thumos*: ardor, anger and also breath, vapor, can, like intellection, be situated in the *phrenes* (*Iliad* 8.202, 13.487, 22.475, 24.321). Let us add that the *nous*, the intelligence insofar as it perceives, understands or projects, may itself be localized in the *thumos* (*Odyssey* 14.490).

9. On this vocabulary as a whole and the problems it raises concerning psychology, the person, and self-consciousness in Homer, James Redfield has recently published a penetrating *mise au point*, all the more useful in that the reader will find in its bibliographical notes a list of the principal books and articles dealing with these questions. The title of his study is "Le sentiment homérique du Moi," it appeared in *Le genre humain*, vol. 12, *Les usages de la nature*, pp. 93-111.

10. Redfield, *ibid.*, p. 100; and further, "organic consciousness is self-consciousness," p. 99; or, in speaking of the epic character, "his consciousness of himself is also a consciousness of his 'me' as an organism," p. 98.

11. Cf. *Iliad* 6.146ff.: "As with the generations of leaves, so with the generations of men: the wind scatters the leaves over the ground and the burgeoning forest makes them grow again when the spring season returns. Thus it is with men: one generation is born at the very instant that another disappears."

12. The gods are defined *hoi aei ontes*: "those who exist forever." On the value of *aei* and its relation to the *aion*, the continuity of being that characterizes the divine vitality, cf. E. Benvéniste, "Expression indo-européenne de l'éternité," *Bulletin de la Société de Linguistique* 38, fasc. 1, pp. 103-13.

13. Cf. Hesiod, *Theogony* 220ff., and Clémence Ramnoux, *La nuit et les enfants de la nuit dans la tradition grecque*, new ed. (Paris, 1986).

14. On the interplay of *brotos*, mortal, and *brotos*, the blood that flows from a wound, cf. the analysis of Nicole Loraux, "Le corps vulnérable d'Arès," in *Le temps de la réflexion*, vol. 7, *Corps des dieux* (Paris, 1986), p. 335.

15. On *to luthron*, mixed blood with dust, cf. J.-P. Vernant, "The Pure and the Impure," in *Myth and Society in Ancient Greece* (New York: Zone Books, 1989), pp. 121-41.

16. Cf. Apollodorus 1.6.3 on Typhon, weakened and conquered by Zeus after having eaten the *ephēmeroi karpoi*, the "ephemeral fruits," instead of the drug of immortality.

17. Herodotus 3.22.19. Having learned what wheat is and how it grows, the Ethiopian Long-Life

(*makrobios*) observes "that he is not at all surprised if, nourishing themselves on the manure [*kopros*], they lived a short span of years."

18. On the *gastēr kakoergos* (the evil-doing belly), *stugerē* (odious), *lugrē* (despicable), *oulomene* (disastrous), cf. J.-P. Vernant, "A la table des hommes," in *La cuisine du sacrifice en pays grec*, ed. M. Detienne and J.-P. Vernant (Paris, 1979), p. 94ff.

19. Cf. Elena Cassin, *La Splendeur divine* (Paris, 1968).

20. *Homeric Hymn to Apollo* 1.151-53.

21. *Iliad* 13.59-61.

22. Cf. the description of Achilles putting on the warrior's equipment that Hephaestus forged for him: "the divine Achilles tries out his armor: Will it fit him well? Will his glorious limbs run easily with it? And then it is as if he grew wings and they lift up the shepherd of men." *Iliad* 19.384-86.

23. Hesiod, *Theogony* 570-85; *Works and Days* 70-75.

24. The care lavished on a god's statue, of course, falls into the same category: at its fabrication, an incorruptible material is selected and it is enhanced with precious stones and metals to make it shine with a thousand fires; as part of its upkeep, its decayed parts are replaced and it is smeared with oil to increase its brilliance.

25. *Odyssey* 6.137.

26. *Ibid.* 6.227-37.

27. *Ibid.* 13.429-35.

28. *Ibid.* 16.173-83.

29. *Iliad* 17.157.

30. *Ibid.* 20.372.

31. *Ibid.* 5.527.

32. *Odyssey* 10.521.

33. *Iliad* 4.314.

34. *Ibid.* 11.668-70.

35. *Ibid.* 23.627-29.

36. *Ibid.* 17.434-35.

37. *Ibid.* 9.413.

38. Cf. J.-P. Vernant, "La belle mort et le cadavre outragé," in *La mort, les morts dans les sociétés anciennes*, eds. G. Gnioli and J.-P. Vernant (Cambridge and Paris, 1982), pp. 45-76.

39. *Iliad* 20.54-65.

40. *Ibid.* 15.361-65.

41. *Odyssey* 5.217-18. In the same way, When Alcinous wonders if Odysseus might not be a god who has come to visit him and his people, Odysseus answers: "Do not have this thought. I have nothing, neither stature nor presence [*demas, phuē*], in common with the Immortals, masters of the vast sky; I am but a simple mortal" (7.208-10).

42. *Iliad* 3.373-82.

43. *Ibid.* 1.197-200. On the episode as a whole and the problems that Athena's appearance poses within the very text of the *Iliad* itself, cf. the excellent analysis by Pietro Pucci, "Epifanie testuali nell' *Iliade*," *Studi italiani di filologia classica* 78 (1985), pp. 170-83.

44. *Iliad* 13.70-72.

45. *Ibid.* 13.62-65.

46. *Homeric Hymn to Aphrodite* 1.167.

47. *Ibid.* 172-75.

48. *Ibid.* 181-90.

49. *Homeric Hymn to Demeter* 1.275-80. Even animals react to the terrible strangeness of a divine presence: in Eumaeus's hut, Athena stands before the door in the guise of a tall and beautiful woman, a skilled craftswoman. She is invisible to the eyes of Odysseus; Telemachus faces her without seeing her; but, like Odysseus, the dogs have perceived the goddess: growling, but without barking, they take refuge, frightened, in a corner of the hut (*Odyssey* 16.157-63).

50. *Iliad* 20.131; *Odyssey* 16.161. If Alcinous on his Phaeacian isle can claim that his people's ancestors in the past saw the gods a hundred times appear *enargeis*, in flesh and blood, it is because in contrast to other men the Phaeacians, like the Cyclopes and the Giants, are of the same origin, the same family as the gods, who therefore do not need to "hide themselves from them" (*Odyssey* 7.201-05).

51. *Herodotus* 2.42.

52. *Odyssey* 13.221.

53. *Ibid.* 13.288.

54. *Ibid.* 13.312-14: "Goddess," Odysseus declares to Athena, "what mortal, however quick-witted he may be, could recognize you at once when he met you: you take all manner of shapes."

55. *Ibid.* 13.295-99.

56. *Ibid.* 1.22-25

57. Zeus's eyes are always open, his vigilance is faultless. Nevertheless, when Zeus is asleep, Typhon takes advantage of the occasion to try to steal his thunder. The attempt goes badly for Typhon; before he is able to lay a hand on the royal weapon, Zeus's eyes have already struck him with lightning. On the gods' sleep as a substitute for their impossible death, one can invoke the case of Cronus

who, since having been dethroned by Zeus, is, according to some traditions, plunged in sleep and dreams. Especially noteworthy is the *kakon kōma*, the cruel torpor that, for the duration of a great year envelopes the gods who are at fault, who are guilty of perjury, "hiding" them (*kaluptei*) as death hides humans. For them there is no more council, no more banquet, no more nectar or ambrosia, no more contact, communication or exchange of words with other divinities. Without being dead, since they are immortal, those who are guilty are bracketed, they are out of the game (Hesiod, *Theogony* 793-804).

58. *Odyssey* 8.552-54.

59. On this theme, cf. Giulia Sissa, "Dionysos: corps divin, corps divisé," *Le temps de la réflexion* vol. 7, *Corps des dieux* (Paris, 1986), p. 355.

From "Corps des dieux," *Le temps de la réflexion*, vol. 7, Paris, Gallimard, 1986.
Translated by Anne M. Wilson.

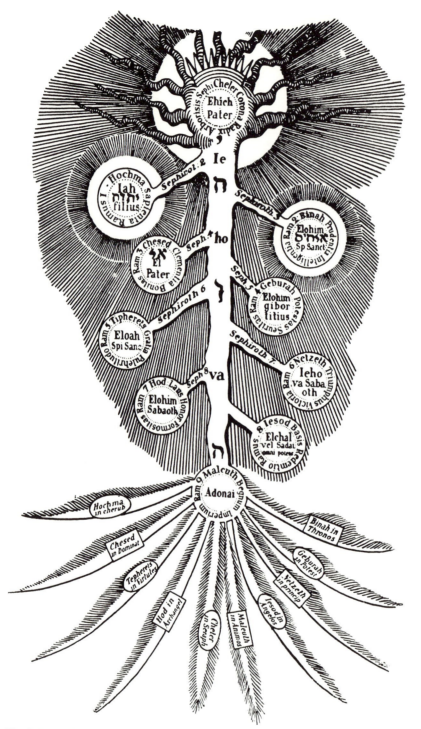

The Sefirotic Tree.
From Robert Fludd, *Philosophia Sacra et Vere Christiana* (Frankfort, 1626).
Republished in Henri Serouya, *La Kabbale* (Paris, 1947).

The Body of Engenderment in the Hebrew Bible, the Rabbinic Tradition and the Kabbalah

Charles Mopsik

The aim of the present article is to demonstrate the unity of Jewish perception, from ancient times to the most recent developments, of what I shall call the "body of engenderment." Why this somewhat odd expression? It is meant to designate a cultural and religious fact, with all its diverse speculative and narrative elaborations, concerning the human body as the subject of filiation and, hence, substantially inscribed in a relation to the opposite sex. Insofar as it concerns their collective and individual survival, the relation of human beings to their lineage is one of the most complex and crucial questions for all societies and for each individual in society. The place of the body within this perspective must be carefully understood. It is through the individual body that the life of a people — and the level of humanity they have achieved — perpetuates itself. Modern societies tend more and more to separate the body that reproduces, a link in an immemorial genealogical adventure, from the body that desires, a lonely object, a consumer of briefly gratifying encounters. Thus, modern man has two distinct bodies, using one or the other as he pleases. This caesura is perhaps merely the persistence of a split opened two millennia ago by the ideological victory over one part of the inhabited world of the Christian conception of carnal relation — and of carnal filiation — as separate from spiritual life and devalued in relation to it.

The intention of this article is to go back before this split took place — not only from a chronological point of view, but by examining several examples of a literature whose roots are in Jewish Antiquity and which extends, independently of Christian representations, throughout history, including the Middle Ages and modern times.

Several possible perspectives presented themselves: one could study the conception of the human body derived from practices linked to worship and sacrifice. These

49

include ritual purification of the "leprous," rules concerning priests who perform sacrifices (the Nazirites), the purification of parturating or menstruating women and men afflicted with venereal discharges. In short, one could address a great number of practices relating to the use of the body and to its sacred dimension, set forth in Leviticus and amplified and detailed in the rabbinic tradition (particularly in the Taharot treatises of the Talmud).[1] These few examples are enough to remind us that in the Bible the body is not understood as a neutral object whose status, at once physiological and social, is indifferent to its relation to God or to the religious community. These biblical texts and their development within the Jewish oral tradition enable the body itself to speak: man, a being of language from birth — from conception? — is a being of language through his body. All rituals that bear directly on the concrete reality of the body — and there are very many of them in classical Jewish religion as well as in other so-called pagan religions — endeavor to make the conflicts and tensions they somatize accede to language and thereby relieve the anguish that results from these conflicts and tensions. But it is not at this level alone that the closeness of the religion of Israel to polytheistic cults is apparent. In Hebrew religious texts, in the Bible and later writings alike, the divinity is presented as having a body of human form. Of course, several Jewish theologians (not least among them Philo and Maimonides) did seek to reduce what they called "anthropomorphisms" to the level of abstract allegories. But this effort at reductive rationalization should not keep us from reading both the biblical text and the writings classified among Jewish esoteric literature as written — like the passage in which God is presented as a giant of fantastic size whose bodily scale is dizzying. The writings said to be from *Shi'ur Komah* (The Measure of Bodily Scale)[2] testify to the great power of the conception of the divinity as endowed with a body, even if this body, human in shape, is gigantic. Therein lie many points which will not be taken up in the present study, but which I will mention in passing if only to give an idea of the great richness of the problematics of the body within the framework of the biblical and post-biblical Hebrew tradition. And there is another reason as well. There has been too marked a tendency to make a radical distinction between monotheism and polytheism, whether archaic or still practiced today. Within the human sciences there is such an absolute division between monotheism and polytheism that theologians have been conceded a virtual monopoly over the three religions that stem from the Bible so that the human sciences can devote themselves exclusively to the elucidation of religions which exercise no magisterium in the West and which have no place in the State. At least where Judaism is concerned, we are able, thanks to the so-called esoteric literature it has produced, to undertake a radical critique of the so-called monotheistic split, a critique that serves the interests of religious reasoning through the theological power of the deepest aspirations of homo religiosus,[3] perhaps the highest form of homo sapiens. For is he not the one who takes on the complexity of organic life in his movement toward humanization, that is to say in his access to language?

A simple look at the text of Genesis tells us a lot about the place of what we have called the body of engenderment. A single notion qualifies cosmogonic becoming and human genealogy: in both cases the text employs the term *toldot*, which can be translated as either "engenderments," "begettings" or "generations." Thus in Genesis 2.4: "These are the *toldot* of the heavens and of the earth when they were created." And in 5.1: "This is the book of the *toldot* of Adam." This linguistic fact is not accidental. The process of creation and the process of procreation, though different, are designated by the same vocable, which implies that the concept of human generation and filiation is rightfully inscribed within the divine creative movement, that procreation merely continues cosmogenesis, that it is a later stage of cosmogenesis. The verb "to create," *bara*, means "to give birth to" as well.[4] Moreover, one of the narratives of mankind's appearance is very eloquent in this regard. "Then God said: 'Let us make man in our image, after our likeness....' And God created man in His own image, in the image of God He created him; male and female He created them. And God blessed them, and God said to them, 'Be fruitful and multiply, and fill the earth and subdue it...' " (Genesis 1.26-28). Although centuries of theological discourse have tried to empty these words of their content, an impartial reading clearly shows the following: first, as in the religious thought of ancient Egypt, man is made after the divine form; thus, in the wisdom of Merikare (around 2000 B.C.) we find this formula: "Men are images of God that issue from His limbs."[5] Second, the same expressions that point out the resemblance of man to God (*tselem* and *demut*) are used to characterize the resemblance of a child to its father: "When

Adam had lived a hundred and thirty years, he became the father of a son in his own likeness, after his image, and named him Seth" (Genesis 5.3). The creation of man and man's begetting are merely two moments of a single movement. Third, man, as the image of God, is a combination of male and female; this is also to be found in Egyptian theogonic speculations, Heliopolitan speculations in particular, in which the principle gods are four male–female couples.[6] Fourth, being the image of God, like God both male and female, mankind is charged with procreation.

It is no doubt through this procreative action that man is in fact made in the image of God, the creator or genitor of heaven and earth. And there can be no doubt that here also is a distinctive feature of the biblical text which has not been sufficiently emphasized by the exegetes: the first thing God said to Adam (that is, to the man and the woman) was not the prohibition against eating the fruit of the tree of the knowledge of good and evil. Following very logically the mention of the likeness to God the Creator, the procreative power of man is evoked. A random distribution of the narrative elements is certainly not the reason. Immediately after man is described as being created male and female in the likeness of God, he is told to be fruitful and multiply, to procreate. There is a direct connection between the image of God in which man was created and his capacity to engender other men. Undoubtedly, God gave man his own image so that man might procreate that which is human. This likeness can only be the power to engender human bodies. Man's survival as human, as a speaking being, stems from this dual divine image, male and female, which gives him organic form. In fact, throughout the biblical narrative of creation, God expresses himself in the second person while addressing his creatures only twice: in the creation of fish (1.22) and in the creation of man, and both times it is tied to their procreative power. This relation between divine direct address and procreation seems highly significant of the Creator's investment in the process of procreation. Thus, cosmogony does not stop in the first chapter of Genesis, it is perpetuated by mankind who is, throughout the biblical narrative, provided with the power to engender derived from the creative power of God. It is in this sense that the celebrated verse must be understood: "Therefore a man leaves his father and his mother and cleaves to his wife, and they become one flesh" (Genesis 2.24). This one flesh is none other than the child they engender. Here it is the plural – the dual to be precise – which begets the unique and the singular. If one recalls that it is from this verse that the New Testament drew its teaching to affirm the indissolubility of marriage (cf. Mark 10.2, 9; Matthew 19.4, 6; 1 Corinthians 6.16; Ephesians 5.31, 33), one can measure the distance that separates this notion from the traditional Jewish reading of this verse, as attested to by Rashi.[7] The one flesh is not the static unity of the human couple, but the fulfillment of its procreative power, the insertion of its geniture in time.

Thus, by reproducing, religious man imitates the divine work of the original organization of the cosmos and his procreative act is perhaps considered as the ritual reenactment of cosmogony. In this way the primary elements which later converge in the medieval Kabbalah to make a sacred ceremony of the sexual union of bodies, indeed, a sort of sacrificial cult,[8] can already be found just beneath the surface of the creation story. However, it must be noted that man himself is not presented as the son or offspring of the divinity. It is only much later that God is qualified as "Father," in Deuteronomy 32.6 and, especially, in the prophet Malachi 2.10 *passim*. However belated this qualification, it provides us with an important piece of information: in all biblical instances (in the Old Testament) where this designation appears — and there aren't that many — God as Father is synonymous with God as Creator.[9] Taking this connotation into account, it is possible to see in the cosmogonic narrative of Genesis that the work of creating the world is assimilated to paternal engenderment: "Father" refers to he who creates something that is perpetuated (see also Genesis 4.21 in which "father" refers to the inventor of musical instruments). The biblical signifiers surrounding a creative activity are often the very ones that speak of engenderment and paternity.

Elsewhere, the biblical book of Genesis may as a whole be considered the narrative of founding marriages and engenderments. The episodes that punctuate the text between the genealogical tables are merely accompanying narratives to the principal matter: the enumeration of begettings and marriages that superintend them. I shall limit my investigations into biblical passages to these few remarks. To summarize briefly: At no point has there been any question of a spiritual filiation so as to reduce its value. On the contrary, it is the engenderment of human bodies that displays the work of creation and which is an integral part of the actualization of cosmogony. The process of human engenderment recounted in Genesis extends the engenderment of the heavens and the earth. The difference between the male and the female that form the human couple is inscribed within the divine image and, therefore, in God himself, and this is not to be taken as a simple allegory, but as a realistic conception of the nature of the divinity and His creative power. Historians of religion have viewed the ancient Hebrews' attitude toward sexual relations and procreation as "naturalistic."[10] But this judgment is rooted in a shortsightedness about biblical texts that must be seen as laden with a message of monotheism. What is characteristically at stake in these texts is above all an attempt to give human engenderment − a conjugal and genealogical relation − a place in speech. In other words, to free the reproductive instinct from its "natural" dimension in order to humanize the act of procreation, thus allowing for the birth of subjects, each of whom occupies a unique and identifiable place in the chain of begettings that is also the chain of likeness to God, its first link.

Thus carnal engenderment, the survival of what is human, which takes place through women giving birth, is valued for itself insofar as it makes the divine image explicit. Israel is first and foremost the promise made to Abraham that he will have descendants, a promise that is fulfilled through sexual union and corporeal engenderment. In the book of Ruth, for instance, one finds the following blessing made by Boaz on the occasion of his marriage to Ruth: "May the Lord make the woman, who is coming into your house, like Rachel and like Leah, who together built the house of Israel" (4.11). The notion of issuing from a single seed, central to the promise made to Abraham, profoundly structured the ancient Hebrew mind for a reason one should not call naturalistic or primitive. Paul's repeated exaltation of spiritual (authentic) Israel over carnal Israel, ardently expressed in his Epistle to the Romans, made possible the indefinite extension of the design of Israel and its universalization. However, it has led us to lose sight of one crucial fact. It is not as the "natural" son of Abraham that the Hebrew feels himself tied to his people, but as the legitimate son, which is to say the son recognized by his father. The newborn's body is inscribed in the genealogical chain, because the law establishes the principle of his legitimization, his recognition as a link in the chain. It is within the framework of fidelity to this law that this inscription is made possible. And what is the lesson of this law that more than any other leads this coupling into the line of generations? Precisely, it is the sacred character of marriage, of the conjugal act: in fact, the strict fidelity of the wife. When the prophets want to condemn the sins of Israel, to denounce its denaturations, its lapses, they show a predilection for the metaphor of the unfaithful woman, the adulteress and the prostitute.

These metaphors are significant on two levels: they reveal a woman's fidelity as a symbol of the bond between Israel and its God, and at the same time they show that this fidelity assures the truth of carnal filiation, that is, of the bond with the fathers and mothers who first bore the consecrated seed. Thus, the engendered and engendering body becomes the vector of the divine image. The body is the multiplier of this image as long as the child's mother is the child's father's wife, as long as he can be recognized as the child of a man who was his mother's husband. To put it in other terms, if he recognizes that he owes his birth to the desire that his progenitors mutually gave themselves to, a mutual desire awakened by the law of fidelity, he is inscribed effortlessly in the chain of engenderments. He becomes a unique moment in the process of creation which he in turn will extend still further. The Pauline split turns precisely on this point: spiritual Israel is instituted beginning with the christology that broke the chain of births: Christ's father is not His mother's spouse.[11] His father presides over the origin of all genealogy, but He is not one of its links. Thus, the son issues directly from the great Reference, without mediation. The chain of engenderments since Adam is broken. The inevitable consequence is that the individual body is no longer the mirror in which the bodies of preceding generations converge and are reflected; it is merely the occasional guise because Christ Himself did not engender other bodies. He is inscribed neither at the end nor at the beginning of a new genealogical series, but cleaves the body of engenderment in order to deliver its spirit out of time and space. And henceforth in Paul's doctrine, this breach opens a gulf between what is known as the carnal relation and the spirit that has been delivered of the flesh, that is, from what is reproduced along family lines. Death had been overcome by the horizontal extension of humanity — generations — but henceforth is replaced by a vertical extension — an ascension. It seems to me that essentially what is at work in the christology of the Incarnation and in the Pauline rejection of the flesh depends on this rupture in genealogy which until then had been considered the extension of divine creativity.

Gnostic elaborations of Paul's teachings clearly and eloquently testify to this. With this in mind, I would like to discuss a passage from the *Book of the Secrets of John*, also known as the *Apocryphon of John*, a work that belongs to Codex II among the writings found at Nag Hammadi. In it the Creator-God of Genesis is considered a usurping archon who, with the aid of the 365 powers of darkness that he himself created, makes Adam "forget his heavenly origin and, so as to assure a wider dissemination and therefore a weakening of the particles of light, creates woman who compromises Adam and draws him into the cycle of engenderments."[12] Here is a brief excerpt from the work in question: "Now up to the present day sexual intercourse continued due to the chief archon. And he planted sexual desire in her who belongs to Adam. And he produced through intercourse the copies of the bodies, and he inspired them with his opposing spirit."[13] For the Gnostic author, the Creator-God, creation, the body and the act of engenderment all partake of the same logic: to distance man from his heavenly origin, to perpetuate the exile of the spark of light in the dark universe of matter. The barely discernible desire one finds in this thought is the desire, beyond the series of generations, for contact with the prime authentic entity, the invisible Spirit, as the *Apocryphon of John* also says, which has no organic link to the genealogical process. Sexual reproduction, reproduction of the bodily image, is a product — and the text emphasizes this — of the logic of travesty. It is not even an imitation or a stand-in for immortality as it is for Plato in the *Symposium*.[14] It is the logic of death itself: according to a celebrated Gnostic logion, Jesus answers the question "When will death disappear?" in this way: "When you women no longer bring forth children."[15] In other words, man is mortal insofar as he prolongs creation and makes creative work of engenderment. The body of engenderment, as elaborated in the Old Testament, is the substratum of mortal causality introduced by the Creator-archon. The body as such is not what is at issue here. Rather, it is the creative concatenation to which it is bound that implies dissemination, dispersal, multiplication, acts of passage. Buddhism has many affinities with this way of thinking. It appears to be more difficult to find anything similar to it in the Essene movement.

In rabbinic Judaism, numerous maxims attest to the development and even to the overvaluation of the act of begetting perceived as that which joins human actors to creative action. Thus, God is associated with the procreative work of the two parents (Nida 31a), the pure conjugal union actualizes the descent of the divine presence between the two partners (Sota 17a). He who abstains from begetting is seen as diminishing divine likeness (Yebamot 63b). Thus, it is not essentially as a function of a natural imperative, nor as a dimension of normal organic life that the sexual act has its place, but, rather, it is intended to perpetuate the relationship between Creator and creation by extending the image of God in successive generations. One can cite numerous maxims in the rabbinic literature that stress engenderment as enabling God to reside on earth. In this respect his fundamental theurgic role is in the conjugal relation. No other natural process — neither the germination of plants, nor the cycle of the seasons, nor meteorological or astronomical phenomena — gives the Creator the opportunity to take part once again in His creation. The conjugal relation is therefore the key element of an interaction between Creator and creation. It actualizes the beginning of the world and demonstrates that this beginning is an act of God. Much of what one finds in the seven nuptial blessings recited in the traditional Jewish marriage ceremony recalls the act of creation. Quite significantly, procreation has been compared to the Temple, the principal function of which was to bring the divine presence and His blessings into the world, like a captor of the divine forces vested in the cosmos: "Rabbi Abin says: The Holy One, blessed be He, has greater affection for fruitfulness and increase than for the Temple" (Jerusalem Talmud, Ketovot 5.6). In this instance, the engendering bodies effect a singular act of worship: they serve God by procreating men who in turn will uphold his presence in the bosom of his earthly creation. For this reason also, coupling requires the ritual purity of the partners, just as the Temple service requires the purity of the officiating priests.

Taking these elements into account, it is not so surprising to find that during the Middle Ages, in the theosophical and mystical movement called "Kabbalah" that was intended to pass on ancient esoteric teachings, this motif of human engenderment is raised to the level of the principal act in the *imitatio Dei*. A veritable theogony is superimposed on the biblical cosmogony: the beginning itself has a beginning. The Kabbalah is devoted to recounting the various moments in the process of divine emanation, that is, the personal becoming of an unspeakable Absolute conventionally known as "En Sof," the Infinite. The kabbalists show a marked preference for describing this process of personalization as sexual act and procreation. The thirteenth-century Zohar (The Book of Splendor) is not alone in developing these

representations at great length, but since the thirteenth century this form of hermeneutics has dominated the various writings of the Kabbalah. Thus, to procreate
is to imitate – in other words, to reproduce at one's own level of existence – the
principal phases of the theogonic process, prior even to the creation of the world.
In this way, the human body as signifier is understood as the structural model of
the divine cosmos. For example, it is not unusual in Castilian literature for the masculine aspect of God to be given an appellation such as "Sacred Body of the King."
This name appears in a passage of the Zohar, in conjunction with the Queen – the
feminine aspect – in order to engender men's souls.[16] The carnal act has become
the model of souls being born of a bisexual divinity. Or, more strictly stated, the
act of mortal flesh only extends and translates a relation of the same order that takes
place within divine dimensions. In the thirteenth century the anonymous kabbalist
who wrote the *Letter on Holiness*, a mystical treatise on sexual relations, ascribes a
double function to the procreative relationship. First, it makes the man who engages
in it "the partner of God in the work of creation,"[17] since procreation makes possible the prolongation of the initial demiurgic act. Second, introducing a strictly
kabbalistic concept, the conjugal act is seen as the translation to a human level of
the union of higher divine entities (for example, that of the *sefirot* Wisdom and Intelligence, called Father and Mother) that results in engenderment, itself viewed as a
prolongation in the human universe of the emanation of the *sefirah* Knowledge,
sometimes called Son.[18]

Before delving further into the kabbalistic universe, some preliminary information is necessary. A few words must be said about the *sefirot* (plural of *sefirah*), a notion
of central importance in kabbalistic theosophy: this word refers to the ten emanations issuing from En Sof, the ineffable Infinite, which form a spiritual structure in
the shape of a human body. The word *sefirah* itself means "number," but kabbalists
often identify it with the word *saphir*, in order to emphasize the function of mediation or of philter that these emanations take on in relation to the superabundant
"light" of the Infinite. What men call God, even the personal God whose actions
are recounted in the Bible and to whom the Bible attributes names and psychological qualities, is none other than this emanative structure. Each *sefirah* has one principal, conventional name: from the first called Keter (Crown) to the last known as
Malkhut (Kingdom) or Atarah (Diadem). The lexicon of their various appellations

is quite extensive. For our purposes, we shall mention only a few types of nominations: the second *sefirah*, Wisdom, goes by the name "Father" or "Father on High"; the third, Intelligence, is also known as "Mother." These two *sefirot* form a couple whose relation is constant. As is often expressed in the Zohar, the *sefirah* Father sows in the *sefirah* Mother the primordial seeds or essences of the entire emanative structure of the *sefirot* that I have already described. The Mother is the seat of a process of differentiation through which these seminal essences acquire a certain quiddity, in the image of an embryo that grows and develops in the maternal belly from miniscule seminal particles. The sixth *sefirah*, Beauty, is the point at which all seminal emanations culminate and condense at the center of the structure. In the human body it corresponds to the spinal column, and it also bears the names Knowledge (the point at which the *sefirot* Father and Mother connect) and Son, their initial engenderment. The last *sefirah*, the tenth or Kingdom, gathers all the emanations and is the mirror in which all the lights issuing from the emanative structure are absorbed. It is known as "Daughter" — the principal feminine aspect — which is in direct contact with lower worlds: the world of angels and the material world where one part of human history is enacted. No doubt it is for this reason that the kabbalists identified the tenth *sefirah* with the Shekhinah in earlier rabbinic literature, the divine habitation or presence on earth. Harmony reigns within this structure, whose fundamental dynamism is understood in terms of both relation and sexual physiology, when the *sefirah* Beauty (Tiferet) or Son, the principal masculine aspect, is coupled with the *sefirah* Kingdom (Malkhut) or Daughter. Thus, these *sefirot* form two sexual poles whose phases of union or disunion punctuate the inner dynamics of the emanative structure and then affect the angelic cosmos and the human world.

I have limited myself to the schematic and partial in order to give a brief idea of the totality of the system of *sefirot*. One should also know that the kabbalists depict the process whereby the *sefirot* essences emerge through the totality of the emanative structure as both an engenderment and a movement of progressive manifestation: each new apparition of a *sefirah* is a birth. Thus, one may legitimately speak of theogony: the arrangement of the ten *sefirot* is the genesis of the human body's form through which and in which the Infinite becomes divine. One may also speak of theophany: the totality of the *sefirot* and each *sefirah* at its own level manifest a previously hidden essence of this divine becoming. Further-more, since all the *sefirot* together constitute a single being — the One of Jewish monotheism from which the ten *sefirot* are essentially indissociable — it is also necessary to speak of self-generation. At first glance the advantage of this eso-teric representation of the biblical God over exoteric theological representations resides in the great flexibility of the system, in the semantic richness of this One, given the extreme abstraction and great poverty of the exoteric One, which often risks petrifaction in what Henry Corbin, in *Le paradoxe du monothéisme*, has called the metaphysical idol of orthodox monotheism. Let us remember that for the kabbalists, the dynamic articulations of this One that manifests itself (the sys-tem of *sefirot*) are principally unions of a sexual nature, copulations and births. It is easy to understand why conjugal relations in the human world have been a permanent object of concern and meditation for the kabbalists, especially be-cause human acts are invested with a theurgic power of intervention in the world of the *sefirot*, where they exercise a harmonizing influence at the center of the theophanic cosmos.

I would like to quote a brief passage from the work of a sixteenth-century kabbalist, Rabbi Moses Cordovero, that summarizes kabbalist ideas quite well:

> No other commandment exists that would have the relation between man and woman resemble the coupling from on high in all ways as does this one. The other command-ments of the Torah allude to the image and likeness from on high in order to unify the *sefirot*. It is, however, a very distant allusion. Whereas the secret of male and female is in truth the secret of the higher *sefirot*, as it is said, "Let us make man..." [Genesis 1.26]. The union and coupling of man and woman is a sign of coupling from on high, as it is said in the Midrash: "The two are not together without the Shekhinah," when coupling is far removed from all unseemliness. It is not without reason that the first instruction uttered in the Torah is, "Be fruitful and multiply." (*Tefillah le-Moshe*, p. 213a)[19]

As a sign and cipher of invisible and divine realities, coupling is unlike anything else. A parallel may be drawn between this concept and the hermetic philosophy that orig-inated in Egypt and was furthered by the worshippers of the Roman god Asclepius.[20] But coupling is still more significant. It harmonizes so well with the intradivine process of uniting masculine and feminine aspects that it serves as the initiating agent of this union. And in return this action makes coupling the vessel of the

Shekhinah, the divine presence. Here again it is the creative nature of physical coupling that is advanced.

Why this extension and passage from the creative human body of engenderment to the emanative divine body of engenderment? As written, the texts we have do not explicitly speak of an *imitatio Dei* at the level of conjugal union. However, we are invited to consider human engenderment as continuing and extending divine engenderment to a greater degree of dissemination, that is, as theogony itself, through which the divinity is made manifest to itself before it is revealed to human beings. In fact, kabbalistic sources lead us to the idea that through human engenderment the divinity accomplishes one more step in the process of its manifestation. After self-generation, the theophany of self to self, the divinity is made manifest to others by borrowing the path of the succession of generations. Thus, mankind does not imitate a parallel process that takes place in a higher world. By engendering, mankind participates fully in the movement of theophanic realization through which the primordial theogony reaches its fulfillment. Indeed, for the kabbalists, man's creation responds to an inner necessity of the divine. It is a crucial stage in the movement that gradually leads the divine to revelation and personal expression. If man has a sense of imitating a higher process (however often the kabbalists refer to it as such), it is in fact merely an illusion. By mating and procreating man furthers the theophanic lineage; he makes it possible for this lineage to progress toward its realization. Each new generation is thus a stage of hiero-history, of the manifestation of God in time. This insertion of the theogonic process into temporality is the exact opposite of an incarnation. God does not fulfill His being in one individual at one unique moment. In order to move toward His fulfillment, in order to be personified, He must pass into time's texture woven by the thread of engenderments. Each new conception, each new birth is inscribed as an indispensable stage on the path that leads to divine manifestation, both eschatological and messianic. The body of engenderment is, therefore, a body of passage. Like the eye of a needle, it allows the thread of theophanic becoming to move through time and weave its fabric. A thirteenth-century kabbalist, Rabbi Joseph de Hamadan illustrates this idea perfectly when he writes:

> He who has children extends as it were the existence of the chain of likeness which is the Chariot [the Divine]. Indeed, the latter is called the "chain of likeness."... He who

is without children lessens as it were the chain of likeness. Thus, every man who has children fulfills the Chariot on high....[21]

This "chain of likeness" here refers to the system of ten *sefirot*, in other words, the primordial theogonic structure. To beget is to enable another link of this "chain" to enter the light. Consequently, to abstain from begetting amounts to depriving this chain of a degree of expression, to diminish the extension of this likeness — the Chariot or self-generated divine structure — in the temporal field which it must enter in order to arrive by degrees at its full actualization.[22]

With these elements in mind, let us take up the question posed at the outset. I would like to point out why I am inclined to believe that the developments of the medieval Kabbalah, numerous and increasingly elaborate and complex, constitute a necessary evolution in the movement of thought initiated by the biblical text and the rabbinic tradition. As esoteric thinkers committed to studying the inner motivations of the text of the Torah, with little interest in its ideological or supposedly ideological background, the kabbalists understood deeply what the notion of creation (which emerges from the relation between the world's creation described in the opening passages of Genesis and the creative process of human engenderment) implies as a conception of the divinity. If, as the biblical text states, man is created in the image and likeness of God, it is because this Creator-God himself — like man — is subject to a creative process whereby he comes into being and emerges from nothingness. Or, if you prefer, this image of God that man offers to scrutiny is the very one that appeared to the kabbalists as His first manifestation, a revelation upon hindsight of creation's initial truth: its seat is in the bosom of the Creator from the beginning. More simply, if God created man in His own image, it is because this image is not created at the same time as man. It existed prior to man and, consequently, we would do well to determine its point of emergence. And to do this we need only follow the logic of the biblical narrative itself: man passes on his image, which in the first instance is the image of God, through the act of engenderment. The implication is that this image has been passed on primordially, has come about through a process identical to that revealed by human engenderment. The creation of this "image," a creation kabbalists often prefer to call "emanation" (*atsilut*), was understandably deciphered from the facts provided by the mode of human generation over time. The kind of interpretation of the biblical text that made such an approach possible, and even necessary, is based above all on a rigorous account of semantemes and the logic of their appearance in the narrative thread, as well as on independence from any artificially applied logic, whether philosophical or theological in nature. This mode of reading is reminiscent of the ideal juridical treatment of a law text. Meaning is discovered in the text itself, strictly within its framework, concealed within the recesses of each of its propositions. No other sphere of meaning should interfere, no intellectual or cultural interest should subordinate the intratextual play of deciphering. In this way, the kabbalists overcame the shock their conception of divinity might arouse in the medieval culture of the twelfth and thirteenth centuries, a culture in which there was anxiety about conformity to the principles of an implacable monotheism. Appearances notwithstanding, the resemblance of certain concepts of the Kabbalah to those of ancient or polytheistic religious systems is not the result of an unlimited interpretive freedom or, indeed, freedom from the biblical text itself. On the contrary, the kabbalists stayed as close as possible to this text and did not impose readings on it that sought to accommodate theological truths elaborated centuries after the Bible was written and whose fundamental ideas it did not share. Hence, they were able to discover the primitive strata of the narrative. Theirs is not the approach of the historian or the archeologist. And it is here that this digression on the kabbalistic method of interpretation returns to our subject: as is known, Kabbalah signifies tradition, reception, transmission. It is not a body of doctrine passed down since Antiquity by Jewish esoteric philosophers, just as it is not merely a corpus produced with each new conception. What is transmitted is nothing other than the power to transmit. The power to adhere to the text, the power to engender: tradition, like the body of engenderment, is the point of passage through which the invisible allows itself to be glimpsed, through which the unspeakable allows itself to be spoken, through which the flux issuing from the Infinite takes form, link by link.

One issue remains. Becoming is here perceived as eminently positive and constructive. The power to engender makes life unfold. However, in Gnosticism becoming is seen explicitly as synonymous with alteration, corruption, death. That which evolves, moves or is disseminated is doomed to disappear, whereas the immutable being who is neither produced nor reproduced enjoys eternity and knows nothing of the shadow of death. These antithetical perceptions must be dealt with. Is engenderment the work of death or life? The answer is not as clear as the question leads us to believe. To declare that engenderment is the propagator of life in the name of a naive vitalism is meaningless in the face of the disconcerting strength of the Gnostic vision, for which the engenderment of a body is the engenderment of a tomb (*sōma-sema*), whereby the soul is chained to a mass of obscure matter. In order to take up this formidable line of questioning, we must turn our attention to the kabbalistic conception of the human soul in relation to the body. We must first describe briefly the manner in which the kabbalists or certain kabbalists have understood the soul. To them the soul is a spiritual entity that issues from the *sefirot* or divine emanations. The Zohar speaks of souls as being engendered by the union of the masculine and feminine aspects, Tiferet and Malkhut, King and Queen. But not all souls proceed from the same celestial region. Each soul's degree of elevation, the spiritual zone from which it is loosed in order to enter the world, is determined by the quality and purity of its parents' sexual relations at the moment of conception. Certain kinds of souls, those of proselytes, are engendered by the postmortem coupling of the just, men and women, in the heart of Eden, an act of copulation that procreates pneumatic lights destined for new converts whose soul is not an inheritance from their parents as it is for those who are Israelites by birth (Zohar 3.167b ff.). In the writings of Rabbi Joseph de Hamadan, souls are spoken of as being assembled in the celestial garden of Eden by family and family groups in a genealogical order nearly symmetrical to that which they knew on earth. The doctrine elaborated in Safed by Rabbi Isaac Louria in the sixteenth century, based on ancient sources, views the totality of human souls — past, present and future — as originating in the mystical body of the first man where they were distributed in each of his organs. Sin caused the dispersal of these souls which, as they pass to earth over generations, gradually repair the damage that was done to them. The lowest souls, those in the feet, indeed in the heels of the first man, will be the last implanted in earthly bodies before the coming of the Messiah (see *Sefer ha-Guilgulim*, chs. 1 and 2). These reminders serve merely to demonstrate the existence of a constant in the various doctrines of the kabbalists: even before it has an earthly destiny, the soul is attached to corporeality, even if there is yet no body with which it is to share an existence. And this corporeality that exists prior to the body is a corporeality of engenderment as well. The realm of the spirit, if it can be distinguished from that of the material body, remains inhabited by the corporeal order that gives it its formal dimensions. The individual body is integrated by rights into the heart of this larger corporeality of which it is a part. It is not an accident of the light but a necessary passage in its propagation. As such, it has played the role of natural text in which a knowledge of higher realities is inscribed.

In order to give the reader an idea of how the kabbalist understood the body as the place of knowing — the site of *gnōsis* — I shall cite several lines from the introduction to the major work of a celebrated Italian kabbalist of the eighteenth century, Rabbi Moses Hayim Louzatto, who commented on several phrases from a passage in the Zohar on the Song of Songs:

The second form of knowledge [which follows the apprenticeship to the theogonic system set out in the preceding paragraph] consists in "knowing one's body, etc." Here begin the essential forms of knowledge which follow the forms of knowledge having to do with the tree [i.e., with the complex structure of emanative configurations and the *sefirot*]. The first consists of the knowledge of the body's secret according to the totality of its form and its organs, of all the elements of its functioning and of how it takes root in the higher *sefirot*, all of which converge toward the level that is Adam's likeness [*demut*]. That is why he was the final creation [in the Book of Genesis], for all things move toward this goal. The truth is that all things converge toward [the body] in order that it may be the sole agent of free choice. Indeed, even the soul can have no free will apart from [the body]. "What is he?" What is man upon whom the whole work of creation is incumbent? [By asking this question] one can easily understand wherein he is the end of all creation; one can understand all the ties between the *sefirot* and him. All parts of the work depend on this knowledge. "How he was created." How this body emerged. Here one understands the pathways whereby material realities emerge, the principal one being the body. "What is he thereafter?" How does his history evolve from the beginning of his being until its end...? "How the body is perfect." Wherein one comprehends the secret of this likeness, what it is according to the intentions placed in it. This is what is treated throughout the *Idra Rabba*, the *Idra Zuta* and the *Tikkunim*.[23] In other words, the relation among *sefirot*, the law of their functioning, is the same as the law of the functioning of the body in all its parts. From this comes our understanding of the verse "Yet in my flesh shall I see God" [Job 19:26], in order to see and comprehend all the doings of man and the whole of his movements, all of which have their roots deep in the *sefirot*. (*Addir ba-Marom*, Jerusalem, 1968, p. 2a)

Among the elements worth remembering are the following: first, it is only when introduced into a body that the soul gains freedom, here considered a positive dimension. Second, the human body occupies a special place at the heart of the material universe. It is not a random assemblage or construction among the elements of matter. Third, the human body is structured anatomically and functions physiologically in a manner perfectly homologous to the system of *sefirot* and the laws governing their relation. Fourth, therefore, studying and learning about his own body enables man to gain knowledge of the divinity, whose system of powers and emanations are governed according to the same characteristics. The soul is not imprisoned in a dark and mortal abode. By passing into a human body it reaches the dimension of free will that paradoxically brings it closer to its divine model. In a body the soul can freely accomplish a task that enables it to reach a higher level. This task is itself a piece of work that is necessary for the full unfolding of the divine emanation. In order to move closer to the kabbalists' conception, when one compares it with that of the ancient Gnostics who in the end did nothing more than radicalize Christian thematics, particularly those of Paul and John,[24] one must remember that in the eyes of the faithful inheritors of ancient rabbinic traditions, the death of the body is not a definitive situation. In this context the concept of resurrection is essential. For us, this is what it implies: to engender a body is not to engender a tomb since this body has a future beyond its ineluctable death. Many kabbalists consider the resurrected body an eternal, imperishable body. Of course, the latter is not engendered by other bodies, by its parents, but it nevertheless results from the former, perishable body; it is a transfiguration of and reconstruction from the dust and bones of the engendered body. Therefore, and in a second degree, procreation initiates an irreversible process within the very order of life, a life that knows a dark passage.

One early seventeenth-century kabbalist, Rabbi Isaiah Horowitz, whose importance cannot be underestimated, clearly describes his fundamental vision of the couple comprising body and soul:

> In one regard, body and soul are both equal, which is to say are both spiritual, as was the first man before the fall and as he will be in the future... even earthly matter will again become spiritual and both will have equal value once again, which is the desired end: [that body and soul be eternal]...." (*Shenei Luhot ha-Berit*, vol. 1, p. 20a, marginal note)[25]

The first couple's sin merely clouded and veiled the essential reality of the nature of matter and, therefore, of the body. It opened a temporary breach within a single spiritual substance. In the eschatological future, the spirituality of matter will be recaptured and body and soul will form one eternal being. The vision of the world implied by such a conception reflects a categorical optimism of which the ancient Gnostics were entirely incapable. It is astonishing in its radicality and in the reversal it urges upon the reader regarding the classification of body and soul within ordinary hierarchies. But it is this very radicality, and it alone, which is provocative and powerful enough to stand up to the equally powerful conception of Christian Gnosticism. It implies all this vis-à-vis the body of engenderment, a body dedicated to life, to eternal life. The taint of death is not its last term nor its final destination. It is a passage.

It is useful here to point out one important fact. However central a place kabbalistic thinkers have given the body — for them the point of acquiring *gnōsis* about the supercelestial worlds, the divine structure itself, a body capable of theurgic action in these sacred realms — this body never became for them an object of plastic exaltation or aesthetic contemplation. In my ventures into the writings of the Kabbalah, I have never come across any evidence of adoration of the bodily form. This bodily form remains above all the bearer of signatures of the divine order; it is the vector of knowledge but it is not the object of visual fascination. This explains the restraint shown in the abundance of drawings and other diagrams produced by the kabbalists to illustrate their at times very complex speculations. They always avoid figurative representations and prefer abstract drawings.

Just as the kabbalists have searched for the beginning of beginnings in the order of the past, so they have set out to find the end of ends in the order of the future. But in essence these elaborations are merely a long detour that leads back to the biblical narrative of the first day of Genesis. With great simplicity, Genesis presents man as having been created in the image of God and, therefore, fundamentally immortal like God, even in bodily form. It is to their great credit that the kabbalists have upheld, as far as possible and often against the readings of fashionable theologies, the calm daring of this verse from Genesis, which has been the source of fertile meditation for generations of esoteric thinkers. Therefore, they enable us, as modern readers of the Bible steeped in learned, abstract and reductive constructions of theological doctrines, to recapture lost glimmers of meaning in an over-explicated, over-commented-upon text which every cause has been quick to make its own without regard for what it leaves unsaid, that is, for what the totality of what is said seeks to express without being either willing or able to do so. The esoteric view of the biblical text differs profoundly from the exoteric view. It is attentive in the extreme to all that is waiting to be revealed. For the esoteric thinker, Revelation is a matter of daily effort, it is not a moment of historical foundation.

This article has been limited to generalities. In order to understand just how many multiple and detailed elaborations have arisen from meditation on the body and its complexity, one must immerse oneself in the nearly six thousand works, printed books and manuscripts that the kabbalistic tradition has produced over seven centuries. For kabbalists, understanding the body as the fated locus of their advance toward knowledge of God has not been a simple formula. They have precisely and unceasingly explored all paths opened to them by the human body with all its organs and humors, its functions and movements. In order to appreciate the extent to which this is true, we need only turn to the diagrams they have left us which establish the correspondences between the various parts of the body and the *sefirot*. Yet there can be no doubt that if the body has been able to occupy such a unique place in a school of thought developed in the West, it is because in the eyes of the kabbalists, the genealogy of bodies makes manifest an invisible chain whose first links constitute the divine order itself, the creative activity brought forth in human procreative activity.

NOTES

1. The Talmud (literally "study") is the redactional sum of the oral tradition worked out in rabbinic circles, in Babylonia or Palestine, between the first and sixth centuries. The treatise in question is devoted to the various problems concerning the pure and the impure and practices of purification.

2. Gershom Scholem devoted a chapter of his book translated into French under the title *Le mystique juive, les thèmes fondamentaux* (Paris: Le Cerf, 1985) to the history and content of the literature of the *Shi'ur Komah*. He was the first modern thinker to recognize its antiquity.

3. This term is taken from Mircea Eliade. See esp. *The Sacred and the Profane: The Nature of Religion* (New York, 1968).

4. The literal meaning of *bara* is "to carry beyond," "to take out." In Aramaic, which is very close to Hebrew, *bar, bera*, comes from the same root as *bara* ("to create"), and means child, offspring.

5. The idea is both one of likeness and one of filiation: men are images of the divinity because they are the issue of his members. Likewise, a child resembles his father because he derives from him. That is all the text of Genesis says: if man is created in the image of God, if he is like Him, it is because he proceeds from Him as His offspring.

6. See C. Desroches Nobelcourt's *La femme au temps des pharaons* (Paris: Stock/Laurence Pernoud, 1987), p. 21ff.

7. Rashi is the name, formed from the initials of Rabbi Salomon ben Isaac, of the first Jewish biblical exegete in the Middle Ages (tenth-eleventh centuries), who often did little more than rein- state the most common rabbinic reading. See also the reading given by Pierre Legendre in *L'inestimable objet de la transmission* (Paris: Fayard, 1986), p. 255.

8. On this last point see my work *La lettre sur la sainteté: La relation entre l'homme et la femme dans la cabale* (Paris: Verdier, 1986), p. 151.

9. This is no longer the case in the New Testament where divine paternity is disconnected from its creative work and connotes a different register.

10. See, for example, G. Parrinder, *La sexe dans les religions du monde* (Paris: Le Centurion, 1986), p. 191. The chapter devoted to Hebrew concepts is an example of the all-powerful influence of righ- teous theological discourse on a study that takes itself to be historical, scientific and impartial.

11. It is not insignificant that a comparable equation presides at the birth of Alexander of Mace- donia three centuries before Christ. He is mystically believed to be the son of the god Zeus-Ammon; indeed, his mother Olympia maintained that Alexander was not the son of her husband Philip, but that he was the fruit of the god with whom she had been intimate (see A. Weigal, *Alexandre le Grand*, Paris: Payot, 1976, pp. 46-56, 97-98, 146, *passim*; P. Jouguet, *L'impérialisme macédonien et l'hellénisation de l'Orient*, Paris: Albin Michel, 1972, p. 17). This would lead one to think that a direct filiation with a god (or God), outside the genealogical route, whereby the mother claims that her child's father is not her husband, plays a considerable role in the production of certain heroic figures in history.

12. *Cahier Evangile*, supp. no. 58, "Nag Hammadi," with an introduction by R. Kuntzman and J.M. Dubois, p. 40.

13. *Apocryphon of John* 1.24.23-27 (trans. F. Wisse), in *The Nag Hammadi Library*, ed. James Rob- inson (Leiden: E.J. Brill, 1978).

14. See 207c-210b. However, the superiority of immortality achieved through procreation is strongly emphasized by a Zoroastrian text. See *Datastan-i dênîk*, in *La naissance du monde*, "La naissance du monde dans l'Iran préislamique," trans. Marijan Molé (Paris: Seuil, 1959), pp. 313-14.

15. Quoted by Clement of Alexandria, *Stromata* 3.9; see *Evangiles apocryphes*, trans. F. Quéré (Paris: Seuil, 1983), p. 61.

16. See, for example, Zohar 1.245b.

17. Mopsik, *La lettre sur la sainteté*, pp. 233-34 n.8.

18. *Ibid.*, p. 231.

19. *Ibid.*, pp. 144-45.

20. See *Corpus Hermeticum*, ed. A.D. Nock, trans. A.J. Festugière (Paris: Les Belles Lettres, 1973), pp. 320-23 (pars. 20 and 21). See also the Coptic text, in *The Nag Hamadi Library*, pp. 300-01.

21. Mopsik, *La lettre sur la sainteté*, pp. 102ff.

22. This expression is borrowed from Henry Corbin. It is worth noting that in the final lines of the *Iggeret ha-Kodesh*, the Letter on Holiness, the ten generations preceding the birth of King David spoken of in the Book of Ruth (4.8) are presented as manifesting the plenitude of the *Shi'ur Komah*, the divine body composed of the ten *sefirot*. Thus, the mystical body of the divinity sung in the hymns of ancient Jewish sources is considered to be made manifest by the body of engenderment, which becomes the source of revelation at the level of the human world and its history of the divine body (Mopsik, *La lettre sur la sainteté*, pp. 256 and 323). It is obvious that this theophanic aptitude of the body of engenderment is conferred upon it essentially through a submission to ritual and ethical practices which preserve its holiness and the sacred of which it is the bearer. Without these protections, the body of engenderment would lose its theophanic and theogonic power, thus forgetting its destiny, it would split into an engendering body and a desiring body and thus obliterate the essential unity of the desire for pleasure and the desire to procreate.

23. Various writings belonging to the literature of the Zohar.

24. This is the general thesis of the work of Simone Pétrement, *Le Dieu séparé, aux origines de gnosticisme* (Paris: Le Cerf, 1984).

25. There is ample material for a study devoted exclusively to the theme of Moses' body in the Kabbalah, which occupies a central place in it. Rabbi Salomon Halevi Alkabets, for example, a sixteenth-century kabbalistic thinker, maintains that the body of the greatest prophet of Israel was already a resurrected body (see *Berit Halevi*, Jerusalem, 1980, p. 42d).

Translated by Matthew Ward.

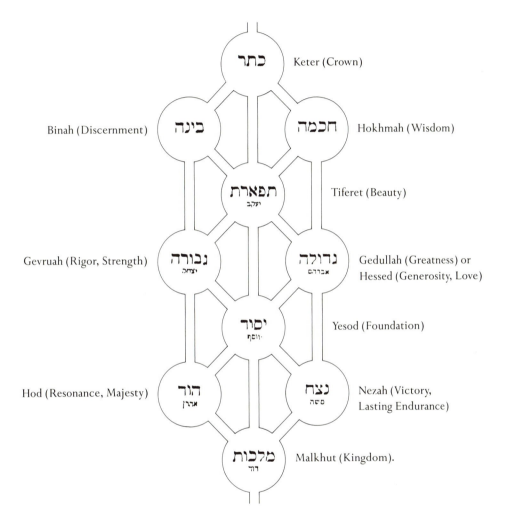

A classic chart of the ten *sefirot* from the *Ketem Paz* (c. 1570) of Rabbi Simeon Labi (Djerba, 1940). It should be noted that the upper and lower extremities are open: the inner structure of the divine constitutes a totality opened by En Sof (the Infinite). The light of En Sof passes through these openings and becomes a seminal flux which takes the form of a genealogical system realized by the main figures of the biblical narrative. The kabbalists most likely called these illustrations the "tree of the *sefirot*" or the "tree of emanation" – since the thirteenth century, that is – with reference to the development at that time of more and more complex family trees.

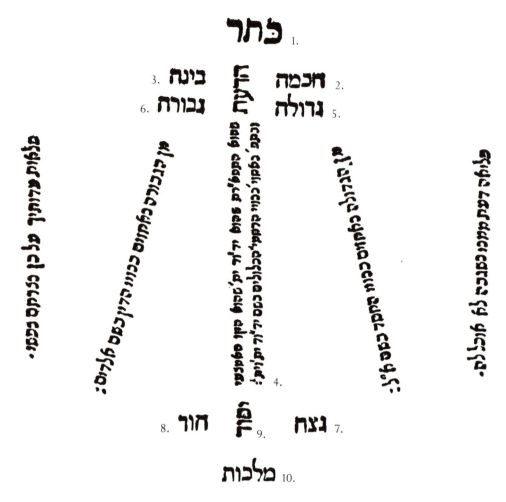

Illustration by Rabbi Joseph Gikatila from his *Sha'arei Orah* (The Doors of the Light), Warsaw 5643/1883, ch. 5. In this illustration of the ten *sefirot*, Da'at (Knowledge) is represented as a vertical axis which connects the summit to the whole of the sefirotic body, to the image of the spinal column through which move the divine influxes like a seed from the head down through the entire organism, according to the ancient physiological representation. The central line of writing reads, "Da'at, which is Tiferet (Beauty), which is YHVH blessed be He, which is the middle line. To Tiferet belong the epithets of mercy in the name YHVH, blessed be He, blessed be He." One can see that Da'at unites right and left, high and low, masculine and feminine: it is the great unifier of the *sefirot*.

Translation of terms: 1. Keter (Crown) 2. Hokhmah (Wisdom) 3. Binah (Discernment) or Tevuna (Intelligence) 4. Da'at (Knowledge) 5. Gedullah (Greatness) or Hessed (Generosity, Love) 6. Gevruah (Rigor, Strength) or Pahad (Dread) 7. Nezah (Victory, Lasting Endurance) 8. Hod (Resonance, Majesty) 9. Yesod (Foundation) 10. Malkhut (Kingdom)

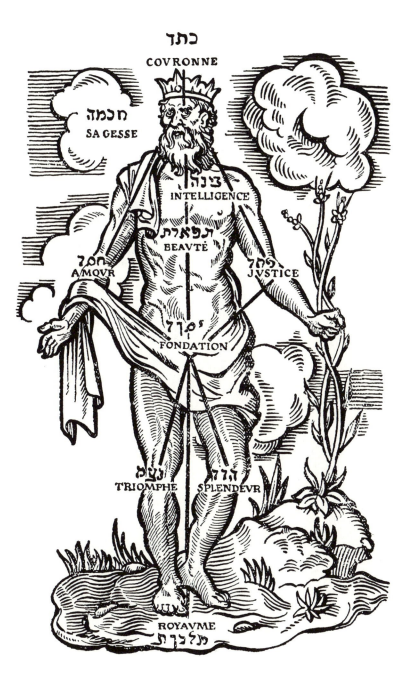

This figure is taken from a modern work, published in 1947 by Henry Serouya entitled *La Kabbale* (Paris: Grasset). It is meant to represent Primordial Man, each of whose members is a particular *sefirah*. This type of figurative representation is not found in the original writings of the kabbalists. It is found in several texts of Christian kabbalism and, more recently, in popularized works intended for a readership of amateur occultists.

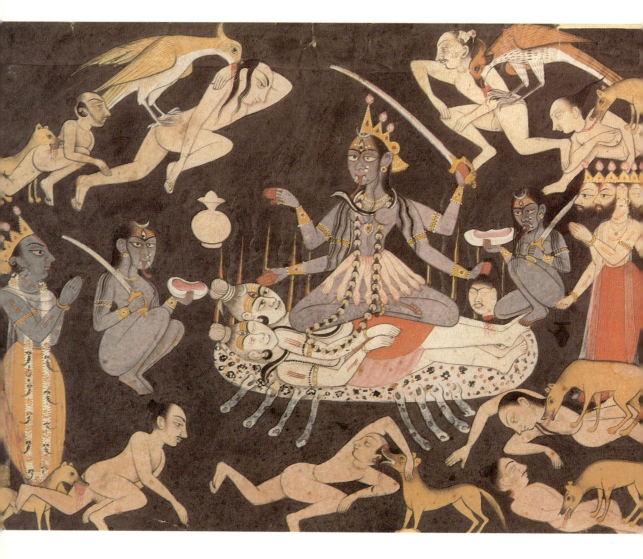

Kālikā on Śiva (London, Victoria and Albert Museum).

Indian Speculations about the Sex of the Sacrifice

Charles Malamoud

The scene is that most sinister of places, a cremation ground, the most impure and most dangerous of sites. The remains of some corpses are being consumed on the fire. Jackals wander around, dragging human limbs which they have snatched from the flames. Vultures wheel in the dark sky. In the central foreground is Śiva. Not the King of the Dance whose sublimely joyful movement is captured in so many bronzes, as he crushes the demon of ignorance (non-savoir) beneath his toe, but Śiva become Śava,[1] also a "corpse," split into two inert bodies, one on top of the other. The first, stretched out on the ground, is the Śiva Niṣkala, "without parts," in other words, indivisible, unjointed, absorbed in his ineffable homogeneity, a figure of the Absolute. Lying on him, as if on a couch, is another Śiva, the Mahākāla,[2] "Great Time," the destroyer, whose posture mimics the contracted immobility, the quasi-nothingness, to which the universe comes in the period separating two cosmic cycles. Yet the fact that he is fixed in such an apparently deathlike position does not prevent Śiva–Śava from having an erection. Seated on the god ("on the heart of the corpse") so that he penetrates her, Kālikā, the three-eyed goddess, naked ("robed in space"), "hips ornamented with a girdle made of dead men's arms," achieves pleasure and triumph.[3]

Another image: The frame is a vast eight-petaled lotus, in the center of which is an entwined couple. Here too the man is lying on his back, his penis penetrating the young woman sitting astride him, clasping his waist between her knees. She is leaning forward; their faces and breasts are touching. What we can make out of their features, and deduce from their posture, shows that in their embrace they are simultaneously absorbed in themselves and in each other. The man is Kāma, Desire; the woman is Rati, Pleasure. Above the couple, treading them underfoot, stands the

75

Goddess;[4] "in the shape of a girl of sixteen, shining with the radiance of ten million suns, with high, full breasts, robed in space, with a collar of skulls about her neck, and snakes like a sacred cordon round her bust."[5] Her upper right hand makes the gesture "which dispels fear" (the gesture known as *abhī* or *abhaya*), her lower right hand the gesture signifying the fulfillment of all wishes (*vara*). Her upper left hand holds a sacrificial knife, and her lower left holds the goddess's own head, the hair dishevelled, red tongue hanging out, teeth menacing. The goddess, in fact, has decapitated herself. A jet of blood spurts from the middle of her neck to the lips of the severed head. Two more streams of blood, this time from the sides of her neck, pour into vessels held by two female figures, one on each side of the goddess: these are Dākinī and Varninī, companions Kālī has provided herself with by making them emerge from her own body.[6]

These images – paintings – are relatively recent.[7] Hardly any of them date from before the eighteenth century. But they belong to a far older tradition, whose origins cannot be dated. Most importantly, the materialized images we find in the albums are no more than mnemonic aids. Theoretically, the scenes they depict should be "visualized" by adepts, constructed mentally through a meditation whose every stage is minutely regulated by texts. In the case of Chinnamastā, the goddess "with the severed head," it is said that if anybody tries to worship her in this form without first having had the correct vision, procured by meditation and contemplation, the goddess will punish the overly hasty worshiper by cutting off his head and drinking his blood.[8]

The tradition we are dealing with here is that of a sect, the Śākta, which forms part of the vast movement known as Tantrism. These figures of the goddess are, therefore, illustrations of a complex theological doctrine. Every detail – the posture of the characters, their number, color, ornamentation, attributes and the framework in which they are set – has a symbolic value and corresponds to a clearly defined point in the teaching of the treatises (*śāstra*) or poems that celebrate the multiform power (*śakti*) of the goddess. I do not propose merely to comment on these images by means of the system of ideas they convey; but it is worth mentioning that as well as engaging the attention of specialists in Tantrism and Indian art, the goddess with the severed head has also attracted the poet Octavio Paz, who goes straight to the heart of the matter in his revealing comparison of the redoubtable Chinnamastā

with Marcel Duchamp's *The Bride Stripped Bare by Her Bachelors, Even*. In both we find,
the separation of the female body into two...the Goddess and her head, the Bride and
her Motor.... The Goddess feeds the world and herself with her own blood in exactly
the same way as the Bride sets her bachelors in motion simply by gratifying herself and
stripping herself bare. In the first case the operation is related to us in terms of myth
and sacrifice; in the second in pseudomechanical terms which, however, do not exclude
the idea of sacrifice.[9]

Paz could have completed the symmetry by adding that the goddess organizing her
own decapitation is also, for her part, a mechanism, a machinery, in which the energy
source creates the receptacles it is destined to keep filled.

For anybody familiar with orthodox Brahmanic texts, these two groups of
images – the goddess sexually enjoying the god-corpse, and the goddess making her
severed head drink her own blood – are highly disturbing because they convey the
impression of a world turned upside-down (in Sanskrit, *viparīta*). And indeed *viparīta*,
"inverted," is the adjective used in Indian eroticism to describe the amorous positions in which the woman places herself on top of the man. The normal procedure
is for the man to lie on the woman, as the masculine sky covers the feminine earth,
or as the masculine melodic air is superimposed on a sequence of words. The inversion of the positions of the bodies is also a sign of the reversal of what in India is
the normal hierarchy of the sexes: man above and woman below. Furthermore, here
it symbolizes the triumph of the active feminine *māyā*, the deployment of the iridescent multiplicity of appearance over the undifferentiated, immutable Absolute,
represented by the immobilized Male. The goddess of *māyā* shows that she is mistress of the game, and also that the game is the master. In the classic Indian form of
this dualism, as embodied in the philosophical school of Sāṃkhya, Prakṛti (or nature
in all its diversity) is developed until it becomes manifest to the eyes of Puruṣa,
"man," insofar as that is a name for the Absolute in its unity: but having provided
him with this spectacle, Prakṛti vanishes.[10] Here, on the other hand, the actress-
character, if we may transfer the Sāṃkhya metaphor to Tantrism, seizes her spectator, dominates him and takes sexual pleasure in him; she integrates the ultimate
reality that he symbolizes and reveals that everything is part of the play of which
she is both author and director. And Chinnamastā, by constructing the circuit of vital
flux around the separation of her body into two parts, provides a feminine version

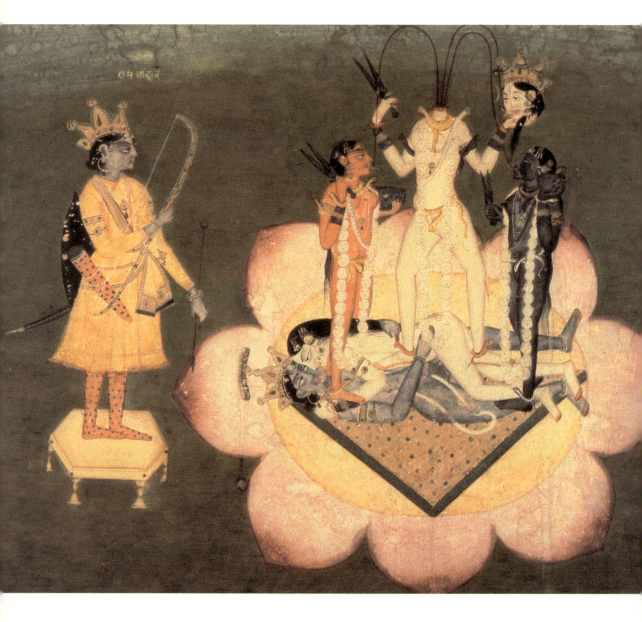

Mahāvidyā Chinnamastā, Kangra School, ca. 1810.
Private Collection.

of the sacrifice, wherein is revealed the most radical and intense manifestation of the desire for feminine domination. In the arrangement of ideas which we find from the Veda onward, in other words, from the oldest Indian texts we possess, whose validity remains unchanged throughout the history of Hinduism, sacrifices and the sacrificial schema constitute the structure that ultimately explains the organization of the cosmos, society, living bodies and all the homologies and interactions between these different levels.[11]

If, then, the goddess with the severed head provides an inverted (*viparīta*) image of the sacrifice, what is the correct, the orthodox image, the one contained in those fundamental Brahmanic texts, the Vedic treatises on sacrifice? Or, to be more precise, for this is the issue that's really at stake here, what is the sex of the sacrifice?

It is quite legitimate to put the question in these terms, as sacrifice in the Veda is personified, and is constantly compared with a body, whose anatomy, physiology and behavior are subjects of study. Sacrifice offers a privileged and constantly exploited site for the metaphor of the body which is used so often in the Veda. And although sacrifice is a machine, a "mechanism," to use Sylvain Lévi's expression[12] — and this will be explained in more detail later — it is also, primarily, a living organism, usually anthropomorphic, but sometimes also viewed as that of a wild deer or a bird. Adventures are attributed to it which cumulatively form a kind of mythology. This mythology relates to ritual, and it is made up of two sorts of narrative: first, pseudo-myths designed to explain how the gods or men discovered a particular form of sacrifice, and what it means or symbolizes; and second, myths whose heroes are rites, elements of the sacrifice that are personified. A difficulty arises if one attempts to sort out these often very brief and allusive narratives, for the definition of sacrifice is unfixed, and the term we have translated as "sacrifice," *yajña*, may be used in either a broad or a narrow sense. In the strict sense, *yajña* is the essential part of the sacrificial ceremony, the culminating moment at which the victim is put to death (by stifling or strangulation in the case of animals; by squeezing, if the sacrifice is an offering of the plant known as *soma*; or by pouring clarified butter into the fire if the sacrifice is of the *homa* type). In its broader sense, *yajña* encompasses all the acts preceding, constituting and following this central moment, and not only the actions, but also the ingredients (oblatory substances, fireplaces and fires, the herbs strewn on the sacrificial ground, altar-bricks and various other vessels), the differ-

79

ent types of texts spoken, and the different ways of speaking them (by chanting them, reciting them aloud, murmuring them or saying them to oneself), the psychical and physical powers (mind and breath) needed to perform the gestures and pronounce the words, the characters both human and divine involved in the ceremony and so forth. The list could be extended: sacrifice, the organizing principle of everything that exists, tends to include within itself everything that it organizes.

But whether it be *yajña* in its narrow sense or in its wider meaning of the ceremony as a whole, whenever Vedic sacrifice is compared to a body it is indubitably and supremely male. Thus, for example, the three sequences known as *anuyāja* (the accompanying offerings), a kind of appendix to the main offering, are likened to the penis (*śiśna*), and the texts discourse about the three penises of sacrifice.[13]

The overall body of the sacrifice is thus composed of the ceremony's constitutive elements, each of which is itself regarded as a living body, even if it is a material object, an event, an action or an abstract idea. One is reminded here of Arcimboldo and those faces collaged from fruits, or even more of the Indian Moghul paintings of elephants or horses that are actually agglomerations of human or animal figures contorted and intertwined in the obscure altercations of love or war.

The individual bodies, which together make up the body of the sacrifice itself, are noteworthy in that they are described as sexed beings and, normally, are associated in such a way as to form couples (*mithuna*).[14] But why in couples? The answer given in the texts each time one of these elemental pairs is mentioned is that they are meant "for procreation" (*prajnanāya, prajātyai*). The aim of the sacrificer is to obtain a huge progeniture, abundant livestock, a fecundity that is prepared and prefigured by the unions arranged or established during the actual process of the sacrifice. The first thing these *mithuna* must give birth to, however, is the internal progress of the sacrifice, its ability to engender each stage from the preceding one. For these *mithuna* to be authentic and effective they must be founded on nonredundance (*ajāmi*),[15] which means that they must establish a contact between partners with different characteristics. In the cases where these partners are living organisms, the salient feature is, of course, their sex.[16] Where inanimate objects and ideas are concerned, the sex attributed to them is determined by the grammatical gender of the name they bear. In Sanskrit (as in Greek, Latin, German and Russian) there are three genders, masculine, feminine and neuter; and entities which have no natural sex are not always designated by neuter nouns, so that the distribution between masculine and feminine is a matter of linguistic arbitrariness. The grammarian Patañjali claimed that as it is impossible to formulate rules governing the gender of nouns, issues relating to grammatical gender simply cannot be taught.[17] Before he reaches this conclusion, however, Patañjali considers alternative points of view, in order to refute them: for some, he says, all entities, whether animate or not, have a sex, and the gender of their names is an indication of this; if we cannot see that a tree is male and a stool female, this is simply because our organs of perception are too weak. Patañjali criticizes this argument for being circular: its adherents argue that the male sex of an entity determines the masculine gender of its name, whereas the male sex is itself induced from the masculine gender of that name.

Patañjali's commonsensical approach differs from that of the doctrinal writers on Vedic sacrifice. The authors of the Brāhmaṇa have no hesitation in systematically assimilating gender to sex, and in reading gender as a symptom of sex: this is one indication, among others, of the supremely powerful place language occupies in this system of thought.

It should be pointed out at this point that in the constitution of *mithuna* the neuter gender is treated as if it were masculine (which is surprising, given that the word that means "neuter" in grammatical terminology is *napuṃsaka*, which literally means "nonmale"), so the partner of the feminine may equally well be masculine or neuter.[18] Thus, the "melodic air" which makes a couple with the "verse" – the feminine *ṛc* – is the *sāman*, a neuter word. Similarly, the neuter word *manas*, "mind," is one of the partners of the word *vāc*, which is feminine. The fact that the neuter should be classed alongside the masculine clearly indicates that we are dealing here with an issue that is more abstract than it appears: two elements form a fertile couple because there is an opposition between them which makes them complementary, not because the one or the other has an organ or a substance which makes it capable of reproducing itself or of contributing to its reproduction. The *mithuna* is fertile in the sense that it sets in motion, acts as a catalyst for, the general fecundity of the sacrifice, not because it may give birth to offspring of its own. Furthermore, we are never told what the "child" of each of these couplings might be. And, as we shall see, there are substitutes for the differences of sex and gender.

Let us examine some examples of these *mithuna*.

Man, Woman, Belt and Cord. When he begins the sacrifice, the sacrificer (*yajamāna*), that is, the man who orders the ceremony, pays for it and hopes to receive its beneficial effects (progeny and livestock, as we have seen, but also, more significantly, heaven after death), has to put on a belt made out of blades of grass called *mekhalā*, a feminine noun.[19] A *mithuna* is established between the male sacrificer and the female belt. The sacrificer's wife (*patnī*) must for her part have a cord called a *yoktra*, a neuter noun, put around her waist by the officiating priest.[20] There is a *mithuna* between the wife and the cord, as also between the belt and the cord.[21] Finally, the texts regard this ceremony, which takes place at the very beginning of the sacrifice, as a specific realization of the general and, in a sense, self-evident *mithuna* between the sacrificer and his wife.

This calls for several comments. In the first place, while the operations of the sacrifice are in progress, the coupling of the sacrificer and his wife, as sexual union, is neither performed nor even hinted at. Their *mithuna* is mentioned not in order to evoke copulation but as a reminder that they are permanently, and especially in the sacrifice, a couple.[22] On the other hand, symbolic copulation, in which sight takes the place of touch, occurs several times between the wife and one of the males present — not including the sacrificer — or one of the male objects of the sacrifice.[23] A very elaborate *mithuna*, very close to actual sexual union, occurs in the Royal Horse sacrifice, in the hierogamy during which the queen lies down against the horse that is about to be put to death and, by using words and gestures, incites it to penetrate her.[24]

However, the cord does not play the same role for the woman as the belt does for the man. Although both serve to separate the upper part of the body, which is suitable to take part in the sacrifice, from the part "below the navel," which is deemed inappropriate for sacrificial operations (*amedhya*), the impurity of the man's lower part is only mentioned in passing, whereas it is dealt with in emphatic terms where the woman is concerned. The principal function of the man's special belt is to increase his power; it consists of three stems, symbolizing the vital breath that is perceived in this situation as threefold.[25] The woman's cord, on the other hand, is primarily designed to act as a screen between her impurity and the sacrifice. The wife, although her presence is indispensable, is "the hinder part of the sacrifice."[26] The cord is meant to hide the most impure part — which, nevertheless, is the seat of her fecundity[27] — of this "hinder" part.[28] It is placed over the skirt, also made of grass, which the wife has to wear. As often happens, there are a number of intersecting interpretations, some containing additional material, jostling to account for this single ritual fact. The same texts that attribute to the cord the function of isolating the woman's sex remind us that the cord (*yoktra*) is also the link which attaches (*yogya*) a draught animal to the yoke (*yuga*).[29] The cord also represents the noose of *Varuṇa*,[30] the god whose role is to punish anybody guilty of transgressing the world order (*ṛta*). The woman is already held in this bond by means of the cord; and in order for the positive aspects of the analogy to be evoked, and at the same time neutralized and moderated, it is said that the grass skirt protects the woman's body against the harshness of the bond, and that, additionally, there is no need for a knot in the cord, as that might give too exact an image — and thereby generate the reality being represented — of the running knot with which Varuṇa strangles those whom he has decided to punish.[31] Finally, and in a different register, this grass cord is, for the duration of the sacrifice, the woman's equivalent of the Brahmanic cord (*yajñopavīta*)[32] which the men of the three principal classes of society wear permanently across their chest (passing over the left shoulder and under the right arm) from the day of their initiation. This initiation is, as it were, a second birth, and gives them access to the Vedic text; it is forbidden to women, this being the most obvious sign and cause of their ritual inferiority. Unable to recite the Veda, relegated to the hinder part of the sacrifice,[33] their status determined by the lower part of their bodies, reduced to their mere physiological birth, women are by nature[34] linked with lies and disorder, *anṛta*, destruction and disorganization, *nirṛti* (*anṛta* and *nirṛti* are two forms of the opposite of *ṛta*).[35] It is thus with a substitute Brahmanic cord, and one whose validity is only provisional, that the wife penetrates into the sacrificial ground, where yet nothing could be done without her.[36]

The Parts of the Body. The body of the human or anthropomorphic persons who figure in the sacrifice is composed of *mithuna*: thumbs and big toes (*anguṣṭha*, masculine), with fingers (*aṅguli*, feminine); ears (*karṇa*, masculine), with eyebrows (*bhrū*, feminine); lips (*oṣṭha*, masculine), with nostrils (*nāsikā*, feminine); teeth (*danta*, masculine), with the tongue (*jihvā*, feminine), etc.[37] Thus, what is described is the supreme body of the cosmogonic god Prajāpati, who can be said to be the sacrifice made body.

Receptacles, Contents, Ingredients and Various Utensils. In the sacrifice where the offering is the juice of the *soma* plant, receptacles (*pātra*) are used, some of which are bowls (*sthālī*, feminine) and others small vats (*vāyarya*, masculine), and there is a coupling between the two sorts of vessels. The draughts of *soma* are also of two kinds, but the difference this time is not one of sex: some are mixed, while others are pure. And the *soma* liquor also exists in two kinds, either well-endowed with the "benedictions" that accompany its preparation, or not. There is an overall *mithuna* formed out of the *mithuna* of the receptacles, the draughts and the *soma*. "He who recognizes it finds in it his birth," that is, a man who has understood the mystery of these relationships between the things involved in the sacrifice becomes a new man, he is reborn.[38] And since what is done in the rite is the origin, model and justification of what is done in ordinary life, we learn that the bowls are discarded after use, but that the small vats are not, and thence that a newborn child can be abandoned if it is a girl, but not if it is a boy.[39] The male, as must now be evident, is more valuable than the female, and in cases of uncertainty, things should be assumed to be male, to be on the safe side: if one destroys an embryo of undetermined sex, one is guilty of the same crime as the destruction of a male embryo. And, besides, the word for "embryo" (*garbha*) is masculine.[40]

Among the officiants taking part in the solemn sacrifice, there is one, called the *hotṛ*, who specializes in reciting "verses" from the Veda. The verses are feminine, from which it must be assumed that the *hotṛ* acquires a feminine nature because at a particular point in the ritual he has to climb onto a swing, which in fact has a masculine name, *preṅkha*, while another officiant, the *udgātṛ*, who is responsible for chanting the "airs" (*sāman*, neuter, thus in the masculine sphere), has to climb onto a wooden seat known by a feminine name, *āsandī*. There is an explicit *mithuna* between these two objects, the male *preṅkha* and the female *āsandī*, and an implicit *mithuna* between the feminized *hotṛ* and his male support, and between the *udgātṛ*, confirmed in his masculinity, and his female support, and finally between the two officiants themselves, one of whom belongs to the feminine side and the other to the masculine.[41]

An altar (*vedi*, feminine) is set up on the sacrificial ground. It couples with Agni, the god of fire, and also with the masculine *veda*, a word that here means not the Vedic text, but the bundle of grass with which the ground is swept, and which is also used to spread out the herbs and grass with which the ground is strewn.[42]

In addition to the material ingredients of the sacrifice, and the sacrificial utensils, some more abstract elements also need to be taken into account, as they too are regarded as sexed and paired, the most significant of these being the consecration and the vow, belief and truth.[43] The consecration (*dīkṣā*, feminine) comprises all the rites, austerities and restraints by means of which the sacrificer makes himself worthy to undertake the sacrifice; the vow (*vrata*, neuter) is a generic term for all the observances the sacrificer pledges himself to respect, the special behavior he undertakes to maintain for the duration of the sacrifice; trust (*śraddhā*, feminine) is faith in the efficacy of the ritual and belief in the competence of the officiants; and the truth (*satya*, neuter) appears to refer to the indisputable validity of the Vedic text.

Masculine Singular, Feminine Plural.

There is an observable tendency to construct *mithuna* in which the male partner is single and the female partner multiple.

To pour clarified butter or any other oblatory liquid onto the fire, several "offering spoons" (*sruc*, feminine) and one "dipping spoon" (*sruva*, masculine) are used; this is why if there is one male, even a small boy, among even a large number of women, he has to walk in front.[44]

Transposed to the sociological level, this grouping of gender and number allows polygyny and forbids polyandry, as the following "myth" of origin illustrates:

First there was the verse and the melodic air. The verse was called "she" and the air "he." The verse said to the air, "Let us copulate for begetting children." The air answered, "No, for my greatness exceeds yours." The verse became two, and spoke. But it did not comply with their request. It became three and spoke. And they united. Because he agreed to be united with [the verses become] three, they intone or chant a single air with three verses...and for that reason also one man has many wives, but one woman has not many husbands at the same time.[45]

When oblation has to be made to the Sun god and a whole group of goddesses, some ritualists are of the opinion that the Sun should be associated with the offering made to each of the goddesses in order to create a single *mithuna* each time.[46] But, says the text, this is not the correct way to proceed. The sacrifice becomes exhausted when one formula is used several times for separate offerings. It must be regarded as a single *mithuna* between the Sun and all the goddesses together, which in practice means serving the Sun first, once and for all, and then the goddesses one by one. A man who has a number of wives forms a *mithuna* between himself, on the one hand, and all his wives, on the other.

The affinity between the feminine and the plural is so strong that when there are two similar sentences, the subject of which is not clear, and which differ only in that one has a singular and the other a plural verb, it is correct to conclude that the plural verb denotes a feminine subject and the singular verb a masculine one. This is the analysis advanced by one Brāhmaṇa to provide a basis for *mithuna* between the implicit subjects of both sentences.[47]

The Adventures of the Sacrifice. Some of the *mithuna* are real love stories and, as such, often have bizarre endings. The Sacrifice (here used in its strict sense, defined above, as the culminating point of the sacrificial process) falls in love with a partner who also has a place in this corpus: sometimes this is Speech, that is, the Vedic texts that accompany the gestures; sometimes the *dakṣiṇā*, the Remuneration of the officiating priests (a stage which is of great importance in the ritual sequence, on a level with the Consecration). According to one of the versions of this narrative,

> the Sacrifice, originally, resided with the Gods, Remuneration with the Fathers [the dead whom funerary rites have transformed into Ancestors]. The Sacrifice fell in love with the Remuneration. The Fathers said to the Sacrifice, "Go and ask the Gods to give us a share of the offering of *soma*." The Gods decided that the Fathers should have the third squeezing. This is why the third squeezing is for the Fathers. [Recompense of the Sacrifice:] Remuneration called and the Sacrifice came running. This is why a man runs when he is called by a woman. This is why the Brahman scholar loves women so much: for it is he who is closest to the Sacrifice. The Sacrifice [thus] joins with Remuneration. The god Indra saw this and thought, "The being born of this union will be [so large that he will entirely cover] the world around." So he slipped into the womb of Remu-

neration, then came out of it to be born. And again he observed and thought, "The being who is born next from this womb will be my rival." So he penetrated once more into the womb, and tore it.[48]

How is this particularly refined form of rape to be understood? The embrace of Sacrifice and Remuneration or, in another version,[49] of Sacrifice and Speech, turns the rite into a closed system. The gods are ousted, the rite becomes self-sufficient and dispenses with myth as an inconvenient and unnecessary third element. Indra, the king of the gods and the most mythologized of all of them (having a sort of biography composed of his heroic exploits), does not allow rituals that might be independent and efficacious without the divine powers having a hand in them. Therefore, it has to be the product of the *mithuna* between the Sacrifice and one or another of the feminine component principles of the sacrificial whole. Thus, Indra finds a subtle and ferocious way for himself, and himself alone, to be the child of this coupling. We have here, in mythic form, a narrative of the competing claims of myth and ritual which, historically, took the form of a very real rivalry between a religion organized around ritual and one founded on the worship of divinities; and, as we know, it was the latter, predictably, which emerged triumphant.

I have presented this list of *mithuna* (and it could easily have been extended) to demonstrate the way in which Brahmanic sacrifice, although male in gender overall, is composed of couples, and thus that half of its substance is feminine. However, that is not enough to render the body of the sacrifice androgynous: the whole is not the sum of its parts. Sacrifice provides an excellent example of Indian-style hierarchy, and more particularly Brahmanic hierarchy, as described by Louis Dumont. The whole has the same nature as the superior part. While the inferior part is encompassed by the superior part, it, nevertheless, is in contrast with the latter. Applications of the same formula can be found in the relationships of men and women, even apart from the real or symbolic relationships between the sexes that in the sacrifice join the masculine with the feminine. The woman is a complete human being, with full rights, and, in her own way, is autonomous. But she is included in man, and in her entirety is only half of him.

Having said this, and having seen some examples of the combinations composed by masculine and feminine in the Sacrifice, we must now look in more detail at the characteristics typical of sacrificial femininity and masculinity, and consider the figures between which they are distributed.

Of all the dramatis personae of the sacrifice, if we leave aside the sacrificer's wife and the goddesses (whose characters are not really developed in Vedic mythology, and who are only invoked in the rite collectively as "the wives of the gods"), the one whom the texts present most emphatically as feminine is Speech. The supreme example of this is the text of the Veda, of course, but it also refers to human and divine speech in general; and the shift in meaning from one to the other is not always easy to discern.

The stereotypes about women are all formulated in relation to Speech; the reason why women are drawn to the pleasures of love, why they like music and songs, is that they model their conduct on *Vāc*, Speech. To attract the *soma* which is found near the celestial beings known as Gandharva, the gods send Speech to them, with instructions to seduce them "because the Gandharva love women." The Gandharva are very keen to keep *Vāc*, and to that end they try to impress her by reciting the Veda. But the gods, more shrewdly, play music and sing songs that ensure her return.[50]

Women lie, and are thus in the sphere of *anṛta*. This is not merely a matter of Speech itself, but a reminder that speech is originally twofold, equally capable of uttering truth and falsehood: it was only after a kind of rearrangement or redistribution that the gods chose what is true in speech, and the demons what is false.[51] Another method of sorting truth from falsehood is to divide Speech into four parts, the three sacred exclamations *bhūr*, *bhuvar* and *svar*, in which all truth is concentrated and which the gods keep for themselves, and a fourth part containing all the lies and falsehood, which is man's share.[52] This division into three and one can also be organized differently: of the four parts of Speech, the first three constitute articulate and explicit speech, while the fourth is implicit, indeed ineffable; this "fourth" (*turīya*) realm of Speech is another name for the Absolute, which is also called *brahman*.[53] (It is noteworthy that this area of speech which lies beyond speech is designated by a neuter noun, rather than a feminine one.) Insofar as it is coextensive with the Veda, Speech is divided into three, as the Veda itself consists of three major groups of texts.[54] (There is, in fact, a fourth Veda, which is traditionally regarded as falling outside the canon of the Triple Knowledge: it is of lesser worth, and is used only in magical rites. Its adepts, however, consider it to be the greatest of the Vedas, the one that corresponds to the *brahman*, the unrevealed, mysterious, unspeakable element of Speech.)[55] Regarded in its phonic substance, Speech is divided into vowels, and occlusive and spirant consonants,[56] although that is far from being an exhaustive list of its fragmentations. What is interesting about these different ways of analyzing Speech is simply the fact that they are analyzable and therefore composite; Speech carries multiplicity within itself, and multiplicity, as we have seen, is one of the characteristics of the feminine. There is also a ritual instruction that confirms this liaison: when a sacrifice is celebrated that lasts for a whole day and continues into the following night, a victim has to be sacrificed to the goddess Speech, because Speech is feminine and so is the night. Moreover the femininity of the night is not related solely to the feminine gender of its name: it is also demonstrated by the great number of stars which provide its light, in contrast with the male day, which is lit by the sun alone.[57]

What, then, within the framework of the sacrifice, are the partners of Speech? We can say a priori that act, mind and silence make a couple with Speech as, singly or together, they constitute its masculine counterpart. To these three concepts must be added the melodic "air," the partner of Speech in its narrower sense of Vedic "verse," and also "breath." These combinations are not just borne out in the texts, they also correspond to what actually happens on the sacrificial ground. In the same way as Speech is represented in the actual sacrificial process by the officiant *hotṛ*, who specializes in reciting verses of the *Ṛg-Veda*, and the melodic "air" by the officiant *udgātṛ*, action — which here means the gestural part of the sacrifice, the comings and goings, and the manipulations — is the responsibility of the *ahdvaryu* and his associates. Not that the *ahdvaryu* is mute, but his speech is composed of *yajus*, Vedic formulas extracted and adapted to the gestures that accompany them; it is, so to speak, the verbal face of action. Silence itself has a concrete presence among the sacrificial officiants in the person of the one known as *brahman* (in this case a masculine word, not neuter like the word that designates the unspoken element of speech), he is the doctor of the sacrifice, and neither acts nor speaks, except to indicate errors that have been made and the ways of compensating for them.

Sacrificial silence is a notion on the same level as that of the spoken word, the chant, and the act which sets the body in motion. It is not mere absence of speech;

and it is endowed with positive values which have been admirably distinguished and defined by Louis Renou.[58] Thus we learn that, on the one hand, there is the silence that makes it possible to evoke the realm of the inexplicable, of things which have not happened or which cannot be explained. To make a sacrificial gesture without accompanying it by speech is to charge the act with silence, and to perform it in thought at the same time as in action; thought occupies the space left empty by speech. On the other hand, there is silence as pause, or as retention of the voice: its function is to enclose the sacrifice, to prevent it from fleeing and becoming dispersed. "Speech draws and sucks in the Sacrifice,"[59] and silence reinvigorates and reassembles it.

Silence of the first type is thus at the service of thought or, more precisely, of "mind" (*manas*, a neuter word), and silence of the second type serves the nonverbal part of the sacrifice, the action (*karman*, a neuter word). A series of correspondences and equivalences makes it possible to regard "breath" (*prāna*, masculine) as the foundation of the physiological manifestation of "mind." Word and breath, and word and mind constitute almost identical and interchangeable couples. The masculinity of silence is thus attested by its name (*mauna*, neuter) and by its proximity to those other entities in the masculine sphere: action, mind and breath. Surprisingly, it also appears in the affinity that exists between silence and sperm:[60] the emission of sperm (*retasah siktih*) happens silently (*upām śu*). There has to be a draught of *soma* (with an inaudible recitation of the appropriate formula) because it symbolizes sperm spilled into a womb; this is especially the case with the draught of *soma* offered jointly to the god Tvaṣṭṛ (the "fashioner" of living beings) and the group of wives of the gods.[61] Any other silent offering in the sacrifice is explicitly designated as the act that consists of pouring Breath-sperm into Speech-womb; there is a *mithuna* between the femininity of the explicit (*nirukta*) and formulaic Speech (consisting of *yajus*) and the masculinity of the sperm, the silent act, related through this silence to the "mental."[62] In practical terms, fertilizing Speech by breath–sperm–silence means dividing one rite into two successive stages, one in which the texts are recited aloud, and one in which they are recited inaudibly.

The sources of this information about the way masculine and feminine traits are distributed among the figures who compose the sacrificial body are to be found in the instructions about ritual, and in the speculations they give rise to. But a more systematic view of them can be obtained by looking at the mythology. In fact, in the texts of the Brāhmaṇa we are trying to understand, the borderline between the two domains is not clear-cut: we are dealing with treatises on sacrifice in which myth only intervenes in order to explain the symbolism of the rites, and thus to provide material for speculation. But then the mythic figures and stories which come most naturally to mind are the ones concerned with cosmogony, and in Vedic mythology this is always presented as a vast sacrifice. The creation of the world is simultaneously the invention and the first performance of the sacrifice.

At all events, gods appear in outline, and while obviously not independent of the rites in connection with which they are evoked, they nevertheless possess more continuity and greater consistency than the divinized forms of the sacrifice we have so far encountered in orthodox Vedism. Among these gods are the figures associated with Agni, the god of fire, and Prajāpati, "Lord of the creatures," simultaneously creator of all that is and, as we have seen, sacrifice incarnate; in the person of Prajāpati, we have a mythological version of the sacrificial body whose contours and composition I have tried to outline with the help of what is said about sacrifice.

Here, in a rather schematic version, is the principal myth about Agni and Prajāpati. In it, both gods are involved with Speech, and their male characteristics appear in contrast to the femininity of Speech.

In the beginning, Prajāpati is alone. He is overcome with a desire to procreate, which is also the desire to "become multiple." In order to realize this desire "he becomes sacrifice,"[63] in which he is simultaneously the sacrificer, because it is his own project; the officiant, because he himself carries out all the necessary operations; and the victim, because the only oblatory material at this stage is his body. Thus, he performs the sacrifice and emits (rather than, strictly speaking, creates) beings, and disperses his person in the infinity of things which thenceforth form the cosmos.[64]

There are several different accounts of the way he went about this. Some texts insist on the solitude of the god. Others teach that Prajāpati has Speech already within him, and that his first act was to bring it out of himself, so that it is, or thereby becomes, his "assistant," his feminine double, with whom he copulates; there are, however, two competing narratives of what happened next. Speech, pregnant, separates from Prajāpati, gives birth to the creatures and then returns not to him but within him;[65] alternatively, the copulation occurs between Prajāpati's "mind" (*manas*) and Speech, but it is Prajāpati who becomes "pregnant."[66] In both variations the parent who is assimilated to the primordial Male, the Puruṣa of the most ancient cosmogonies, yet contains a trait of femininity. He includes within himself, and reintroduces into himself, Speech-woman; or else he takes into himself the sperm he has poured into Speech, or else Speech itself, and himself becomes pregnant and gives birth. These are not the only signs; on several occasions we find mention of the two breasts of Prajāpati,[67] and of the gods milking them.[68] Yet Prajāpati is not androgynous: he is the totality of man and can either encompass woman or keep her at a distance, as he wishes. He can either make her part of himself or make her the "other" with whom he copulates.

In any event, Prajāpati emerges exhausted and dislocated from his act of creation. Faced with this emptied, suffering body – or, conversely, one already swelling up like a corpse – the gods he has created take fright and decide to restore him, literally to reconstruct him.[69] The story of Prajāpati's reconstitution by the gods, at the initiative of Agni, the one among them most gifted with the ability to go "forward,"[70] corresponds to the recreation of the father by his son, who thereby becomes his father's father.[71] This story merges, in our texts, with the description of a magnificent ritual, the "Piling Up the Fire." This rite, which is, in fact, a complex sequence of sacrifices, is designed to commemorate and reactivate this second stage of the genesis. Analyses and speculation, drawn from the network of correspondences on which the symbolism of Piling Up the Fire is based, occupy hundreds and hundreds of pages of the Brāhmaṇas.[72] These treatises, which date from the eighth or ninth century B.C., contain the beginnings – and some of the high points – of Indian philosophical thought, in the form of subtle, systematic, slightly finnicky reflections on similarity and difference, the one and the multiple, continuum and discontinuity.

Piling Up the Fire (*agnicayana*) consists, briefly, of building an altar of five superimposed layers of bricks. A fire is to be lit on the altar. The single bricks, their groupings within each layer, and the relations between the layers, correspond to the elements that compose the reconstituted person of Prajāpati and to their combinations and mode of action. One fundamental idea is that the reconstruction of Prajāpati is also the foundation of cyclical time,[73] symbolized by the year and made up of discrete unities capable of being organized in different kinds of regular sequences, and sequences of sequences, particularly the seasons. (The Sanskrit word for "season" is *ṛtu*, a term which also means "period," sometimes menstrual period, sometimes the period propitious for conception. Yet another of Prajāpati's feminine traits is that he perceives these moments in himself.)[74]

What role does fire play in all this? The god Agni is in charge of building this edifice. He is also its material. In order to restore body and life to his prostrate father, Agni goes back into him and gives him his own substance. The texts repeat time and again that the clay from which the Fire-altar bricks are made is itself solidified fire, so that piling up the bricks of this edifice is really piling up fire, an image of Prajāpati ignited.[75] Prajāpati and Agni are thus consubstantial, in myth as well as in its ritual replica. And like Prajāpati, but more uniformly, Agni is clearly male, as can be seen from his way of being creator, from the frequently reiterated identity between fire and sperm, and by his suitability as sexual partner of Speech.

Before going on to describe the modalities of the *mithuna* between Fire and Speech, we need to define the masculinity of Prajāpati and Agni in more detail. Basically it relates to their fecundating power, the action proper to them in the *mithuna* in which they are engaged. Insofar as Prajāpati is concerned, we must also add that he is associated with those other expressions of masculinity: silence and unexpressed thought. But both Prajāpati and Agni eject their sperm, and at the same time *are* sperm.[76]

However, there is more to Indian maleness than this. Further components are *vīriya*, the "heroic force," and *indriya*, "virile worth," which are displayed in combat, but also in a passion for conquering women and in the art of making oneself loved by them. Being heroic and being prolific are separate things, as can clearly be seen in some of the prayers pronounced at the offering of *soma*:

> In accordance with [the draughts called] *śukra* and *manthin* are offspring born: [there are] the eaters and the eaten.... Engendering heroic offspring, come forth, Śukra, with your pure radiance.... Engendering prolific offspring, come forth, Manthin, with your mixed radiance.... The eaters are those who are heroic, the eaten those who are prolific. The offspring of him who knows thus becomes an eater, not eaten.[77]

The most well-known example of the heroic type of male god is Indra, King of the gods and patron of the warrior class, the *kṣatriya*. He accumulates exploits, kills monsters and crushes the enemies of the gods, though not without taking risks and suffering in the process. His thunderbolt and his sex are equally irresistible. He is a bull among the gods. His liking for women gets him into strange and dangerous adventures, but his role as father, as male partner in a fertile couple, is negligible. Is there thus nothing of the feminine in him, no tendency toward femininity? He actually loves women so much that he disguises himself as a woman in order to gain access to them, and the imitation is taken to such a degree that it becomes a genuine transformation, causing Indra acute embarrassment.[78]

What is feminine in Prajāpati, on the other hand, is the power he has to assume the feminine role in procreation. Agni himself is feminine, is actually a womb at the moment in the sacrifice when sperm, in the form of the juice of *soma*, is poured onto the oblatory fire.[79] The special affinities that Prajāpati and Agni have with humans are therefore not with the *kṣatriya* but with the caste of brahmans, who specialize in ritual rather than war.

Here again, though, the Indian concept of hierarchy supervenes. In Indian society, brahmans are superior to *kṣatriya*, in that they have warrior-like potentialities and so dominate *kṣatriya* and, in a sense, encompass them. We have seen, in connection with the loves of the Sacrifice and Speech (or Remuneration), that the brahman scholars were also "extremely fond of women." Once more, it is the hierarchical system that explains the rule that brahmans may have four wives and *kṣatriya* only three:[80] in both cases the first wife is "for *dharma*," for the "religious law" and procreation, and the others "for *kāma*," for "pleasure." This is an entirely theoretical rule, contradicted by the evidence of numerous literary texts and by common sense, as it is perfectly obvious that it is the *kṣatriya*, the kings and princes, who have harems, whose vocation it is to devote themselves to love as they do to hunting. The ritual of Piling Up the Fire provides us with an illustration of this inclusion of the inferior in the superior, the quantitative aspect of the hierarchy: Agni is not the only one to take part in the composition of the reconstituted Prajāpati. Indra also gave himself to him.[81] Thus, the new body is part Agni and part Indra, but in total it is Agni. Similarly, in the Fire altar, the bricks are Agni and the mortar binding them together is Indra, but the edifice as a whole is fire. Agni is essentially brahman, Indra purely *kṣatriya*, but, we learn, Agni contains within him both *brahman* and *kṣatra*, the principles of both classes.[82]

As he appears in myth, Prajāpati, either alone or in association with Agni, or merged with him, is supremely the partner of Speech. The dominant ritual discourse treats as autonomous entities the forms of masculinity that are united within him as attributes of his personality. Thus, he can be said to be silence, the ineffable and spermatic fertility. Yet in his recreated form he is also the arrangement of Time in connected parts and, by the same token, the unfolding of multiplicity, the explication. But this aspect of himself he owes to Speech, with whom he again copulates and then integrates. Indeed, in the tenth book of the *Śatapatha-Brāhmaṇa* the mystery of the Fire altar, its esoteric equivalent (*upaniṣad*), is revealed to us as Speech:

> For it is with Speech that it is built, with the verses of the *Ṛg-Veda*, with the formulas of the *Yajur-Veda* and with the words accompanied by melodic airs of the *Sāma-Veda*: it is the divine speech. And when [the officiant who directs the sacrificial operations gives his instructions and] speaks with human speech, "Do ye this, do ye that!" then also it [the altar] is built therewith. Now, this Speech is threefold...and the altar also is threefold inasmuch as three kinds of bricks are put into it — those with masculine names, those with feminine names and those with neuter names. And the parts of the human body are threefold, for there are those with masculine names, those with feminine names and those with neuter names. But all the bricks have the generic name *iṣṭakā* which is feminine, for they are Speech and Speech is feminine.[83]

Another side of this mystery is that Prajāpati's reconstituted body "is made entirely of *mithuna*"; *mithuna*, first of all, between the body of Agni and the vital fluid that flowed from Prajāpati's dislocated body, which Agni was able to collect; and *mithuna* in the altar, which replicates the body of Prajāpati, between the first and second layer of bricks, between the third and fourth, and between the fifth layer and the fire that is lit upon it when the construction is complete; and finally, *mithuna* between the totality of the edifice, which is entirely Speech (as each brick is itself Speech), and Breath (*prāṇa*), which is the esoteric equivalent of the fire lit on the fifth and last layer.[84]

In brief, then, the difference between the direct and the esoteric interpretation of Piling Up the Fire is that the former places the stress on the masculine singular, the reconstituted body of Prajāpati–Agni, whereas the second attributes ultimate significance to the feminine plural, the articulated multiplicity of Speech-bricks.

The feminine plural is also what characterizes the Tantric sacrificial scene organized around the goddess with the severed head. Chinnamastā dominates the *mithuna* of Love and Pleasure; and in this *mithuna*, it is the feminine that has the upper place and occupies the dominant position. The two feminine figures who flank the goddess are projections of her own person that is thus multiplied. She herself is fragmented. The distinction between the roles she simultaneously assumes, like Prajāpati — sacrificer, executioner, victim and, in this case, additionally, the divinity for whom the offering is destined — is represented spatially by the severance that affects her. Prajāpati is remade by reassembling himself in such a way that his constituent elements can join together and give him an unbroken body. The goddess, on the other hand, completes the circle of the sacrifice by the jets of blood which travel across, but do not cancel, the distance she has created and likes to maintain between the different parts of her being.[85]

The assemblage of objects, characters, gestures and speech which composes the Indian sacrifice derives its form and intelligibility from the metaphor of the body. Because it is described as a body that is itself made up of conjunctions of many bodies indefinitely rearranged, the sacrifice provides both the prime locus and the material for sexual symbolism. All the elements in this arrangement and all the sequences of the event are so many illustrations of the combinatory of the sexes, and reminders that the process by which sacrificial energy proceeds is a series of couplings. The metaphor of the body implies the preexistence of the body, and indeed the precosmic world is in the beginning a body which is both monstrous (with a thousand heads and eyes) and, by definition, human: genesis according to the Veda is the process by which Puruṣa, primordial man, is dismembered so that each part of his body may become one of the elements of the natural, social and ritual world that is thenceforth the dwelling place of men and gods.[86] The aim and purpose of the sacrifice is to reconstitute the image of this original, precreation body.

Puruṣo vai vajñaḥ: "[I]n truth, the sacrifice is a man [or is Man]."[87] This Brahmanic formula, which is both a definition and a metaphor, is thus a program. It initiates a long list of local identifications, the sum total of which is precisely that human configuration which the sacrificial construction has to make manifest. In fact, the two carts that are used to transport the stalks of *soma* together form the head of the sacrifice; the offertory fire (*āhavanīya*), its mouth; the roof (*sadas*) that shelters the secondary hearths, its stomach; the "dominical" fire (*gārhapatya*) and the cooking fire (vrataśrapaṇa), its foundation; the officiant brahman is its "mind" (manas, i.e., the psychic life); the chief chanter (udgātṛ) is the intake of breath; the second chanter (prastotṛ), the exhalation of breath; the third chanter (pratihartṛ), the transversal breath; the hotṛ, the specialist in reciting Vedic verses, is its speech; the adhvaryu, its eye; the hotṛ's assistants, the different limbs; while the sacrificer, yajamāna, constitutes the ātman of the sacrifice, that is, the torso, the essential and central part of the sacrificial body. This last identification is worth commenting on: ātman, which is sometimes, not incorrectly, translated as "soul," is not here the noncorporeal element of the person as contrasted with the material body (tanū, sarīra or deha). Ātman is that in the body which is contrasted with the limbs (and the head), as the center to the periphery, or else it is the whole as distinguished from the parts it encompasses. In this sense, ātman is the "person himself" (not my leg, nor even my heart, but "me"), and thus the body, to the extent that it supports reflexivity (ātman, like its synonym tanū, is used as a reflexive pronoun for all persons).

If we now turn our attention to the sacrificer, who is thus the center and the "self" of the sacrifice, we find that the metaphor is paralleled by a metamorphosis. The Brahmanic doctrine is that the sacrificer, in constructing the sacrifice, is also constructing himself, and providing himself with a body in which the constituent elements of the sacrifice take the place of the organic materials of his profane body. Just as the fatty membrane that encloses the victim's intestines (the vapā, i.e., the epiploon) is its ātman, so the verse called āprī is the ātman of the sacrificer.[88] But at a more general level, by virtue of the sacrifice he reaches heaven with a "body" made of verses, formulas, melodies and offerings.[89] He has incorporated the sacrifice, and thenceforth consists of chandas, metric schemes of the poetry of the Veda; he has become chandomaya. The body of Man is the model for, and the origin of, the sacrifice and is therefore both its departure point and its effect. But the sacrifice, for its part, in the guise of Speech — which is its final form — is what gives the body its ultimate substance.

This article is based on a paper presented to Jean-Pierre Vernant's seminar at the Collège de France on March 1, 1982. I am grateful to him for his hospitality. As usual, his questions, his short comments and his final summary enabled me to clarify what I had to say.

ABBREVIATIONS

AitĀ	*Aitareya-Āraṇyaka*	*RS*	*Rk-Saṃhitā*
AitB	*Aitareya-Brāhmaṇa*	*ŚaṅkhĀ*	*Sāṅkhāyana-Āraṇyaka*
ĀpŚS	*Āpastamba-Srauta-Sūtra*	*ŚB*	*Śatapatha-Brāhmaṇa*
JB	*Jaiminīya-Brāhmaṇa*	*ṢB*	*Sadvimśa-Brāhmaṇa*
KB	*Kauṣītaki-Brāhmaṇa*	*TA*	*Taittirīya-Āraṇyaka*
KS	*Kāthaka-Saṃhitā*	*TB*	*Taittirīya-Brāhmaṇa*
MS	*Maitrāyani-Saṃhitā*	*TS*	*Taittirīya-Saṃhitā*
PB	*Pañcaviṃśati-Brāhmaṇa*	*VŚS*	*Vaitāna-Śrauta-Sūtra*

NOTES

1. Punning on Śiva–Śava is commonplace in sectarian literature. Cf. H. Zimmer, *Myths and Symbols in Indian Art and Civilization* (Princeton: Princeton University Press, 1946), p. 206.

2. Again, a play on *kala*, "part" (here, as the masculine ending *-kala*), and *kāla*, "time."

3. *Karpurādi-Stotra* 7. This verse of the hymn to Kālī ends with the line: "O Mother, even a dullard becomes a poet who meditates upon Thee." For a chaste version of this posture, see Bhuvaneśvarī, tutelary goddess of the mahārājā of Mysore, who is represented in the palace temple, seated on the extended body of Śiva. In her hand she holds a sugar cane, symbolizing victory over sensual desires. The recumbent body of Śiva itself rests on the back of Brahmā, who is supporting himself on the ground by his hands and knees.

4. On "the" Hindu goddess, of whom the figures described here are only a few of many aspects, see esp. M. Biardeau, ed., *Autour de la déesse hindoue*, Collection *Puruṣārtha* 5 (Paris: Ecole des Hautes Etudes en Sciences sociales, 1981).

5. *Tantrasāra*, p. 115.

6. *Ibid.*; *Karpurādi-stotra* 4. For the myth of origin of Chinnamastā, the goddess with the severed head, see *Prāṇatosiṇī*, p. 728. For bibliographical references, see T. Goudriaan and S. Gupta, *Hindu Tantric and Sākta Literature* (Wiesbaden: Otto Harrassowitz, 1981), pp. 68ff., 71, 81. See also W. O'Flaherty, *Women, Androgynes and Other Beasts* (Chicago: University of Chicago Press, 1980), p. 85.

7. Not surprisingly, these images are often reproduced in books for the general reader on Indian art or mythology. See, for example, *Hymnes à la déesse*, trans. into French from the Sanskrit by Ushâ P. Shâstrî and Nicole Menant, with comments on the iconography by C.B. Pandey (Paris: Le Soleil Noir, 1980).

8. *Tantrasāra*, p. 115.

9. Octavio Paz, *Marcel Duchamp, or the Castle of Purity*, trans. Donald Gardner (London: Cape Goliard Press, 1970), p. 16.

10. *Sāmkhya-Kārikā* 59: "Just as a dancer ceases to dance after she has shown herself to the public, so the Prakṛti comes to an end after it has been manifest to the Puruṣa." Cf. G.J. Larson, *Classical Sāmkhya* (Delhi, 1969), pp. 171-79.

11. See M. Biardeau, *L'hindouisme, anthropologie d'une civilisation* (Paris: Flammarion, Collection Champs, 1981); and M. Biardeau and C. Malamoud, *Le sacrifice dans l'Inde ancienne* (Paris: Presses Universitaires de France, 1976).

12. Sylvain Lévi's book, *La doctrine du sacrifice dans les Brāhmanas* (1898), reprinted with a preface by Louis Renou (Paris: Presses Universitaires de France, 1966), still remains an indispensable guide to the analysis of the Vedic sacrifice.

13. *ŚB* 11.1.6.31 (see the key to abbreviations which precedes the footnotes).

14. Cf. H. Oldenberg, *Vorwissenschaftliche Wissenschaft, Die Weltanschauung der Brahmana-Texte* (Göttingen: Vandenhoeck and Ruprecht, 1919), p. 172ff.; A. Minard, *Trois énigmes sur les cent chemins II* (Paris: De Boccard, 1956), s. 148. See also M. Eliade, *Le yoga, immortalité et liberté* (Paris: Payot, 1954), pp. 257 and 259; J. Gonda, *The Dual Deities in the Religion of the Veda* (Amsterdam: North Holland Publishing Co., 1974), pp. 92-112. On the correspondence between the grammatical notion of *samdhi*, "linkage," and the mystical pairing of *mithuna*, see *AitĀ* 3.1.5, and L. Renou, "Les connexions entre la grammaire et le rituel en sanskrit," *Journal asiatique* 112 (1945). See also J.C. Heesterman, "Kauṭalya and the Ancient Indian State," *Wiener Zeitschrift für die Kunde südasiens* 5.12-19 (1971).

15. On "redundance" (*jāmitva*) as opposed to the "possibility of forming a couple" (*mithunatva*), see L. Renou, *Etude sur le vocabulaire du Rg-Veda* (Pondichéry: Institut Français d'Indologie, 1958), p. 49ff.

16. For coupling and procreation to take place, the woman has to be characterized by the lack, the less (*nyūna*) evinced by her lap (*upastha*), and man by the addition, or super-addition (*aitirikta*) of the penis (*prajanana*). Cf. H. Oertel, *Widersprüche zwischen grammatischen Genus und Sexus in der Symbolik der Brāhmanas* (Munich, 1943), p. 3, n.3.

17. Patañjali, *Mahābāsya* 14.1.3. Cf. O. Strauss, *Festgabe Garbe*, p. 84; and L. Renou, "Connexions," p. 164.

18. This is all the more remarkable because in the speculation about the sex of things, the distinction between masculine and neuter is just as important as that between masculine and feminine or between feminine and neuter. Thus we read in *ŚaṅkhĀ* 3.7 that man, by virtue of his breath (*prāṇa*), which is masculine because it has a masculine name, comes to know the masculine names of the god

Brahmā; by virtue of his speech (*vāc*), which is feminine, he comes to know the feminine names; and by virtue of his mind (*manas*), which is neuter, he comes to learn the neuter names. Cf. also JB 2.291ff., and s. 155 of the *Auswahl* by W. Caland (Amsterdam, 1919).

19. *TS* 4.1.3.3ff.

20. *ŚB* 1.3.1.12ff.; 5.2.1.8; *ĀpŚS* 2.4.1.5.2 and 10.9.13; *VŚS* 2.6.

21. *KS* 23.4.

22. E.g., *Āp Dh S* 2.6.13.

23. See C. Malamoud, *Annuaire de l'Ecole Pratique des Hautes Etudes, Ve section*, 1983-84, p. 167ff. Cf. J. Gonda, *Eye and Gaze in the Veda* (Amsterdam, 1969), pp. 2 and 21.

24. Cf. M. Winternitz, *Die Frau in den indischen Religionen* (Leipzig: Curt Kabitzsch, 1920), p. 11; P.E. Dumont, *L'Aśvamehda* (Paris: Paul Geuthner, 1927), p. 177.

25. *TS* 4.1.1.3.

26. *ŚB* 1.3.1.12.

27. *Ibid.* 5.4.2.9.

28. *Ibid.* 1.3.1.13.

29. *Ibid.*

30. *Ibid.* 14.

31. *Ibid.* 15.

32. *TB* 3.3.2ff.

33. That is, in concrete terms, in the western part of the sacrificial area. Cf. *ŚB* 5.2.1.8, and Eggeling's note. (The woman does not stay there all the time. At certain moments in the ritual she has to be led forward by an officiant called the *neṣṭṛ* or "guide.") In Sanskrit, the West is behind and after, while the East is in front and before. The fact that the woman is associated with what is "behind" can be seen again in this prescription for beheading the victim in animal sacrifice: the *jāghanī* or "tail" of the victim reverts to the wives of the gods, because it is from the hind part (*jaghana*) of the female that her progeny is born. Cf. *ŚB* 3.8.5.6.

34. There are, however, some aetiological narratives which set out to demonstrate that women are only inferior because they have been emasculated. In their gradual and sometimes fragmentary discovery of the procedures of sacrifice, it was revealed to the gods that a share of the liquor of *soma* was to be reserved for their wives. This "wives' draught" gives them a vision of the celestial world. But the *soma*, which is also the god Soma, may not be consumed by women. So the gods had the idea of mixing clarified butter with the wives' share of the *soma*. The clarified butter acts on the *soma* like a thunderbolt, striking it and taking away its virility. By drinking the weakened *soma* the

wives of the gods are themselves struck and deprived of their virile qualities. In the somic sacrifices offered by men to the gods, the same procedure is followed, which is why human women are also powerless, cannot control themselves and may not inherit. Cf. *TS* 4.5.8.1ff.; *ŚB* 4.4.2.13.

35. There are numerous references to this in Lévi, *La doctrine du sacrifice*, p. 156ff. On the notion of *nirṛti*, see L. Renou, *L'Inde fondamentale* (Paris: Hermann, 1978), pp. 127-32.

36. The social and religious status of women in Brahmanic India is very well described in Winternitz, *Die Frau in den indischen Religionen*.

37. *ŚB* 10.1.1.8ff.

38. *KS* 27.7.

39. *MS* 4.6.4.

40. *Ibid.*, and *ŚB* 4.5.2.10.

41. *AitĀ* 1.1.4. Cf. also *ŚB* 4.3.2.3: "the *udgātṛ* is Prajāpati, and the *hotṛ*, being the verse, is feminine. When he chants, the *udgātṛ*-Prajāpati pours his sperm into the *hotṛ*-verse.

42. *ŚB* 1.2.5.15, 9.2.21ff. Cf. Oertel, *Widerspruche*, pp.23-5. *Mithuna* between pots (*kumbha*) and jugs (*kumbhī*) is mentioned in *TS* 5.6.2.3, 6.5.11.3; *MS* 4.10.

43. *SB* 12.8.4.6.

44. *ŚB* 1.3.1.9, 5.3.15.

45. *AitB* 3.23.

46. *AitB* 3.48.

47. *ŚB* 1.5.3.15.

48. *KS* 23.4.

49. *ŚB* 3.2.1.1ff.

50. *Ibid.* 3.3.4.3.

51. *Ibid.* 9.5.1.12.

52. *KS* 6.7.

53. Cf. Renou, *L'Inde fondamentale*, p. 86 ff.

54. *ŚB* 10.5.1.2.

55. On the fourth Veda, the *Artharva-Veda* and the tradition which regards it as the Veda of *brahman*, see M.Bloomfield, *The Atharvaveda* (Strasburg: Karl J. Trübner, 1899), pp. 29-34.

56. *PB* 20.14.2.

57. *ŚB* 4.2.5.14.

58. Renou, *L'Inde fondamentale*, pp. 66-80.

59. This expression (Renou, p. 79) means simply that Speech exhausts the Sacrifice. It is linked

to the one cited above about the way the Sacrifice can become tired if a formula is repeated too often. Speech, furthermore, can also become tired. On the procedures to be adopted in order to reinvigorate the sacrificial Speech, see C. Malamoud, *Le svādhyāya, récitation personnelle du Veda* (Paris: De Boccard, 1977), p. 78. The avidity of Speech does not prevent it from being frequently compared to a milk-cow, particularly in the hymns of the *Ṛg-Veda*; the comparison reappears in the Brāhmaṇa, for example in *ŚB* 11.3.1.1, where the Speech-Cow is described, accompanied by her calf, Mind, *manas*; and in other parts of the same text (*ŚB* 6.1.3.6, 3.3.1.16) Speech and Mind form a *mithuna*: it would seem more likely that this represents a lack of internal coherence, the autonomy of two metaphors, rather than a conscious desire to suggest an incestuous *mithuna*.

60. E.g., *AitB* 2.38.

61. *AitB* 6.3.

62. *KS* 6.5. Cf. H.W. Bodewitz, *The Daily Evening and Morning Offering (agnihotra), According to the Brāhmanas* (Leiden: E.J. Brill, 1976), p. 80ff.

63. *MS* 1.9.3.

64. *ŚB* 2.1.8.2.

65. *KS* 12.5.

66. *ŚB* 4.1.2.6ff. Other examples of pregnant men in mythology are cited in J.J. Meyer, *Sexual Life in Ancient India* (London, 1952), p. 372ff.

67. *PB* 13.11.18.

68. *JB* 1.225.

69. *ŚB* 13.4.4.6.

70. *Agni* is the first born of the gods. He is also their guide. The Brāhmana abound in wordplay on the name Agni and *agre*, "in the first place," and *agram*, "in front." See esp. *SB* 1.4.1.10-17.

71. *ŚB* 6.1.2.26.

72. Principally, *ŚB*, bks. 6-10.

73. Cf. L. Silburn, *Instant et cause* (Paris: Vrin, 1954), p. 50.

74. *PB* 10.3.1.

75. Cf. C. Malamoud, "La brique percée," *Nouvelle revue de psychanalyse* 11 (1975), p. 212.

76. *ŚB* 10.4.1.1.

77. *TS* 6.4.10.4ff.

78. *ŚB* 3.3.4.17; *SB* 1.1.16.

79. Cf. Minard, *Trois énigmes*, vol. 2, s. 881.

80. Cf. for example the "Laws of Manu," *Mānava-dharma-śāstra*, 3.12ff.

81. *ŚB* 10.4.1.12.

82. *Ibid.* 11.4.1.16.

83. *Ibid.* 10.5.1.1ff.

84. *Ibid.* 10.1.1.8.

85. The critical moment in the process of inversion that takes place between the Brahmanic version of sacrificial sexuality and the Tantric version may well, therefore, have been the "esoteric" elaboration of Vedic doctrine. In fact, when the Tantra claim to be part of the Vedic tradition, they like to refer to the *Āraṇyaka*; and it is in the *Āraṇyaka*, the "forestlike" appendices to the Brāhmaṇa, that the "secret" teachings of the Veda are concentrated.

The interplay of masculine and feminine (or rather nonfeminine and feminine) in the Indian sacrifice seems, in many other ways, to fit in with traditional Western stereotypes: the feminine speaks (or chatters), whereas the masculine acts and thinks (witness his silence); unity and unicity belong on the masculine side, diversity and plurality on the feminine. But the most remarkable aspect of Indian speculation is that Speech is a figure of femininity, while women have no right to this Vedic Speech. And also that because Speech is multiple, fragmented and explicit, it is also articulated; similarly, femininity, to the extent that it is expressed by Speech, is not confined within matter, but becomes capable of generating form.

86. *RS* 10.90.

87. *KB* 17.7.

88. *KS* 26.9.

89. *ŚB* 11.2.6.13.

Translated by Ian Patterson.

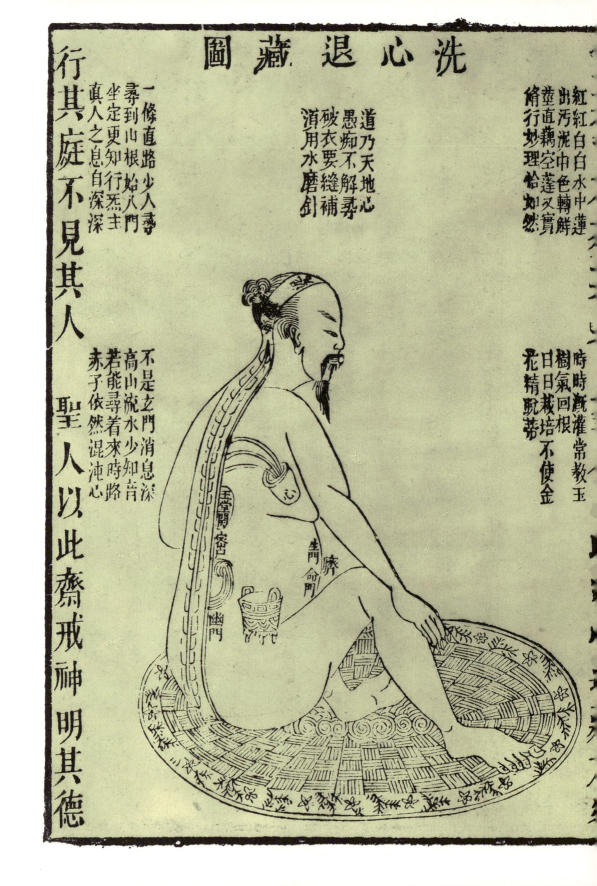

洗心退藏圖

紅紅白白水中蓮
出汙泥中色轉鮮
整直藕空蓬又實
修行妙理恰如然

時時煎灌常教玉
樹氣回根
日日栽培不使金
花精脫蒂

道乃天地心
愚痴不解尋
破衣要縫補
湏用水磨針

一條直路少人尋
尋到山根始入門
坐定更知行炁主
真人之息自深深

不是玄門消息深
高山流水少知音
若能尋着來時路
赤子依然混沌心

行其庭不見其人
聖人以此齋戒神明其德

玉堂關宴寜
幽門
心
膂
生門命門

The Body: The Daoists' Coat of Arms

Jean Lévi

The Body as Representation of the Cosmos

In China the body is perceived as a replica of the universe. Whereas during the imperial period – the third and fourth centuries B.C. – philosophers essentially derived from this a political principle,[1] starting in the following century this equation of the two orders was articulated in a veritable cosmogonic system. The emblems structuring the universe, the numbers cataloging the intimate and pertinent relations among things could be found in the human body, whose organization was marked by the same algorithmic formulas:

> His round head is the celestial vault, his square feet are in the image of the earth; his hair is the stars, his eyes the sun and moon, his eyebrows the Great Bear, his nose resembles a mountain, his four limbs are the four seasons, his five internal organs the five elements.[2]

The Daoists were the ones to pursue the most extreme implications of this widely held theory. To them, the body was not merely constructed on the basis of the celestial model and norm, it was the universe, it contained the universe in its totality. The equivalence between microcosm and macrocosm in the *Wufuwu* (*Book of the Five Talismans*), for instance, is absolute:

> Man contains the entire universe: the sun, the moon, the Great Bear, the pole star, the jade scales, the five peaks, mountains and streams, rivers and seas...grains, mulberry and hemp, domestic animals, horses, cattle, birds, quadrupeds, fish and tortoises, trees and plants.

In the body one discovers not only flora and fauna, but the whole of society and the buildings in which it lives:

> There is also the emperor, the three dukes, the nine ministers, the twenty-seven high

105

officials, the eighty-one gentlemen. There are the larger administrative divisions with the nine provinces, the 120 commanderies, the 1200 prefectures, the 18,000 cantons, the 180,000 villages with their palaces, their houses, which in their turn possess hearths, windows and doors, wells and implements.[3]

Once the human body exactly replicates and includes the whole of the cosmos – while still being an element itself – cosmogenesis merges with embryogenesis, as is shown by a text from the fourth century A.D. which works with these two systems:

> The breaths from the ninefold heavens descend and mingle in the form of yin and yang – red breaths and yellow breaths, each of which deposits its seed and sets an embryo by divine transformation, corresponding to the model of the nine skies. The celestial breath spreads down below: it condenses and solidifies into seed in the gateways of destiny [the loins]. After nine transformations, it forms the three fields of cinnabar [corresponding to the brain, the thorax and the lower part of the abdomen] where, by transformation of the transcendent elements and coalescence of the earthly elements, man is formed. Man in the first month of his embryonic life receives breath, in the second month his soul…in the fourth month his essence is set…in the sixth month, by transformation, he takes form; in the seventh month the sites of the gods are there.[4]

This text echoes the *Huainanzi*, written in the second century B.C., which describes the nine-stage process leading from the embryo to the finished form of the human being:

> We receive our spirit from heaven and our body from the earth. This is why it is said: the one produces the two, the two produce the three, the three give birth to the 10,000 beings, the 10,000 beings turn their backs on the yin and embrace the yang, while the spouting of breath gives birth to the central harmony which is man. Thus, in the first month, it is like a ball of fat, in the second month like a tendon, in the third month the fetus appears…and the child is born in the tenth month[5] with a complete body possessing the five internal organs.[6]

There are nine months of gestation, there are nine transformations through which the genesis of the world is accomplished, issuing from the divine body of Laozi exalted into a hypostasis of the Dao in its activity of creation.[7] In certain versions, the world is compared to the body of the dismembered god-man; or rather, one recognizes in the cosmos, underlying it or inscribed implicitly in it, the body of Laozi, the body of man par excellence:

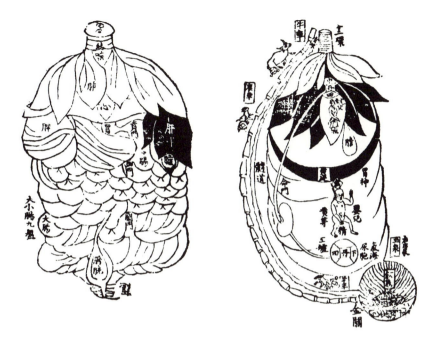

Interior Landscape, Front View

This engraving depicts the principal organs in a summary way that is more physio-logical than emblematic. The leaves in the upper part represent the lungs, half hiding the heart in the center. To the right, in black, is the liver, and hanging from it the spleen, while the entire lower part is occupied by the large and small intestines.

Interior Landscape, Right Profile

At the top is the heart, and inside it the figure of the "father." Above the heart lies the middle field of cinnabar, connected by a canal to the kidneys (the right kidney is known as the substance of destiny). The figure in the middle, above the lower field of cinnabar, is none other than the child of immortality – the "real self" which the adept develops through fusion of breaths and circulation of the essence. Above, to the right of the child, is the god of the stomach and below, to the right, at the level of the lower field of cinnabar, lies the sea of breath in which the primordial tortoise frolics. The spinal column allows the essence to move from the seminal vesicles to the brain. Up and down it run a series of animals in harness.

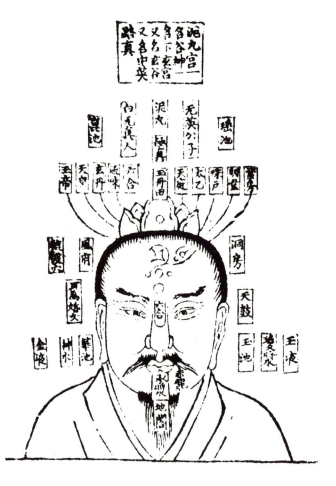

The Divine Structure of the Head

Representation of the head with its gods and mystical components. It is made up of nine palaces corresponding to the nine heavens: one inch in, between the two eyebrows, is the "palace of lights," in which dwells the divinity of the Great One, flanked left and right by the purple room and the vermilion cross. One inch farther in is the palace of the three immortals. Three inches into the skull is the palace of the upper field of cinnabar; four inches in, the palace of moving pearls; five inches in, the palace of the Jade Emperor. In addition, above these dwellings, we have the celestial courtyard, the palace of the Highest Summit, the palace of the mysterious cinnabar and the palace of the August Heaven.

The ears are known as the celestial drum, the mouth is the jade lake and the base of the nose is the six harmonies.

Laozi transforms his body: his left eye is the sun, his right eye the moon, his head becomes Mount Kunlun, his beard the planets, his bones the dragons, his flesh the quadrupeds... his belly the sea, his fingers the five peaks, his hair the vegetation, his heart the Flowering Dais and his two kidneys, joining together, the essential real Father and Mother.[8]

This myth is lifted from an undoubtedly earlier tale in which the world is born of a cadaver, the cadaver of the demiurge Pangu (who, for the Daoists, is one of the many guises of Laozi). We will not cite the oldest version of this myth, but that of the Daoist cosmogonies in which it is inscribed in the process leading from nonbeing to being:

When the primordial breath burgeoned forth, the heaven and the earth divided and formed the trigrams *qian* and *kun* [male and female], yin and yang came into force by dividing. It was then that the primordial breath engendered the central harmony which is none other than man. It gave birth to Pangu, who, at his death, transformed his body. His respiration yielded the clouds and the wind, his voice the thunder, his limbs the four extremities of the world, his left eye the sun, his right eye the moon, his internal organs the five peaks.... And all the vermin he carried, roused by the wind, metamorphosed into humans.[9]

Being a reproduction of the cosmos, and having issued from the divine transformation of the divine breath or from a secret alchemy taking place in the crucible of the maternal belly, the body is thoroughly divine. It appears in the center of the world as the most precious of beings, and together with the sky and the earth it forms a triad which sums up the universe in its single and multiple aspect.[10]

The Body as Principle of Death

This divine body, however, is marked from before its birth by the stamp of decrepitude and death, unlike the macrocosm it replicates. Herein is contained the whole paradox of the homology between the body of the universe and the human body, whose priority is nonetheless affirmed. Through obstructions and entanglements within the womb, man forgets his celestial origin at birth; he is preyed upon, attacked, by principles of death[11] resulting from the mother's diet of grains, the putrefaction of which soils the embryo's nature. Far from elevating man to the divine rank for which he is destined, the body debases him to the level of corruption and ordure, which cause him to lose his divinity: "What misfortunes I would

zone

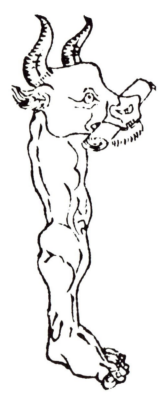

Cadaver of the Lower Field of Cinnabar

It is called "*Pengjiao*" (or *Li xi*), dwells in the stomach and attacks the lower part of the body. It spoils the sea of breath, causes all sorts of illnesses and is responsible for our bad thoughts and sexual desires. Because of it the marrow dries up, the tendons knot, the flesh hardens, the mind grows tired, the body wastes away, the waist thickens, etc. Its only desire is that man should die so that he might become a demon and be entitled to sacrifices. The scroll that the cadaver holds in its mouth is the book in which this spy records mankind's faults before ascending to heaven to report to the Director of Falc, who will curtail each person's life by a certain number of years in proportion to his sins.

suffer if I did not have a body," certain people lament, "for the form I have been given is only a dwelling place wherein I live but is not me, for he who has obtained the Dao has no form."[12]

Pernicious agents act on three levels: on the physiogical level, first, as within the body the grains nourish three worms (also called "Three Cadavers") which gnaw at the organism and render it vulnerable to disease. These essential components of the body which are excremental in nature and which lodge in the three central regions of the organism (the three fields of cinnabar constituted, as previously mentioned, by the brain, the thorax and the lower part of the abdomen) will obstruct the internal organs, hamper the circulation of breath and the passage of light which, by bathing the organs, confer on them a truly divine character.[13] On a moral level, in texts of Buddhist inspiration, they act on the three spheres of desire (corresponding to the fields of cinnabar where they operate): wealth, food and lust.

Yet it is essentially on the divine level that their action turns out to be most pernicious: the Three Cadavers are censuring divinities. After the manner of the god of the household stove, who comes up once a year to make his report to the director of fate, they go to heaven on the *gengsheng* days of the sexagesimal cycle to expose the sins committed by the organism that feeds them.[14]

But there exist in the organism other censuring divinities whose spying action cuts short existence by causing years of life to be struck from the little green book of the powers of fate; such are the divinities of the loins, the divinities of the cycle of the hours and especially the vegetative and chthonic spirits: the seven *po* spirits whose perverse character is expressed by the graphic representations and their epithets ("cadaver dog" is a grimacing demon, as is "stinking lung"; "flying fish" is a one-footed monster; "bird's sex" sports a bird's head surmounting a single leg; etc.). These genies have only one desire, to hasten man's end in order to return to the dark earth to which they belong:

> On the first, the fifteenth and the last day of each lunar month, the seven vegetative spirits, with libidinous appetite, go and roll in mire and ordure, either joining with the gods who consume bloody food, and strolling about with demons and ghosts, or associating with the principles of rot and death, or soiling ourselves and ruining the dwelling of the body by traitorously attacking it. Or they ascend to expose the sins to the three offices, to the Count of the River and to all the officials in charge of punishments; some-

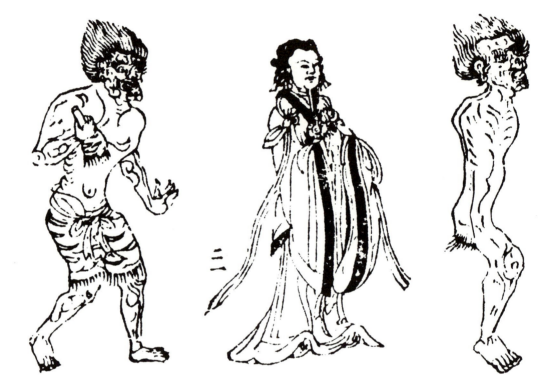

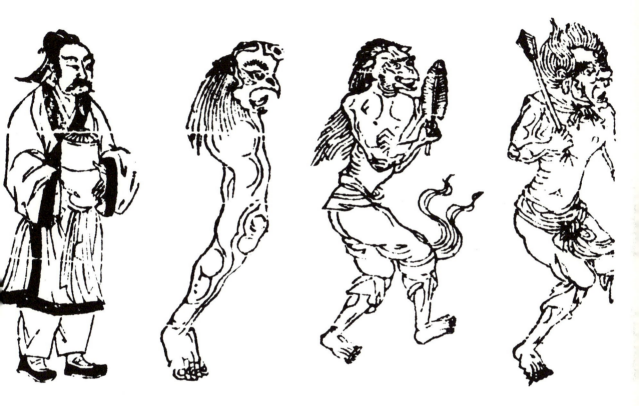

The Seven Bodily Souls, *po*

"The seven bodily souls which cause disturbances in the organism are produced by the yin and take the form of demons; it is they who produce desires and worries. They delight in filth and turn their back on life, fixated on death. They give rise to lechery, and hasten the end of the organism."

Right to left, we see: dog cadaver, flabby piss, bird's sex, the gluttonous thief, flying fish, filth, stinking lung.

times they transform themselves into specters who infect men, sometimes they invite the demons to enter the organism and summon all the miasmas so that they may sap our vitality and diminish our substance.[15]

The Three Cadavers also correspond physiologically, or are the organic manifestation of, the little genies which populate the countryside. And if these cadavers, like the souls, want to leave the dwelling of the body in which they are imprisoned, it is because once they are free, they become gods, gods richly fed with bloody sacrifices.

And upon the death of the individual, cadavers and souls wander over the earth, display efficacy, power, which must be rendered propitious by offerings of animals, as is indicated by the Daoist texts as a conclusion to the profanatory and criminal mastication of cereals:

> Of all living beings, man is the most sacred of creatures, but he does not know it, and, incapable of safeguarding his gods, in order to repel the miasmas he seeks the help of outside divinities, without stopping at his own body.[16]

These outside divinities result from the transformation of spirits and cadavers, sanctioning the mortality of the body. As for the sacrifices which are reserved for them, they are in no way distinguishable from the other sacrifices: what the presence of these elements in the body implies is, in fact, the ancestor worship that structures the whole society, and that consists in bloody offerings to the divinities which are the spirits of the departed. Every god primarily expresses a function filled by a dead person. And every cult is a sacrifice to spirits, the latter acquiring power through the very act of sacrifice. Thus, these murky and disquieting elements within the body, the cadavers, represent the common practice of sacrifice — a practice refused by the Daoists in order to establish "pure contracts" with the gods.[17] The bloody sacrifice to the *gui-shen* (demons), which sanctifies the loss of the divine by ratifying it, must be banished from the organism (in the corresponding form of the three worms) by virtue of the identification of the microcosm and the macrocosm.[18]

The cadavers and souls are therefore only physiological representations of the cult of the gods. The sacrifice commemorates the distance between men and gods; it is the gesture which, by referring to the mortal part, maintains it. In order to return to his original nature, to the divinity of his body, man must establish a different relation with the gods, that is, with his organism.

The Body as Alchemy of the Divine

Once the cadavers have been eliminated by various techniques (the ingestion of drugs, visualizations, recitations, etc.) the body becomes delicate and light and, most importantly, the gods which populate it manifest their presence again. The adept must thenceforth reunite with his divine nature by reconstructing his body through a sort of mental "bodybuilding." But this "spiritual body" is not distinguishable from his physiological body, and the murmuring of the gods mingles with the rumbling of his organs. The Daoist is listening for the mystical voices which sing in him and which rise from his viscera. He visualizes ethereal breath produced by the distillation of the juices of his entrails: it is at the paroxysm of the organic and at the lowest and most quotidian level that the body is decanted, that matter is transmuted into essence and that sublimation takes place. But this is made possible only because the organic functioning is sacred: because the inside of the body, where crude secretions are developed, is the vessel of delicate spirits. The humors are actually essences which, when refined, metamorphose into primordial breath — the special site of this celestial transmutation being the internal organs, whose number, five, signals their central position. Just as the world is organized on the basis of five cardinal directions, the body is structured on the basis of its internal organs: heart, liver, kidneys, spleen and lungs, each of which, according to the system of correspondences, refers to an element and its movement, and governs a color, a space and a cardinal direction. They are granaries, reservoirs of humors and breaths corresponding to their specialization on the space–time axis. It is therefore fitting that they be fed with an adequate breath — which is only a hypostasis of the unique, primordial breath, particularizing itself in the body in quintessential liquors. It is fitting that they be refined through visualizations and breathing exercises so that they become ether, a divine substance. The body therefore has something in common with an alchemical crucible whose raw materials would consist of its own secretions. But once again, if it is similar, this is because the organism reproduces the spontaneous movement of the cosmos, representing the course of the planets, the succession of the seasons and the alternation of yin and yang in the distillation of its juices: in the manuals devoted to strengthening the breath, the internal organs are paired with a trigram (the basic graphic building blocks of *The Book of Changes*) and a direction.

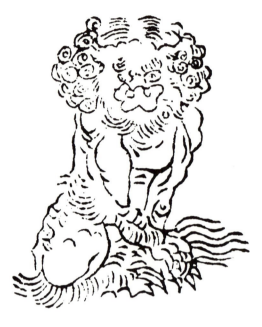

Spirit of the Lungs

The lung is the concrete form of the breath of the trigram *kui*, the essence of the metal. Its color is white, its form is that of a collection of suspended resonant stones; its emblematic animal is the white tiger. The lungs give birth to the *po* bodily souls and their spirit changes into a little jade boy nine inches high, whom one can see coming and going through this organ.

The lungs are the breath of the trigram *kui*, the aggregate of metal; their color is therefore white, their form that of a carillon of suspended sounding stones and their guardian spirit the white tiger. They give birth to the earthly spirits, *po*, whose manifestation is "a little boy made of jade" seven inches high, holding a stick, who wanders around in the lungs. Through visualizations and the appropriate guidance of a breath, one would cause divinities to descend into this organ, while preserving those who are already present.

The heart is the breath of the trigram *li* and the aggregate of fire; it is red and takes the form of a lotus; its guardian spirit is the red bird. The manifestation of the spirit to which it gives birth is "a girl made of jade" eight inches high, holding jade blossoms.

The liver is the breath of the trigram *zhen*, which is a sign of spring and is the aggregate of wood: it takes the form of a suspended gourd; the ethereal spirits, *hun*, are based in it; its guardian spirit is a dragon, the heraldic animal of the east; and the spirits it harbors manifest themselves as two "jade girls," one in white clothes, the other in green.

The spleen, associated with the earth, is yellow; its eponymous guardian spirit is the phoenix, while the emblem of the black kidneys, associated with the north, is the dark tortoise, because they are the aggregate of water.[19]

These organs/guardian spirits/breaths bear names as fundamental as the form in which the parts of the body are visualized; their sounds evoke pulsations, winds or organic throbbings — *hong-hong* (of the lungs), *ju-ju* (of the heart), *lin-lin* (of the liver).[20] Furthermore, the five main internal organs also correspond to a type of breathing called the six breaths, with characteristic noises: *xu, he, che, qi, hu, xi*. They strengthen and look after the internal organs, each of which, by resonance, presides over a sense organ and a type of illness:

> Thus, *qi* appertains to the lungs, which preside over the nose. If one is too hot or too cold, and if one is very tired, one breathes in and out using *qi*. *He*, on the other hand, appertains to the heart, which presides over the tongue: a dry mouth, a raspy tongue, fetid breath or difficult respiration are remedied by breathing of the *he* type.[21]

The Daoist therefore auscultates his body's palpitations, while at the same time contemplating the efflorescences colored by his interior vision, his attentive gaze on the functioning of his entrails. Rumblings, throbbings accompanying glandular secretions, colored images symbolizing the refinement of the waxlike emissions produced by the mucous membranes...such is, on the basis of the representations of the internal organs, the Daoist vision of the body.

But these viscera contain another dimension, in this case formed by the emblematic relationship with the cardinal number that governs the elements (see above, its equivalence on the space–time axis). By virtue of the system of correspondences, the viscera are exalted into cosmic entities since they replicate, in the organism, the collection of beings and things placed under the rubric signifying *five*. They are therefore congruent with the five elements — water, wood, fire, metal and earth — and one can compare them to the five emperors, transferring the cardinal directions onto the temporal axis, as well as to the five guardians:

> Above, they correspond to the five planets; on earth, they are identified with the five peaks. In their external manifestation, they are the five virtues; in their internal manifestation, they are the five kings. When they rise to the heavens, they form clouds of five colors; when they transform themselves, they are like five dragons.

On the administrative level, they are equivalent to the workings of the imperial court: the spleen is the Son of Heaven, prince of the Dao; the gallbladder is the Empress, the heart is the Minister of War, the left kidney the Minister of Public Works.[22]

The organs are also ruled by emblematic signs, or rather their value in the body is determined by their heraldic function. It is this function — this signifying and classifying value — which, in fact, authorizes the mysterious sublimation of the organic humor into divine essence.

The Body, Vessel of Divine Images

Daoism sees the body as immortal, and this immortality is achieved when all the organic gods are present, restored to their existence through meditation on their forms and names. In order to evoke the gods or to visualize them, it is necessary to represent them to oneself. Thus, a large part of Daoist literature consists simply of catalogs of gods who are the objects of meditation. And no treatise shows more clearly the emblematic nature of the gods than the Central Canon of Laozi.[23] It can be defined as a mystical calendar showing the moments and hours of visualizations appropriate to each divinity. What is involved, then, is a veritable dissertation on the human body as a space adorned with heraldic bearings.

On the vertical axis, the three parts of the body correspond to the three forces animating the cosmos – the heaven, the earth and man – while at the same time expressing the three stages of human development – the embryo, the child and the adult – which mark the passage from chaos to order by division. Since each of the parts is a whole, the parts also correspond to the triad of three unities which shows that man is one, formed of these three totalities.

On the horizontal axis, the Central Canon of Laozi works with symmetry (the reflection on the anatomical level of the yin/yang alternation). Thus, a series of couples is set up which multiply into triads in order to reproduce allegorically the formula of Laozi: "The Dao has produced one, one two, two three, whence have issued the 10,000 beings." This formula will sometimes be expressed in cosmological terms (by the yin/yang alternation), sometimes in astronomical terms (by the sun/moon opposition). But it can also be represented in mythological language by the characters of the Queen Mother of the West and the King of the East, her husband and counterpart, these two legendary figures referring in their turn, by symbolic resonance, to an infinite number of oppositions (life/death, spring/fall, right/left, green/white, etc.).

But these oppositions are resolved in the center by their product, which includes them and sums them up: the child, that is, the real self. Metaphorically, it also manifests the creation of the embryo of immortality and the return by involution to the primordial chaos, sign and vessel of all divinity.

The King of the East and the Queen of the West inhabit the eyes, which will then be sun and moon. But the divine couple – flanked by their offspring Brilliance – may dwell in many other places, places which then become sun and moon. In the breasts, they will mark morning and evening, accompanied by their eponymous animals, the dog and the cock. In the kidneys, they are opposed through colors (white/black) and functions (Minister of Public Works/Minister of Punishments). In the spleen, they give birth to the embryo of immortality.

The binary opposition that operates on the horizontal axis is taken up again on the vertical axis, where the tripartition is also projected. The first god with which the treatise opens evokes the mountain of the man-bird, endowed with a bird's head and the form of a "cock with the five colors of the phoenix," and is as much an incense burner as the distinguishing mark of the meditators or a mountain or a

Gymnastic Postures

Six of the eight postures of the Zhongli gymnastics:

1) In the first, you grind your teeth thirty-six times in order to call the gods together, then you encircle your head (known as Mount Kunlun) with your hands and "beat the celestial drum" twenty-four times — which consists of pressing your ears with your palms and tapping the back of your neck with your fingers.

2) Then you bend your spine to the right and left.

3) You collect your saliva by moving your tongue around, rinse your mouth thirty-six times, then you divide your saliva in three and chew it as though it were a solid food before swallowing it. After this, you can make fire circulate through your body.

4) You massage your kidneys with both hands thirty-six times.

5) You rotate your wrists alternately thirty-six times.

6) You rotate both arms together thirty-six times, etc.

These "gymnastic postures" protect against illnesses and demons, and constitute a preparation for breathing and meditation exercises. By controlling the breathing, they also allow one to eliminate obstructions, etc.

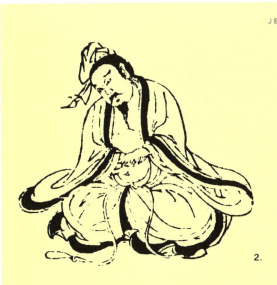

2.

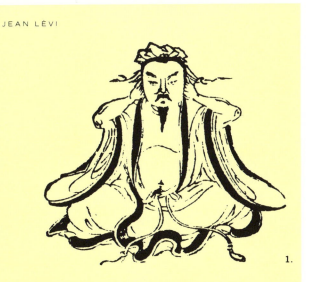

1.

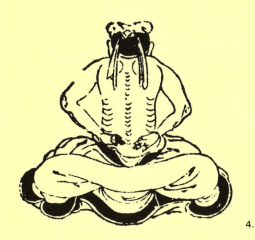

4.

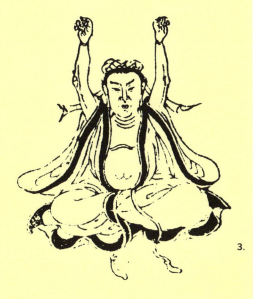

3.

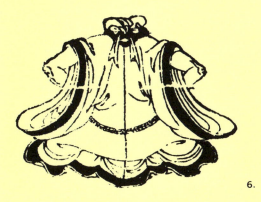

6.

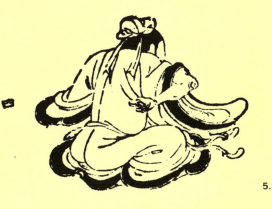

5.

labyrinth.[24] It must be connected with its counterpart and aquatic opposite, the tortoise who frolics about in the sea of the two kidneys and evokes (like the mountain of the bird-man) the sacred mountain of the *Kunlun*,[25] the embryonic respiration and the totality of the cosmos. Here we have two antithetical and symmetrical illustrations of high and low, of water and fire, since they operate according to the system of metaphorical transpositions: bird/tortoise, south/north, high/low, yang/yin. And these two images of the bird and the tortoise evoke — in the classification by two on the heaven/earth opposition axis (to which man is added) — the pentavalent structure of space.

This spatial structure is recalled to mind by the five cities of the navel, which are equivalent to the five cardinal directions and replicate the royal hillock of the god of the soil, with five colors, each associated with one direction.[26] The navel, or capital of the body, condenses the emblems and the numbers of the universe: one finds in it the eight ministers (corresponding to the eight trigrams), and the saints of the twelve pavilions, which evoke the twelve lunar months. But in this median center, space can retract, be torn in two, spread: it then composes the five internal organs, which, like the five cities, mark cardinal directions. In the red heart dwells the old man of the south pole; in the green liver, Laozi, image of spring and the east, with his grass of immortality and his green flag. The yellow spleen houses the Queen Mother, and so on.

Thus, cardinal rubrics carve out this space, break it up or recompose it into a field adorned with heraldic bearings in which numbers (like colors, figures and orientations) have an ordering value that is expressive of the cosmos. As in a kaleidoscope, a symbolic algebra displays its changing combinations, combinations governed by multiples or sums of three, five or two. The prince of the Dao has nine heads, wearing a cap of nine colors. Laozi measures nine-tenths of an inch; and there are nine divinities of the two kidneys (3 x 3).

There are five emperors, rectors of the cardinal directions, as there are five internal organs, cities of the navel, and colors worn by the prince of the Dao. Three inches above the navel lies the second field of cinnabar: three is the sum of the One-Earth, the One-Heaven and the One-Man. The circumference of this field is four inches: four is the number of the seasons reproduced by the four members — which, with the center, compose the five cardinal directions.

This center, the navel, reduces to a series of numbers whose sum yields the triad cubed: there are the five cities of the five emperors, the eight ministers of the eight trigrams, the twelve pavilions of the twelve months of the year, inhabited by the twelve dolphins and the twelve high officials, whose total number is raised with the gods of the three cooking pots to $24 + 3 = 27 = 9 \times 3$. The total number of gods dwelling in the four limbs/seasons corresponds to the eighty-one gentlemen (9×9).

Decked out in its armorial bearings and its images, characterized by colors, defined by numerical relations, the body is a space governed by the laws of the cosmos. The network of correspondences encloses it in a symbolic area, a ritual place which is none other than the sacrificial platform surrounded by enigmatic effigies of the divinities. The gods are coats of arms or breaths which, in their turn, refer back to colored images. The child of immortality (the true self) is visualized in order to be fed by the colored secretions of the organism that merges with astral efflorescences. This child is born in the spleen of the empress mother of the Dao – "girl of jade of the dark luster of the great yin" – and of her partner, the old yellow man. He is sustained by the visualization of the yellow breaths of the sun and the red breaths of the moon, circulating from the breasts (sun and moon) into the fields of cinnabar: he rises into the esophagus in order to eat his fill; and, resting in the stomach on a bed of pearls and jade, protected by a baldachin of yellow clouds, he suckles greedily at a liqueur-like source, the saliva.[27]

The gods only acquire substance and form in the movement that makes them present, through the melting of the humors, just as the latter can only be decanted because the substance from which they are produced is of the same kind as the symbols or the coats of arms expressing the configuration of the cosmos. In other words, the crudest physiological substance assumes a heraldic value because its secretions are integrated into a symbolic system in which they correspond to divine effigies.

NOTES

1. In the *Guanzi*, a text about kingdoms at war dating from the fifth–fourth century B.C., a prince asks his sage counselor where one must begin in order to establish confidence. The other answers: "One begins with one's own body-person, one continues with one's country and one finishes with the whole empire" (*Guanzi*, vol.1, ch. 8, pt. 19 *zhongkui*, Shahnghaai: Commercial Press, 1936, p. 96).

In another text from the beginning of the Han, the Yellow Emperor questions his counselor, asking, "I want to extend the five ordinances to the empire. Where should I begin and where should I end?" and obtains from him more or less the same answer: "Begin with your own body. When you have governed your heart, you will be able to govern the affairs of others, when the inside and the outside are in harmony, the regulation of the affairs of the State will be in order" ("wu-zheng," in *Mawangdui hanmu beishu*, Beeijing: Wenwu Chubanshe, 1973, p. 65). The body is, in fact, the image of a country and the body's senses are like the functionaries of the State, the same word, *guan*, designating both. Translator's note: The pinyin system has been used to transcribe Chinese words and names. Thus, Daoist is used for Taoist, Laozi for Lao-tzu and Shahnghaai for Shanghai.

2. *Huainanzi*, a Daoist encyclopedia from the second century B.C. (Shahnghaai: Shangwu yinshuguan, 1936, p. 213); the text adds: "The heaven has its four seasons, its five elements, its nine divisions, its 366 days; man has his four limbs, his five internal organs, his nine orifices and his 366 joints.... His bile is cloud, his lungs are breath, his spleen is wind, his kidneys are rain, his liver is thunder...."

3. "Wufuxu" (Daoist text from c. fourth century A.D.), in *Daozang*, Hanfen lou (photographic reproduction, Shahnghaai, 1924, 183.1.19-21b).

4. "Wushang biyao" (Daoist encyclopedia from the sixth century A.D.), in *Daozang* 768-79.5.1a-b.

5. The Chinese include the full term in their count.

6. *Huainanzi*, ch. 7, p. 212.

7. On the question of Laozi deified transforming his body nine times, cf. A. Seidel, *La divinisation de Lao-zi dans le Taoïsme des Han* (Paris: Publications de l'EFEO, 1969, pp. 92-98). Cf. also the "Hunyuan shengji" (eleventh century), in *Daozang* 770.2.37a-b.

8. This is a lost passage quoted by a Buddhist sutra in an anti-Daoist polemic, the "Xiao dao lun," from the sixth century A.D. Cf. A. Seidel, *La divinisation de Lao-zi*, p. 93.

9. The *San-wu liji* (third century A.D.) says: "Heaven and earth were intermingled, like an egg. Pangu was born in the midst of them. After 18,000 years, when heaven and earth separated, pure yang formed the heaven, murky yin formed the earth. In the midst of them Pangu transforming himself nine times in the course of one day... every day the heaven became ten feet higher, the earth ten feet wider...." (in "Yu-han shanfang" 63.1a-b). The *Shuyi ji* gives only a truncated version of it ("Hanwei congshu" 1.1a). The passage we cite is taken from "Yuanqi lun," in "Yunji qiqian" 56.1a-b (*Daozang* 677-702).

10. On the question of the three forces — man, heaven and earth — cf. A. Cheng, "La conception de la triade Ciel-Terre-Homme à la fin de l'antiquité chinoise," in *Extrême-Orient, extrême Occident* 3 (1984), pp. 11-22.

11. "Wushang biyao," in *Daozang* 5.2a, describes the occlusions of the womb which cause the newborn to lose his awareness of his divine origin. The "Yuanqi qiqian" (*Daozang* 81.15a, 83.10b) describes the worms of grains present in the mother's belly that feed parasitically on the fetus.

12. "Wushang biyao" 5.5a.

13. On the question of the grains and their excremental nature, cf. Jean Lévi, "L'Abstinence des céréales chez les Daoistes," *Etudes chinoises* 1 (1983), pp. 6-14. The elimination of fecal substances occasioned by the mastication of grains constitutes the sole preoccupation of a treatise of the breath: they are the opaque and gummy substance that prevents interior vision ("Taiqing zhonghuang sheng-jing," in *Daozang* 568.1.14a-b).

14. On the relation between the Three Cadavers and the three *klesà* (desire, anger and attachment), cf. Jean Lévi, "Vers des céréales et dieux du corps dans le Taoïsme," *Le temps de la réflexion* vol. 7, *Corps des dieux* (1986), p. 105. On the action of the three worms on a religious level, cf. *ibid.*, pp. 106-09.

15. "Yunji qiqian" 54.7a.

16. "Wushang biyao" 5.6b.

17. On the question of different sacrifices, other than those advocated by the practice of ances-tor worship, cf. Jean Lévi, "Vers des céréales et dieux du corps," pp. 111-12. And on the implications of sacrifice, in relation to the loss of divinity and the invention of cooking fire, cf. Jean Lévi, "L'abstinence des céréales," pp. 12-40.

18. Jean Lévi, "Vers des céréales et dieux du corps," p. 112.

19. There exist a number of treatises – which hardly do more than repeat one another – on this subject. Cf., among others, the "Shanqqing huangting wuzang liufu zhenren yuzhou qing," in *Daozang* 1050.2a-10a.

20. "Wufuxu" 1.21a.

21. "Songshan taiwu xiansheng qijing," in *Daozang* 569.9a-b. On the processes of guiding the breath, cf. also H. Maspéro, "Les procédés de 'nourrir le principe vital' dans le religion taoïste ancienne," in *Le Taoïsme et les religions chinoises* (Paris: Gallimard, 1971), pp. 532-35.

22. "Wufuxu" 1.21a.

23. This work probably dates from the second–third centuries A.D. Cf. K. Schipper, "Le livre du centre de Lao-tseu," *Narischten der Gesellschaft für Natur und Völkerkunde Ostasien* 125, pp. 75-80. It is recorded in the Daoist encyclopedia of the Song, the "Yunji qiqian," chs. 18-19.

24. This mountain is compared to the Kunlun, Daoist paradises in the "Wuyue zhenxing xulun" (*Daozang* 1005.11a-b) and also the "Xuanlan renniao shan jingtu" (*Daozang* 196), where it appears in the form of a labyrinthine diagram. As for its relation with the perfume burner, on the mountain grows

a tree the sap of which yields a gum of such powerful fragrance that it revives the dead. Cf. also K. Schipper, *Le corps taoïste* (Paris: Fayard, 1982), p. 19.

25. The navel, gulf and mountain, whose hollow summit has its roots in the depths of the ocean of breaths, in the lowest field of cinnabar in which frolics a great tortoise; it breathes in and breathes out the primordial breath that it causes to circulate even in the four limbs. The tortoise is also a representation of the cosmos with its four feet (the four directions), its square breastplate (the earth), and its rounded carapace (the sky). The Kunlun are the islands in the middle of the Western sea. The paradises of the Eastern sea, which are also mountains, are held up by a great tortoise.

26. L. Vandermeersch, *La voie royale* (Paris: Publications de l'EFEO, 1980), vol. 1, p. 441.

27. Cf. "Laozi zhongjing," in "Yunji qiqian," 18.7a-b.

Translated by Lydia Davis.

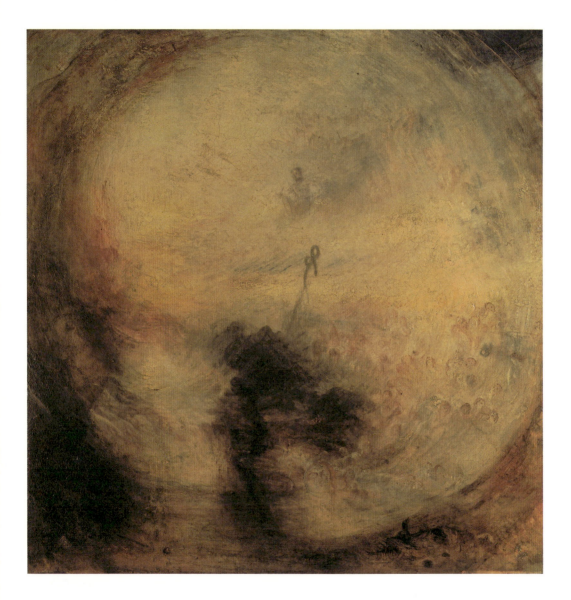

J.M.W. Turner, Light and Colour (London, Tate Gallery).

Divine Image – Prison of Flesh: Perceptions of the Body in Ancient Gnosticism

Michael A. Williams

Introduction

The third-century Neoplatonist Plotinus "seemed ashamed to be in the body."[1] Yet Plotinus knew late antique contemporaries who were driven by an even hotter embarrassment, contemporaries who, in his words, positively "hate the nature of the body" and "censure the soul for its association with the body."[2] These acquaintances of Plotinus were "Gnostics," persons convinced of the soul's desperate need for a divinely revealed *gnōsis*, "knowledge," in order to be awakened from a lethal amnesia as to the self's origins and rescued from submersion in an alien, material world.[3]

There may be no movement in late Antiquity more identified with the renunciation of the physical body than Gnosticism. It is true that Christian monasticism produced some star ascetic athletes, whose achievements in devising ever more eccentric tortures for their own bodies might seem to have eclipsed all competition in body renunciation. Yet the ancestry of this orthodox Christian monasticism itself may, at least in part, derive from earlier Gnostic asceticism and mark the latter's domestication.[4] And, in any case, Gnosticism's peculiar edge in body renunciation has never been credited so much to any specific feats of Gnostic ascetic praxis (for which we have much less historical description than in the case of later, orthodox monasticism), as to Gnosticism's shocking *mythological* devaluation of the human body. We will turn to examples of this in a moment.

And, as we shall see, one thing that these and other examples reveal is that Gnostic perceptions of the body were actually more complex than is often recognized. Discussions of Gnostic attitudes toward the physical body have been too frequently content with summary statements about the "radical rejection of the body." There was that in Gnosticism, to be sure. And it is understandable that it has been Gnostic renunciation of the body that has captured the interest of scholars. For Gnostics went further than to stress the weakness, the perishability of the flesh. As we shall see, they spoke of the material body not as a garment designed and bestowed by a benign Creator (and then soiled by sin), but as a "prison," a "cave," devised in desperate malice by invisible monsters who created and control the cosmos. Any account of Gnostic perceptions of the body must consider such language.

Nevertheless, Gnostic body *renunciation* is only part of the story. Odd as it may seem, Gnostics who called their bodies prisons were at the same time making a more positive claim on the body. I hope to demonstrate in what follows that Gnostic perceptions of the body in late Antiquity manifested a certain ambivalence that is not often appreciated. On the one hand, the human self is quite completely distinguished from the physical body, and ultimately must be rescued from it; but on the other hand, according to many Gnostic sources, precisely in the human body is to be found the best *visible* trace of the divine in the material world.

Our Sources for Gnosticism

What we call "Gnosticism" seems to have flourished particularly during the first three or four centuries of the Common Era. We are not talking about a single organization, but a religious trend, characterized by certain recurrent themes and a typical jargon. There were many different Gnostic sects during this period. Some were part of the larger Christian movement; others were separate from it. Some of the sects were genetically related to another, schools branching out from common origins; other similarities seem to be the result of no more than different groups having read similar literature. We do not always know what such people called themselves. Sometimes it must have been simply "Christians"; sometimes they were named, at least by their critics, after their supposed founders (Valentinians, Basilideans), or after mythological figures prominent in their literature (Sethians after Seth, Naasenes after Naas, "the Serpent"); some may actually have called themselves *gnōstikoi*, "knowers."

Part of our evidence for Gnosticism comes from secondhand sources, and part from actual Gnostic writings. We have descriptions of Gnostic teaching and behavior provided by Christian writers such as Irenaeus of Lyons, Tertullian of Carthage, Clement of Alexandria, all from around the late second century A.D., or Hippolytus of Rome in the early third century A.D. and Epiphanius of Salamis in the late fourth. None of these can be said to be sympathetic accounts, and virtually all are sharply the opposite. Nevertheless, we do know that they provide much reliable information, for we also have writings from Gnostics themselves with which to compare such secondhand descriptions. The last generation of scholars has had the benefit of a large collection of Coptic manuscripts, found near the town of Nag Hammadi in Upper Egypt in 1945, whose contents include fourth century A.D. copies of many writings from various Gnostics. Greek originals of some of these Gnostic works were probably composed at least as early as the second century A.D., and a few could go back even earlier.

There are documents surviving from this period that are Gnostic without question, and there are documents that contain just enough traces of gnostic-like language to raise the possibility that they were written by Gnostics who, had they wished, could have been more explicitly Gnostic, and there are a range of documents in between. Here we will primarily concentrate on the first category of writings, the works that most modern scholars would consider Gnostic.

Gnostic Myths of the Body's Origins

"If one does not understand how the body that he wears came into being, he will perish with it."[5] It is in Gnostic myths about the origin of the first human bodies that we meet the essential understanding of what the body is — and is not. There are few Gnostic writings that illustrate this more clearly than the *Apocryphon ("Secret Book") of John*. We have four separate manuscripts of this writing, a rarity among surviving Gnostic texts. Three of these manuscripts come from three different books in the Nag Hammadi group — and always as the first tractate copied into the book — and a fourth manuscript, of roughly the same date, comes from still another Coptic book from a separate find. Two of the four manuscripts contain a somewhat longer version of the *Apocryphon of John* than that found in the other two. In addition, the anti-Gnostic Christian bishop Irenaeus seems to have had access in the late second century A.D. to a work very similar to the *Apocryphon of John*. Thus, there is some reason to conclude that this text, undergoing several different revisions during its history, represented a relatively popular version of gnosis.

The *Apocryphon of John* contains (in essentially the following order) revelations about: the nature of the true God, the invisible structures in the divine realm, how the original perfection of the divine realm was interrupted, how this led to the emergence of subdivine entities and their creation of the material world in which we live, how human beings were created and thus entrapped within the cosmos, and how salvation from the world is achieved. All of this is framed in a dialogue between the apostle John and Christ, after the latter's Resurrection. For our purposes here, we need not provide detailed description of the entire myth in the *Apocryphon of John*, and can instead focus directly on those dimensions most revelant to questions of the human body.

Above all, our attention is drawn to the portions of the myth describing the creation of the human being. The first Human in the myth is not a physical being at all, but rather the true God's perfect image — mental self-image, that is. The true God in this text is usually called the Invisible Spirit, and the Spirit's personified self-image is called Barbelo. An entire entourage of mythopoetically personified eternal divine attributes ("aeons") eventually unfolds, climaxing in the appearance of the Perfect Human, Adamas, an unflawed distillation of the divine image, and his son Seth.

Then, the serenity of the divine world is shattered by the self-willed behavior of Wisdom (*Sophia*), one of the divine attributes. Abandoning the carefully balanced patterns of harmony and authority that had prevailed in the divine realm, Wisdom produces her own thought. But this thought, far from being a proper reflection of the Divine, comes forth grotesque and unformed, unlike its mother and unlike any of the other divine entities. This creature is theriomorphic rather than anthropomorphic, resembling a lion-headed serpent. Wisdom calls him Ialdabaoth, and hides him in a cloud far from the immortal, divine realm.

Ialdabaoth is clearly identified with the Creator in Genesis, although many of his mythological features are also adapted from other religious and philosophical traditions of the day. Ialdabaoth begets various other rulers (*archontes*), henchmen to help him control the realm of darkness, and then organizes the created world in a pitiful attempt to imitate the first, divine order (*kosmos*) of immortal entities. Ialdabaoth's ludicrously mistaken arrogance in proclaiming, "I am God and there is no other God beside me,"[6] is a parody of similar assertions by God in biblical scripture (e.g., Isaiah 45.5; 46.9). As a correction of this ignorant proclamation, a voice

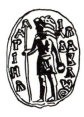

"Lion-headed figure on gemstone of uncertain date and provenance, which may have been a gnostic amulet. Beside the figure are the names Ialdabaoth and Ariel, 'Lion of God.' Names of some other gnostic archons appear on the reverse." From Jean Doresse, *The Secret Books of the Egyptian Gnostics* (New York: Viking Press, 1960).

from the divine realm announces, "The Human exists, and the Son of the Human,"[7] and Providence allows the divine Human image to reflect on the waters beneath Ialdabaoth and the other archons.

The archons' response to this apparition is to attempt to create its likeness. "Come," Ialdabaoth urges his archons, "let us create a human after the image of God and after our likeness."[8] The two manuscripts of the *Apocryphon of John* that contain a shorter recension of this work have a slightly different reading at this point: "Let us create a human after the image of God and after *his* likeness."[9] The allusion, of course, is to Genesis 1.26ff.: "Let us make man in our image, after our likeness.... So God created man in his own image...." The plural in this verse had already been an exegetical puzzle for generations of monotheists.[10] The author of the *Apocryphon of John* obviously takes the plural as a literal reference to a plurality of archons.[11]

The created human's body thus constitutes the arena for the decisive convergence of the divine and material realms. The body is supplied by the archons, but somehow bears a resemblance to the Perfect Human. In fact, while the shorter version of the *Apocryphon of John* simply refers to the human's creation after the image and likeness of God, the wording of the longer recension, "after the image of God and after *our* likeness," seems designed to underscore the created human's dual resemblance to both God (i.e., the invisible, immortal Perfect Human) and the archons. The same idea is found elsewhere: in the Nag Hammadi treatise *On the Origin of the World*, the luminous heavenly Adam's appearance in the world below leads the chief archon to say to the other archons, "come, let us create a human from the earth after the image of our body and after the likeness of that one...."[12] Then later we are reminded that "from that day, the seven archons have fashioned the human, his body being like their body, while his likeness is like the Human who appeared to them."[13] Similarly, in the closely related *Hypostasis of the Archons*, found in the same Nag Hammadi codex, the archons are said to have fashioned the human "after their body and [after the image/likeness] of God."[14]

Irenaeus mentions a similar teaching in his description of the Gnostics whom later heresiologists came to label "Ophites," although this version contains an additional ironic twist. The divine announcement of the existence of a Divine Human higher than Ialdabaoth was heard by all the archons. Ialdabaoth, in an amusing attempt to distract attention from the divine voice and its embarrassing revelation, and to divert it to himself, quickly says, "Come, let us make a human being after *our* image." Yet, as the archons proceed to accomplish this, Wisdom causes them to think of the Divine Human rather than of their own image, "so that by this means she might empty them of their original power."[15] The created human, "immense in breadth and length," thus served as the instrument through which any residual intimation of divinity remaining in these lower, illegitimate gods was extracted from them and distilled in the human vessel. Though this human was only a copy of the Divine Human, the very form of the created human rendered it superior to its archontic creators.

From this perception of the human body as fateful intersection of divine image with defiled matter, Gnostic commentary on the body was to embrace interestingly divergent themes.

The Body Negative: Victimization and Disassociation

The creation of Adam's body in the *Apocryphon of John* actually takes place in two stages: first the creation of a psychic ("soul") body, and only later the creation of a material body. Thinking of Adam coming into being in two stages was not without precedent, as we can see from a distinction made in some Jewish exegetical circles of the day, between a material human whose creation is narrated in Genesis 2.7, and an immaterial, ideal Human inferred from Genesis 1.27.[16] In the *Apocryphon of John* the psychic body is given psychic bone, psychic sinew, psychic flesh, psychic marrow, psychic blood, psychic skin and psychic hair, each of these seven psychic bodily elements being supplied by a different archontic power.[17] The creation of these bodily parts by the offspring of Ialdabaoth is a Gnostic interpretation combining elements from Plato's *Timaeus*, where the Demiurge assigns the creation of the material body to the "younger gods,"[18] with late antique traditions that associated various regions of the human body with each of the seven planets.[19]

The long recension of the *Apocryphon of John* continues at this point with an extensive section having no parallel in the shorter version. Here we find an even more detailed listing of the psychic bodily anatomy, and the names of the various archontic powers responsible for the manufacture and control of each part: Raphao makes the crown of the head, Abron the skull, Meniggesstroeth the brain, Asterekhme the right eye, Thaspomakha the left eye, and so forth.[20] Over seventy such parts are listed, proceeding generally from the top of the head to the toenails. We are told the names of the powers that control the heat, cold, dryness and wetness of the body, and a list of demons in charge of the individual passions of pleasure, desire, grief and fear, and the vices that spring from these.

The distinction between psychic body and material body is more blurred in the longer version than in the shorter. The anatomical listing found in the longer text is concluded with the remark that a total of 365 angels labored on the human until, "limb by limb, the psychic and material [hulikon] body was finished."[21] Yet it is not until later on in the narrative that the archons, in an attempt to counteract the superior knowledge possessed by the human being, make a material body from the four material elements of earth, water, fire and wind in which to imprison the human.[22] The psychic human is dragged by the archons, called here "the robbers," into "the cave of the refashioning of the body in which the robbers clothed the human, the chain of forgetfulness."[23] As Bentley Layton has pointed out, this is an allusion both to the dark cave where, in Plato's allegory, people are chained so as to be able to see only shadows of reality, and to caves typically used by robbers of the day.[24]

In the shorter version, the two stages of the psychic and material bodies are not confused at all. But, in any case, the difference between the two bodies is evidently only in their substance, not their form. The "Ophite" Gnostics, whose myth is described by Irenaeus, also taught that there were two stages in the acquisition of material bodies by the primordial humans. Having been cast out of Paradise into this material world by a frustrated and angry Ialdabaoth, the bodies of Adam and Eve became material: "Now, previously Adam and Eve had had the nimble, shining and, as it were, spiritual bodies that had been modeled at their creation; but when they came hither, these changed into darker, denser and more sluggish ones."[25] Neither here nor in the *Apocryphon of John* is any change of form mentioned, only a different, material substance for the body, and the latter's insidious effects. Encased within its cortex of flesh, the human image is trapped as though in a prison.

The orphic–platonic metaphor of the body as prison had served to characterize reincarnation as punishment.[26] So also in the *Apocryphon of John*, at the death of the person who has not attained gnosis in one lifetime, the archons seize his soul and "bind it with chains and throw it (back) into the prison."[27] In the poem toward the end of the longer version of the *Apocryphon of John*, we hear of the Revealer's descent to bring deliverance:

And I entered the midst of their prison,

Which is the prison of the body.

And I said, "O listener, arise from heavy sleep."

And that person wept and shed tears, heavy tears;

And wiped them away and said, "Who is calling my name?"

"And from where has my hope come, as I dwell in the bonds of the prison?"[28]

The *Book of Thomas the Contender*, a Nag Hammadi work that may have originated in Syrian Gnosticism, includes this same cluster of metaphors in its sharply ascetic renunciation of the body's desires: "Woe to you who put your hope in the flesh and the prison that will perish.... Woe to you who are captives, for you are bound in caves."[29]

The motif of victimization that is expressed in such descriptions of the body as a prison is also conveyed in some Gnostic myths through the theme of rape — particularly in the rape, or attempted rape, of Eve by the archons.[30] The attempt is foiled by the departure of the spiritual Eve at the last minute, leaving only her material "shadow" — that is, her body — for the archons to defile.[31] Karen King has called attention to the way in which such a motif may express how the Gnostic in the body seems often to have felt subject to oppression, humiliation, physical abuse, pollution and exploitation from the nefarious forces in control of the cosmos, and how escape from such oppression required a psychological disassociation of oneself from the body.[32]

The material body is something with which the "robber" archons of the *Apocryphon of John* are said to have "clothed" the human being. The body as a "garment" was a widely used metaphor in Antiquity.[33] Gnostic writers, too, often made use of the image, to underscore the disassociation of the person from the physical body. It might be noted that the idea of the body as garment did not in itself have to suggest to ancient men and women any sharp alienation of the self from the flesh. For example, in the widely read collection of general moral maxims known as the *Sentences of Sextus* (a copy of which appears among the Nag Hammadi writings, though it contains no distinctively Gnostic features), we find the admonition: "Say with your mind that the garment of your soul is the body, and keep it pure, since it is sinless."[34] Here, though the body is to be thought of as no more than clothes worn by the self, nevertheless the clothing is viewed as important, not irrelevant to the self's sense of well-being, its purity. The clothes are to be kept clean. A version of the metaphor with a more typically Gnostic tone is found in the famous "Hymn of the Pearl" in the *Acts of Thomas*. The redeemed son, lost in the sleep of forgetfulness in a foreign kingdom, has been awakened from amnesia by a revelatory letter from his parents. Remembering once again his royal identity, he rips off the clothing which he had put on upon arrival in this alien land: "And their dirty and unclean garment I took off and left in their land."[35] The story reads as an allegory of the soul's descent to and ascent from the body. But here the bodily garment is not something that one can keep pure in any meaningful sense.

As we have noted, metaphors of the body as "prison" or "garment" were not peculiar to Gnostics in Antiquity. They receive their distinctively Gnostic timbre only from their context within the Gnostic mythological devaluation of material existence. It is because one is convinced that the human body has actually been molded by malevolent archons that its description as a "prison" carries a pathos not quite equaled when non-Gnostic contemporaries called it the same thing.

The Body and Beasts

As was mentioned earlier, sometimes the created human is said to be modeled not only after the likeness of the Divine Human, but also after the image of the archons. And, as some of these same texts inform us, archons look like beasts. Because of the circumstances of his emanation, the Demiurge Ialdabaoth did not inherit the countenance of the Perfect Human. He appears in the form of a lion-headed serpent in the *Apocryphon of John*,[36] and with leonine features in other texts as well.[37] Nor are we surprised when this Demiurge's archontic offspring also turn out to be theriomorphs.[38] We are supposed to recognize their inferiority in this regard to their own creature, whose body has a human form. This point is made explicitly in at least one text, *On the Origin of the World*, where we are told that when they created Adam and Eve, after being enlightened with knowledge sent from the divine realm, "looked at their creators, who were beastly [*thērion*] forms, they despised them."[39] Yet the bodies of these humans themselves must somehow also resemble their beastly creators. The same Gnostic author had said that the physical body of the human was formed by the seven archons, and that "his body is like their body, his likeness like the Human who appeared to them."[40] The author is not very explicit here about exactly how the human body is like the beastly bodies of the archons. Nevertheless, we really do not have to look far for a suggestion as to the probable implications.

"The human being became like the beasts when he began to practice sexual intercourse."[41] So Clement of Alexandria quotes certain of his opponents, and the context suggests that some Gnostics were among those who shared this viewpoint. Certainly, the notion that sexual intercourse is a subhuman, beastly use of the body was expressed by more than one Gnostic author. According to Hippolytus of Rome, some second-century Gnostics, whom he calls Naasenes, taught that intercourse was something appropriate for pigs and dogs rather than humans.[42] The *Gospel of Philip*, another Gnostic writing in the Nag Hammadi collection, speaks of two trees that grow in Paradise, one producing beasts and the other producing humans. Adam ate of the first tree, became a beast and begot beasts.[43] In the *Book of Thomas the Contender*, the human body is said to be something that is "beastly," which will perish like the bodies of beasts, and which can never beget anything different from what beasts beget, since it itself was produced through sexual intercourse, just like the bodies of beasts are produced.[44] And still another writing from the Nag Hammadi collection, the *Authoritative Teaching*, describes the soul as having abandoned knowledge and fallen into "beastliness," which in this text refers to the passions associated with bodily existence.[45]

Even so orthodox a bishop as the fourth-century Ambrose asserted that among those virtues that constitute the human's peculiar worth is "chastity" (*pudicitia*), "which separates us from animals and unites us with the angels [*quae nos separat a pecudibus, angelis jungit*]."[46] Similarly, Gnostic authors of earlier centuries had seen in the ability to deny the body's animal craving for sexual intercourse a distinctively human characteristic.

The Body as Divine Image

The denial of sexual desire was the assertion of humanity *in spite of* the human body's urges. But Gnostics recognized something about the human form itself that set it apart from beasts and archons.

Although the archons in the *Apocryphon of John* create the human body, whether psychic or material, in the likeness of the Perfect Human, this likeness is enhanced through an element which the archons are in no position to provide. For their human is unable to stand upright and lies motionless for a long time, until finally Ialdabaoth, coaxed by representatives from the immortal realm above, unwittingly breathes into the creature whatever portion of Spirit he had inherited from his mother, Wisdom. Immediately the human stirs to life.[47]

This is evidently an old motif. A very similar version is attributed to the "Ophite" Gnostics,[48] although there the creature is able at least to wriggle around on the ground, rather than lying motionless before receiving the Spirit. The early second-century Gnostic Satornil of Antioch is said to have taught that seven demiurgic angels created the world and everything in it, including a human whom they formed "in the image and likeness" of a divine figure whose shining image was revealed from above, much as in the *Apocryphon of John*. But the created human could not stand erect, was able only to crawl like a worm, until a spark of life was sent from above.[49] In the *Hypostasis of the Archons*, the archons breathe soul into their created human but are not able to make the creature rise up off the ground, in spite of their ferocious persistence "like storm winds," in an attempt "to capture that likeness which had appeared to them in the waters."[50] And in the treatise *On the Origin of the World*, the chief archon is so afraid that the Human might actually enter the molded imitation (*plasma*) which the archons have fabricated "and gain mastery over it," that he gives no soul to it, but instead abandons it for forty days, leaving it like a lifeless aborted fetus on the ground.[51] In this text, the raising of Adam to upright posture takes place in two stages, with first a breath sent from a Wisdom figure called "Wisdom-Life" (*Sophia-Zōē*), which causes Adam to move on the ground, and then instruction from Life (=Eve), which allows Adam to rise up from the ground.

What all of these Gnostic traditions have in common is the theme that the ability to stand upright is a human feature which the archons were unable to imitate when they created their own human. The created body came to possess this uniquely human ability only by divine gift.

Other Gnostics evidently saw the same divine feature in the upright human stance, even though they did not always convey this through the specific mythic motif of the archons' inability to make the created human stand up. According to Hippolytus, the Naasene Gnostics taught that the first physical human, made by the archons, at first "lay without breath, immovable, unshakable, like a statue, being an image of that one above, the Human Adamas who is praised in song."[52] In this case, the initial perfect stillness of the protoplast, its statuelike stability, is actually viewed positively, and the loss of this stillness is a loss of one of the very similarities between the protoplast and the heavenly Adamas. For when the archons wish to enslave this image of Adamas, they give it a soul and bring it to life and movement, so that it "might suffer and be punished."[53] If Hippolytus's account is to be credited, the Naasene source on which he is drawing was an attempt to show, among other things, how the esoteric truths of the sect's teaching could actually be discerned in the myths and rites of various Hellenistic-Roman cults. Thus, the Samothracians really pay homage to the primal Human Adamas, since in their temple two statues of naked men stand upright, with hands stretched up toward heaven and with phallus erect. The two statues are "images of the primal Human and the spiritual human who is reborn."[54]

The upright stance is commonly mentioned in Hellenistic-Roman literature as a distinctly human trait, allowing humans to gaze upward and contemplate the orderly movement of the heavens.[55] Now Gnostic writers like those who composed the *Apocryphon of John* or the other works mentioned would hardly have found much noble about contemplation of any heavenly order. Indeed, it was most of all the "chaos" of Creation rather than its order which they seem to have noticed.[56] Yet they do seem to find the upright stance of the created human to be an important feature. Of course, they also saw in the "raising" of the human something more important than an erect posture: it signified spiritual illumination, the reception of *gnōsis*, the awareness of one's spiritual roots and therefore of one's superiority over even the creator of one's body, the god of the material world. But the metaphor surely drew its power, in the first place, from the perception of an actual and significant difference between animal and human bodies. The characteristic upright stance was a feature of physical human bodies in which even Gnostics, who gained reputations as "haters of the body," saw something extraordinary, a sign of divine power, setting human bodies apart from those of the animal world.

Anatomy and Revelation

We have seen that Gnostics renounced the body's substance, though they found a certain reassurance in the image traced by its form. Its substance — crude matter — subject to mutilation, disease, inevitable decay, shared in the instability of all mat-

ter, all bodies.[57] Its substance was doomed. Yet its form was a mirror of the divine.
Somehow, even the physical human form recalled divinity, in spite of the imperfect
and defiled material medium in which the shape had been cast. It was different from,
more excellent than, the form of beasts, a nagging reminder to the theriomorphic
archons that there were mysterious powers transcending the ugliness of their tyrannical control and deformed understanding.

It is striking how frequently Gnostic mythology actually brings in the human
anatomy — and especially the sexual anatomy. It is as though many Gnostics saw in
the body not only an intimation, a reflection, of a divine Human identity, but a
kind of map of reality. The Gnostics whom Hippolytus calls the Peratae are said to
have appealed to the anatomy of the brain, "likening the brain itself to the Father,
because of its immovability, and the cerebellum to the Son, because of the fact that
it moves and is serpent-like in appearance."[58] Hippolytus says that the Naasenes speculated about the mystical congruence between, on the one hand, the biblical description of the Garden of Eden and the four rivers flowing out of it (Genesis 2.10-14),
and, on the other hand, the human brain and the four senses.[59] Another, even more
elaborate, allegorical/anatomical interpretation of Eden and its four rivers is found
in Hippolytus's account of a work called the "Great Exposition," which he claims
to have been the composition of Simon Magus, but which probably comes only from
later Simonians.[60] Since God is said to form humans in the Garden, then the Garden is the human womb, Eden is the placenta, the "river which flows out of Eden
to water the Garden" (Genesis 2.10) is the navel, which is divided into four chan-
nels — two arteries and two veins, etc. But the four rivers of Eden are also interpreted as an allegory of the four senses possessed by the unborn child in the womb.

Now there has been some scholarly debate about how much we ought to rely
on every detail in Hippolytus's accounts of the teaching of these Gnostic sects, since
there are indications that the accounts tend suspiciously toward homogenization at
points, and may sometimes — so it is argued — be closer to tendentious paraphrases
of Gnostic sources than accurate quotation.[61] But the extent and diversity of speculations ascribed here to Gnostics concerning the allegorical significance of the human
anatomy is unlikely to have been entirely a fabrication.

Evidence from other Gnostic sources also encourages that judgment. For example, in their mythology about the invisible, true God and the primordial elabora-

tion of eternal divine aspects, or "aeons," Valentinian Gnostics tended to organize
the initial stages of the myth in numeric patterns which reflect the influence of
Pythagorean speculation. Thus, the primordial source of all things is to be found in
the pair Depth and Silence. Depth deposited a first thought like sperm in the womb
of Silence, and from this were conceived Intellect and Truth. This Tetrad multiplied
to form an Ogdoad, which produced a Decad and then a Duodecad. The Ogdoad
plus Decad plus Duodecad constitute the primordial thirty aeons, the Triacontad.[62]
Valentinians delighted in pointing to ways in which this numerical pattern and other
features of Valentinian myth were encoded in scripture and leapt with stubborn persistence before the exegete, once they knew to look for them. And at least one
Valentinian, Marcus, noted that the code was written in the human body itself:

> [T]he man formed after the image of the power above has in himself the power from
> the one source. This is situated in the region of the brain. From it there proceed four
> faculties, after the image of the Tetrad above, and these are called sight, hearing, smell,
> and taste. The Ogdoad is indicated by means of man in the following way: he has two
> ears, the same number of eyes, two nostrils and a twofold taste, of what is bitter and
> what is sweet.... The whole man contains the total image of the Triacontad as follows: in
> his hands he bears, by means of the fingers, the Decad; in his whole body, which is
> divided into twelve members, [he bears] the Duodecad, for [the Marcosians] portion
> out the body, just as they divide up the body of truth.... The Ogdoad, being unspeak-
> able and invisible, is understood as hidden in the viscera.[63]

Above all, it is the sexual anatomy that comes before us so often in the symbolism of Gnostic myth. A famous Valentinian Gnostic adage cautioned that, while baptism is the moment when one passes beyond the force field of Fate, it is not just
the washing that frees, but the knowledge of: "Who were we? What have we
become? Where were we? Where have we been thrown? Whither are we hurrying?
From what are we saved? What is birth? What is rebirth?"[64] Birth and rebirth – *gnōsis*
involved an understanding of the mystery of both. Sentiments such as this no doubt
account for the fact that one of the most recurrent anatomical images is that of the
female womb, and the womb's features as commonly understood in the medical literature of the day.[65] For example, some schools of ancient medicine taught that both
men and women produced semen. However, the female seed was weak and unable
by itself to produce a perfect fetus.[66] Miscarriages, or the ejection from the uterus

of tumerous growths related to fetal miscarriages, were often considered growths from the female seed alone, lacking the completion provided by the male seed. The ugliness of such abortions sometimes prompted their description as inhuman, monstrous things. Gnostic myths that account for the origin of the material creation by describing Wisdom's attempt at solo conception, the resulting "abortion" (beastlike and named Ialdabaoth, according to some Gnostics), and the creation of the world by this aborted, inhuman being, clearly drew some of their inspiration from speculation about the spiritual significance of current medical knowledge of the female anatomy.

Whatever we imagine when we speak of Gnostics renouncing their bodies, or despising the flesh, we should not ignore how intrigued they seemed to have been with their own anatomy, how often they seemed convinced that truths, both pleasant and unpleasant, about their origin and their destiny could be traced within its form and functions.

Conclusion

Gnostic mythology about the body's origin articulated, on the one hand, one of the more brutal symbolic devaluations of the body in the history of religions, and on the other hand, ironically, a conviction that the human form somehow mirrors the divine world. The created human body is not the work of the transcendent and beneficent God, as most contemporary Jews and Christians believed, and as Plato had suggested in terms that Jewish and Christian writers had often appropriated. Instead, it was the crude work of archontic pirates, literally "capturing" the Human (=Divine) image and polluting it with beastly qualities and urges. But if the human body is not the work of the transcendent God, it nevertheless bears the divine image like nothing else in creation.

The ambivalence is perhaps brought into greater relief if we contrast Gnostic myths such as those discussed above with what we know of the teaching of Marcion of Sinope, a second century Christian. Though Marcion is sometimes categorized in modern scholarship as a Gnostic, his dissimilarity to the Gnostics we have described here is nowhere more obvious than in the area of anthropology, including the question of the body. Marcion also taught a distinction between the creator of the world and a good God, the Father of Jesus. And he adopted a sharply ascetic attitude toward the human body, which he described as "full of excrement."[67] But Marcion produced no myth that connected the human image with the good God. Marcion taught that the good God was completely alien to creation, and by his grace alone chose to redeem humanity from creation by sending his Son. Marcion seems to have taken the first chapters of Genesis more or less at face value, as the description of the creation of the world by the God of the Jews, a just but harsh divinity. Marcion's Creator was not, like Ialdabaoth, an aborted castoff from a higher realm, and was not trying to replicate the image of a Perfect Human higher than himself when he created the first human. The human creature is simply the product of the Creator. Compared with the Gnostic writers we have mentioned, Marcion was entirely unambivalent in his anthropology. Unlike them, he pointed to nothing about the human body that intimated the divine.

NOTES

1. Porphyry, *Vita Plotini* 1.

2. Plotinus, *Enneads* 2.9.17.1-3, 2.9.6.60.

3. For general introductions to Gnosticism, see Kurt Rudolph, *Gnosis: The Nature and History of Gnosticism*, English trans. and ed. R. McL. Wilson (San Francisco: Harper & Row, 1983); Hans Jonas, *The Gnostic Religion*, 2d ed. (Boston: Beacon, 1963). For English translations of principal Gnostic writings, see Bentley Layton, *The Gnostic Scriptures: A New Translation with Annotations and Introductions* (Garden City: Doubleday, 1987); Werner Foester, *Gnosis: A Selection of Gnostic Texts*, English trans. and ed. R. McL. Wilson, 2 vols. (Oxford: Clarendon, 1972); James M. Robinson, ed., *The Nag Hammadi Library in English*, 2d ed. (Leiden: Brill, 1987).

4. Henry Chadwick, "The Domestication of Gnosticism," in *The Rediscovery of Gnosticism*, Bentley Layton, ed., *Studies in the History of Religions* (Suppl. to *Numen*) 41 (Leiden: Brill, 1980), vol. 1, pp. 3-16.

5. *Dialogue of the Savior*, Nag Hammadi Corpus 3.134.11-13 (hereafter cited as NHC).

6. *Apocryphon of John*, NHC 2.11.20ff.

7. *Ibid.* 14.14ff.

8. *Ibid.* 15.2ff.

9. *Ibid.* 22.4-6; BG 48.11-14: "after the image and likeness of God."

10. R. McL. Wilson, "The Early History of the Exegesis of Genesis 1.26," *Studia Patristica* 1, ed. K. Aland and F.L. Cross, *Texte und Untersuchungen zur Geschichte der altchristlichen Literatur* 63 (Leipzig: Hinrichs, 1957), pp. 420-37; Birger Pearson, *Philo and the Gnostics on Man and Salvation*, Center

for Hermeneutical Studies in Hellenistic and Modern Culture, Protocol of the Twenty-Ninth Collo-quy (Berkeley: University of California, 1977).

11. R. van den Broeck, "The Creation of Adam's Psychic Body in the Apocryphon of John," *Studies in Gnosticism and Hellenistic Religions*, ed. R. van den Brock and M.J. Vermaseren (Leiden: Brill, 1981), p. 43, has correctly pointed out that in the *Apocryphon of John*, Ialdabaoth stands more apart from the seven lower archons than is the case in other Gnostic texts, and does not himself take direct part in the creation of the body, but leaves this to the seven.

12. *On the Origin of the World*, NHC 2.112.33-13.1.

13. *Ibid.* 114.29-32.

14. *Hypostasis of the Archons*, NHC 2.87.30-32.

15. Irenaeus, *Adversus haereses* 1.30.6, Layton, *The Gnostic Scriptures*, p. 176.

16. E.g., Philo of Alexandria, *Opera* 134ff.; see Pearson, *Philo and the Gnostics*.

17. *Apocryphon of John*, NHC 2.15.13-23.

18. Plato, *Timaeus* 42d-e; 69cff.

19. See R. van den Broeck, "The Creation of Adam's Psychic Body"; and cf. Michael A. Williams, "Higher Providence, Lower Providences and Fate in Gnosticism and Middle Platonism," in *Neoplatonism and Gnosticism*, eds. R.T. Wallis and Jay Bregman, *Studies in Neoplatonism Ancient and Modern* 6 (New York: SUNY, forthcoming).

20. *Apocryphon of John*, NHC 2.15.29-18.13.

21. *Ibid.* 19.2-6; but a few lines later, in 19.10-12, we find a second summarizing remark that men-tions no material body: "And all the angels and demons worked until they had constructed the psy-chic body." Such awkward superfluity suggests the existence of a literary seam, resulting from the interpolation into the long recension of the lengthy anatomical description. In the process, the edi-tor has either forgotten momentarily that it is the psychic, not the material, body being described, or is no longer really so interested in any significant distinction between psychic and material body.

22. *Ibid.* 20.28-21.13.

23. *Ibid.* 21.9-12.

24. Plato, *Republic* 7.514a; Layton, *The Gnostic Scriptures*, p. 45, n.21b.

25. Irenaeus, *Adversus haereses* 1.30.9; Layton, *Gnostic Scriptures*, p. 177.

26. Plato, *Cratylus* 400c; see Jaap Mansfeld, "Bad World and Demiurge: A 'Gnostic' Motif From Parmenides and Empedocles to Lucretius and Philo," in *Studies in Gnosticism and Hellenistic Reli-gions presented to Gilles Quispel on the Occasion of his 65th Birthday*, ed. R. van den Broeck and M.J. Vermaseren, Etudes préliminaires aux religions orientales dans l'Empire romain 91 (Leiden: Brill,

1981), pp. 291ff.; K. Corrigan, "Body and Soul in Ancient Religious Experience," in *Classical Mediterranean Spirituality: Egyptian, Greek, Roman*, ed. A.H. Armstrong (New York: Crossroads, 1986), p. 365ff.

27. *Apocryphon of John*, NHC 2.27.7ff.; cf. *On the Origin of the World*, NHC 2.114.20-24.

28. *Apocryphon of John*, NHC 2.31.3-9; Layton, *The Gnostic Scriptures*, p. 326.

29. *Book of Thomas the Contender*, NHC 2.143.10-22; Layton, *The Gnostic Scriptures*, p. 407.

30. Gedaliahu A.G. Stroumsa, *Another Seed: Studies in Gnostic Mythology*, Nag Hammadi Studies 24 (Leiden: Brill, 1984), esp. pp. 42-45; Anne McGuire, "Virginity and Subversion: Norea Against the Powers in the *Hypostasis of the Archons*," in *Images of the Feminine in Gnosticism*, ed. Karen King, *Studies in Antiquity and Christianity* 3 (Philadelphia: Fortress, forthcoming).

31. *Hypostasis of the Archons*, NHC 2.89.19-30; *On the Origin of the World*, NHC 2.116.8-17.15; cf. *Apocryphon of John*, NHC 2.23.35-24.15.

32. Karen King, "Deciphering the Feminine: Toward a Typology of Images of Gender in Gnosticism," paper delivered at the American Academy of Religion/Society of Biblical Literature, Boston, 1987.

33. See Dennis R. MacDonald, *There is No Male and Female: The Fate of a Dominical Saying in Paul and Gnosticism*, Harvard Dissertations in Religion 20 (Philadelphia: Fortress, 1987), esp. p. 23ff.

34. *Sentences of Sextus* 346, NHC 12.30.11-14.

35. *Acts of Thomas* 111; Edgar Hennecke and Wilhelm Schneemelcher, eds., *New Testament Apocrypha*, English trans. and ed. R. McL. Wilson (Philadelphia: Westminster, 1964), vol. 2, p. 501.

36. *Apocryphon of John*, NHC 2.10.9.

37. *Hypostasis of the Archons*, NHC 2.94.15ff.; *On the Origin of the World*, NHC 2.100.5-26; Ophite diagram described by Origen, *Contra Celsum* 6.30ff.; see Howard M. Jackson, *The Lion Becomes Man: The Gnostic Leontomorphic Creator and the Platonic Tradition*, Society of Biblical Liberature Dissertation Series 81 (Atlanta: Scholars Press, 1985); Michael Williams, *The Immovable Race: A Gnostic Designation and the Theme of Stability in Late Antiquity*, Nag Hammadi Studies 29 (Leiden: Brill, 1985), p. 111 n.7.

38. *Apocryphon of John*, NHC 2.11.26-35: Athoth, sheep's face; Eloaiou, donkey's face; Astaphaios, hyena's face; Yao, serpent's face with seven heads; Sabaoth, dragon's face; Adonin, ape's face; Sabbede, shining fire-face. Compare the theriomorphic forms of the archons in the Ophite tradition in Origen, *Contra Celsum* 6.30-33.

39. *On the Origin of the World*, NHC 2.119.16-18.

40. *Ibid.* 114.29-32.

41. Clement, *Stromata* 3.102.3ff.

42. Hippolytus, *Refutatio omnium haeresium* 5.8.33.

43. *Gospel of Philip*, NHC 2.71.22-26.

44. *Book of Thomas the Contender*, NHC 2.138.39-39.10.

45. *Authoritative Teaching*, NHC 6.24.20-22.

46. Ambrose, *Enarrationes in XII Psalmos* 61.21, *PL* 14.1233.

47. *Apocryphon of John*, NHC 2.19.13-33.

48. Irenaeus, *Adversus haereses* 1.30.6.

49. *Ibid.* 1.24.1.

50. *Hypostasis of the Archons*, NHC 2.88.3-9.

51. *On the Origin of the World*, NHC 2.115.3-11.

52. Hippolytus, *Refutatio* 5.7.6ff.

53. *Ibid.* 5.7.8; see Williams, *The Immovable Race*, p. 32ff.

54. Hippolytus, *Refutatio* 5.8.10.

55. Antonie Wlosok, *Laktanz und die philosophische Gnosis*, Abhandlungen der Heidelberger Akademie der Wissenschaften, phil.-hist. Klasse 2 (Heidelberg: Winter, 1960).

56. Williams, *The Immovable Race*, pp. 132-35.

57. *Ibid.* pp. 44ff., 114, 121ff.

58. Hippolytus, *Refutatio* 5.17.11.

59. *Ibid.* 5.9.15-17.

60. *Ibid.* 6.14.7-15.4.

61. Klaus Koschorke, *Hippolyt's Ketzerbekämpfung und Polemik gegen die Gnostiker: Eine tendenzkritische Untersuchung seiner "Refutatio omnium haeresium,"* Göttinger Orientforschungen: 6. Reihe: Hellenistica 4 (Weisbaden: Harrassowitz, 1975).

62. Irenaeus, *Adversus haereses* 1.1.1-3.

63. *Ibid.* 1.18.1; trans. from Foester, vol. 1, p. 214.

64. *Excerpta ex Theodoto* 78.1ff.

65. On this, see the exceptionally useful discussion and collection of evidence in Richard Smith's, "Sex Education in Gnostic Schools," in *Images of the Feminine in Gnosticism*, from which the examples I cite here are drawn.

66. E.g., Galen, *De usu partium* 14.7.

67. Tertullian, *Contra Marcionem* 3.10.

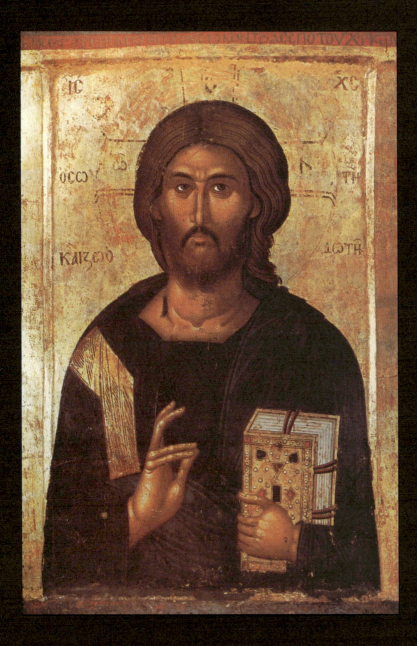

Christ as Savior and Creator of Life, 1393/1394, Skopje.

The Face of Christ,
The Form of the Church

Marie-José Baudinet

The subject is the face of Christ. More specifically, it is an examination of what was said about it at that moment in history when Christians split into two camps. For one group, in Constantinople, adopting the imperial line, the representation of Christ's face and its cult were henceforth forbidden and to be considered blasphemous. For the others, who saw themselves as faithful followers of the tradition, this face would be painted and adored despite all the bloody military repressions that the iconophiles suffered. I am, of course, referring to the iconoclastic crisis. This paper, however, will examine only that aspect which concerns the legitimacy of the iconic representation of Christ's face — the face of God's son, also known as the Father's Economy. For one camp, this economy was restrictive, for the other, it authorized the proliferation of an image whose paradigm should not be questioned. Economy, that is *oikonomia*, in Greek reads as *ikonomia*. To the Byzantine ear familiar with the iconoclastic debate, the law of the icon and the law concerning the administration of goods are one and the same thing. In either case, the supreme administrator, the great economist, is God the Father *who gave His essence in order that it be distributed in the visible world through His own image* — the natural image of His Son.

At stake in the iconoclastic debate is a face that, far from being a false pretext or mere cavil, is of capital interest to the relationship between power and vision. By reading the texts in favor of icons, it is possible to understand what the traditional Church, on the one hand, and the emperors, on the other, wanted to possess exclusively. Traditionally the iconoclasts were known to be as iconocratic as the iconophiles. For them, it was never a question of abolishing all images and governing without them. They were content to ban the representations of Christ's face and the Virgin's and to replace them with their own.

To understand the question in all its complexity, it is necessary to look at a short text by Nicephorus the Patriarch, the exiled champion of the iconophiles. In the second volume of the *Antirrhetics*, Nicephorus claims that his iconoclastic opponent is unable to distinguish between inscription and circumscription. What is the real meaning, both in its assumptions and consequences, of the figuration of a face within an iconic space? According to Nicephorus, the iconophile does not see the pictorial inscription of a face as a circumscription imprisoning and limiting that face. For the iconoclast, however, such an inscription automatically circumscribes, and therefore limits, divine infinity — the endless openness of the Word. This is why the only visible sign he accepts as a memorial of the Incarnation is the Cross. How can one understand the iconoclast's figureless space, this open, cruciform and faceless territory?

To have a clearer idea of the true meaning of this ecclesiastical meditation, it is necessary to return to the iconic inscription of the facial outline. We must understand how the line, this incision that divides and cuts the iconic plate in two, can impose a formal illusion on its viewers without violating or disfiguring the essence of its model. The line is the border where being begins, the edge of the finite thing. Inscriptions allow the statement of a name. The image is homonymous; it has the right to partake of the name of its referent without making any claim of its essence. It does not divide; it entertains a double relationship with its model in time, in the form of a memorial, as well as in space, in the form of a trace, because it purports to re-present a God whose absence it respects. Thus, form delineates a conceptualizable area within a homogeneous space, but it does not enclose or contain it. But what remains within the line, what is outlined by it? Is it meaning or merely emptiness? Does the line generate a full, differentiated space or does it mark, like a furrow, the visible limits of emptiness? The function of the icon constantly goes beyond the perimeter of its vision. The face of Christ — also known as *morphē, eidos, schēma* — resembles its image by virtue of a *mimēsis* that must be clearly distinguished from the *perigraphē* that was His lot during His earthly life. To engrave (*graphein*) is not the same as to encircle (*perigraphein*). Christ is not encircled in His image; He is not circumscribed by it because the image is not a being or an absolute but, rather, a *relative* term. The incarnation of an absence, the flesh of the image is as supernatural as Christ's flesh after His Resurrection. Iconic mimesis establishes a resemblance that is neither an essential identity nor a realistic reproduction (*homoiōma*). It is a *homoiōsis*, a formal resemblance that points to and stresses the direction of the gaze rather than indicating a place of recognition. The image of Christ is empty of His presence and full of His absence. What could be more faithful to the Incarnation, which the Greek Fathers also called *kenosis*, evacuation or emptying? To incarnate. To empty. When the Word became flesh, divinity did not fill up with matter nor did matter fill up with divinity.

As a memorial of the Incarnation, the icon is, therefore, a memorial of *kenosis* that poses the problem of the line's infinity. For some, *kenosis* is only an act of divine condescension designating the Messiah's humility, poverty and nakedness. In short, *kenosis* is, in the context of the great economist's expenditure, the sacrifice of the Father who exiles His Son from His glory during His earthly life. This does not mean that the Son ceases to participate in the Father's glory, but, rather, that He renounces making it visible. The *akmē* of *kenosis* undoubtedly occurred at the moment of Christ's supreme triumph and absolute dereliction, the moment of His death on the Cross when He cried out, "Why hast thou forsaken me?" Thus the line, the tear, that incarnates and outlines the sign of that moment must be darker, bloodier, more terrible. A line divides space, just as Christ's coming divided time into the old and the new alliance. The Church understood this well when it announced that from that moment on it was no longer necessary to represent the Messiah symbolically as a lamb. Suddenly, because of the new law, Christians had a right to Christ's face. And the iconoclasts could be reproached for failing to understand His Incarnation, and, therefore, for denying His Resurrection. To keep only the Cross without allowing access to the face amounted to an anthropomorphism of Christ's person that limited its inscription to the form of His human misery. But Christ was resurrected, His face, His person (*prosōpon*) did triumph over the Cross: the Transfiguration of His body must, therefore, continue in the icon. Transfiguration, *metamorphosis*, this is the name that designates both the glory of the resurrected body and the work of the spectator's gaze on the icon. Both emptiness and fullness are foiled. The line on the surface cannot imprison any more than the Cross could annihilate. Christ's *uncircumscribability* is the sign and the pledge of His Resurrection, just as circumscribability is the sign and pledge of His Passion. The image of Christ's face frames Christ, just as His absent grace frames the eyes of the spectator who, in an act of faith, metamorphoses this absence into a presence.

In the third *Antirrhetics*, Nicephorus asks whether Christ is on the plate of an icon the way the griffin is on the calyx it decorates. The answer is no: the griffin is a mere ornament, in other words, a complete resemblance. The ornament encloses an appearance and renders it visually pleasing. The image of Christ on an icon is not visually pleasing because He is not an ornament. In other words, He is not visible but He can see, since the icon establishes a relationship between two who gaze upon one another. And He is audible for His name must be inscribed on the icon according to the *epigraphē* that, as a literal inscription, vouches for the homonymy between the image and the model. Indeed, in an icon everything is exteriority. As a material object, the icon itself is obviously outside the spiritual realm it invokes. The enclosed space of Christ's body, nose, hands, ears and hair is a series of grooves bled into the plate. What Saint John Damascene identifies with the *skiagraphein* is the effect of shadow that outlines essence without enclosing it in the expectation of color's grace. Just as the drawing is the trace left by the body that has disappeared so the chromatic range is the *tupos*, the image imprinted on the onlooker. Like line, color is an agent of transfiguration. It is applied in successive layers, from the darkest to the most transparent. Each of the iconographer's gestures is a memorial to the progressive redemption of the flesh that offers itself to the eyes of the viewer only as a surface suitable to the passage of the Spirit. The face of Christ in an icon outlines His essence and reiterates the Incarnation but does not represent them.

Thus, one can see how Nicephorus, in a veritable tour de force, succeeds in persuading his audience of the radical difference between the spatiality of the icon and that of perception. The law of the icon rests on its "territorial" autonomy, on its capacity to establish a relationship between periphery and content that this very periphery transfigures. Its existence is purely liminal; the limen, the threshold, it marks is free from all closure because it is the threshold of infinity. Idolatry is averted because the eyes cannot find anything to "graze upon" in this blessedly vacant object that respects the uncircumscribability of its model. The iconic line is a fault that designates Christ's body as God's temporary, but voluntary because salutary, default. The icon is a kenotic practice. In Byzantium, the aim and meaning of Christ's face is quite different from the sumptuary glorification of Christendom practiced in Western art. Indeed, what does the iconographer do? He encloses, he traces, he follows the indications of *homoiōsis* with his pen and his stylus. Economy can guarantee negotiation, mediations between the infinity of the model and the finitude of the image, because it once was the science par excellence of borders that produced these contiguities. Economy presides over every incarnation, over every productive insemination of meaning into an empty form. Economy thus takes place in a uterine dimension. This matrix, whose value resides only in its borders, and to which everything visible owes its form, is none other than the mother's body. The first icon came into being at the moment of the Annunciation, when Mary received the Word that she had been chosen as the abode of infinity. The icon, in turn, produces the implantation of the Word within the virginal frame — the uterine *Chōra* traversed by divine breath and confirmed by the harbinger's voice that institutes the device of homonymy. The work of the Holy Spirit is a fecundating voice that, in turn, guarantees the icon's fecundity. Even the Church has entrails. The Virgin is the body of the Church, and the Church is full of God without containing Him.

This should help us understand why it was so important to anathematize those who maintained that Christ was preformed and had simply passed through His mother as if she were a funnel. Gregory of Nazianzus vehemently insists on the naturalness of the Virgin's pregnancy. Christ's human face is the fruit of the maternal womb, which was able even before the advent of the icon to "draw" it without enclosing it. The Virgin's womb is full of Christ's form, and yet it remains essentially empty insofar as it is the place of *kenosis*.

This is also true of both the icon and the Church. An image has the speculative status of an abyss and the contractual status of an enclosed space. This is how the Church was able to found the fullness of representation on a theology of *kenosis*. The icon generates surreptitiously a space where the temporal and the spiritual empires coalesce. Christ's infinity is respected in order to allow ecclesiastic thought and actions to reach beyond the narrow boundaries of human monarchy. The emperor governs within frontiers; the Church, on the other hand, has a universal vocation from which it draws its diplomatic and ecumenical ideas. The image of Christ's face is its first emissary; many more will follow. The icon is a net or, perhaps, a chessboard where emptiness and fullness find their metaphors — a complete system, governed by disciplinary canons. It is the universe of the rules of the game that institutes the infinite world as a world of constantly trespassed boundaries. Black and white are ultimately inseparable. Binarism originates in Christ's double nature and continues in the double nature of the icon. But the icon itself plays the role of the third term whose mediation makes resolution between opposite poles both possible and sensible. Matter and spirit: the image is double; but, like the Trinity, it makes communication between opposites possible by joining them without fusion in a woman's body, thanks to the work of the Holy Spirit.

The discourse of the iconophiles is theoretically binary. But a closer look at the way it works reveals that the third term that was excluded from the logical contradiction is implied in the reality it constructs. The iconoclast Constantine V seems firmly attached to the binary logic of exclusion. Every time Nicephorus invokes the iconoclastic discourse, it is to stigmatize its principle: everything must be one thing or the other. For the iconoclast, the image does not constitute a valid mediation between man and God just as the Church is not a valid mediator between God and the emperor. For Constantine V there can be only idolatry or invisibility, whereas for the iconophile the image dissolves the alternative and resolves the opposition just as Christ's face, under the virginal cloak, becomes the sign of communication between the world and God. "Those who refuse the image refuse the economy," writes Theodore of Studios, another iconophile. Without mediation there is no access to the symbolic universe of substitutions. Thus, what might be called the semiotics of emptiness is radically different from the vantage point of the iconophile or of the iconoclast. The iconophylic Church, having triumphed under the aegis of the mediating icon in the name of the Incarnation, elaborates a metaphorical space where both emptiness and fullness meet in representation. According to the iconophiles, the iconoclasts, a horde without metaphor, clearly demonstrate through their military violence an inability to enter a symbolic universe. In fact, they did try to contest the Church's hegemony over the universe of symbols. But, as Christians, they refused to broach the question from the angle of a secularization of power and, instead, took the same stance as their opponents: one of faith. The battle was lost from the start.

The iconoclast counters the iconophile's spatial metaphors by maintaining that, far from being as empty as it pretends, the icon, by means of the *perigraphē*, takes possession of the entire space the moment it is made sacred. For him, any illusion of plenitude is defeated by a graph that does not enclose anything — a truly open form that breaks up space without outlining it. Emptiness cannot assume the form of content, nor can form cope with emptiness.

Thus, iconoclasm developed a cruciform semiotics that, from the very start, placed both Christ and the emperor at the same direct intersection of the spiritual and the temporal worlds, at the crossroad of all directions that generate territory. It is at such a crossroad that the emperor erects his statues. The Cross is not just a memorial to divine suffering, it also marks a strategic space that does not speak the language of mediation, but rather bespeaks the punctual and effective presence of generals and guards destined to control and conquer the territory they oversee. The power of the image is well known to the iconoclastic emperor who is quick to replace Christ's face with his own, or with his son's on the other side of his coins, for the transmission of power also occurs dynastically at a human level. It was imperative for the Church that the image triumph. And triumph it did. For the Christian world, from that moment on, the theology of the face is the key to power.

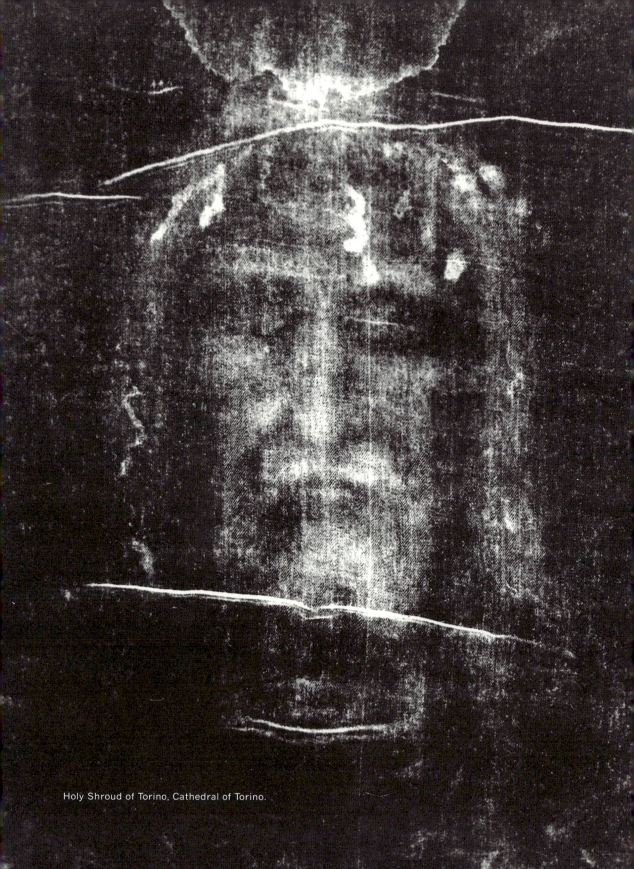

Holy Shroud of Torino, Cathedral of Torino.

Antirrhetic II

Nicephorus the Patriarch

356A Anyone endowed with even a moderate amount of good sense should be able to distinguish between inscription and circumscription. First of all, it should be pointed out that inscription, the simpler of the two, can have two meanings. Its first meaning concerns the characters of those elements that are printed according to a sequential order, proceeding from the syllable, and used by logographers. The second meaning concerns the operations of mimetic representation, which involves the outlining and figuration of a particular model.

356B This second meaning will be the object of our investigation. The first kind of inscription constitutes, by means of the words one utters, the message contained in an articulate discourse. The second kind reproduces, in appearance, the likeness of the person it has chosen as a model. It is not our purpose here to examine the means necessary to reproduce the appearance of certain forms and certain objects. In both instances, those involved or specialized in this sort of graphic activity are commonly known as "graphists," whether they are dealing with verbal or with pictorial inscription. Indeed, in ancient times, the verb "to inscribe," signifying "to engrave," was not so removed from this meaning. And yet the iconoclasts maintain that circumscription is a product of inscription, when in fact circumscription can only occur in space, time or understanding, by virtue of the very nature of the circumscribed object.

356C Spatially speaking, all bodies are circumscribed, since circumscription is a quality of everything that is contained within spatial limits. As for time, everything which, having no prior existence, starts to exist in time is circumscribable. This is the case with angels and with those spiritual faculties that are said to be circum-

356D scribed. As for understanding, all that can be encompassed by thought and knowledge is circumscribable....

357A Thus, it can be said that the angels' relative knowledge of their reciprocal nature is a form of circumscription. For one finds circumscription in the perimeter and determination of a contained and defined object, in the delimitation of everything that is endowed with a beginning and movement, in the understanding of an object of thought and knowledge. Whatever does not fit these categories is uncircumscribable. It therefore follows that Christ, having truly taken on a body like ours, is circumscribed by His humanity. Nor is it an illusion that this incorporeal being is circumscribed in space, He who, having no beginning but having subjected Himself to a temporal one, is circumscribed in time. By condescending to become corporeally a part of humanity, incomprehensible divinity also accepts enclosure within the boundaries of comprehension.

Circumscription can be understood in a number of ways. It is therefore very important that we be able to distinguish one from the other.

357B   In truth, he who constructs the image of a man — by which I mean the painter, since it is of him we must now speak — he in no way circumscribes the true identity of the person he paints. It is wrong to believe that by determining someone's limits we imprison him within a space that contains him, when in fact he is absent from it. For if it is true that somebody is necessarily present in his real circumscription, this is not at all the case in the instance of his graphic inscription. Quite the contrary: strictly speaking, the painter does not circumscribe anything even though there are reasons for believing he does. Generally speaking, as far as corporeally circumscribed things are concerned, their localization in space is the form of their most immediate circumscription. I have already defined what this place is. Conversely, it would be wrong to say that when we circumscribe someone corporeally, to speak as they do, we automatically inscribe him, that is to say, we represent him in an image. This does not necessarily follow since, as I shall demonstrate, there is no evident connection between these two notions.

357C   We commonly say that a man is figured in such and such a space, whether on a wall or on a canvas, but in fact no soberly intelligent being would ever assert that a painted space puts us in the presence of the actual circumscription and delimitation of the model. A man is inscribed in the image that represents him, but he is not circumscribed by it. He is only circumscribed by his own spatiality — the space of his own circumscription. There is a vast difference between these two sorts of space. Depending on the case, a man can be represented with colors on a canvas or in a mosaic. He can be figured with different materials and in a number of forms that play with light. But never, I insist, never can a model be circumscribed in such a way, because, as we have already mentioned, circumscription is something completely different. What's more, each graphic inscription refers to the corporeal form of

357D the model, to his outline, his sensible shape...which it reproduces in its external likeness. An image is always the image of a model, this is how the term is defined; this image, being separate from its model, exists on its own, in its own temporality. Circumscription, on the contrary, has nothing to do with resemblance, nor with its opposite. It is not a fashioned form. We do not say of it that it is the circumscription of an archetype, nor that it is related to it. It is inseparable from it, since it is not relative. Its existence is the very existence of that which it limits, and this unity cannot be broken. Man always exists in space, time and comprehension, and since his nature is circumscribed, it follows that it cannot be traversed by any emptiness. Thus, insofar as spatial circumscription is concerned, we can state that the contiguity of two bodies

360A constitutes the very limits of the visible manifestation of each. Indeed, in a case such as this, mass, size and, therefore, place, are apprehended simultaneously. Graphic inscription, instead, is completely independent, even though, wherever it is, graphic inscription remains determined by its role as figuration. Circumscription, on the contrary, encloses in a simple though not figuratively determined fashion all that is by nature circumscribable. More simply put: graphic inscription does not circumscribe man, even if he is circumscribable, any more than circumscription figures him, even if he is figurable. Each notion has its own rationale.

Translated by Anna Cancogne.

zone

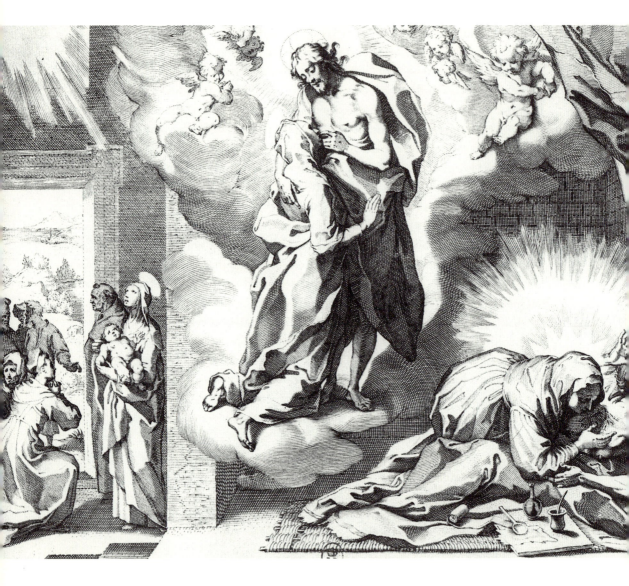

M. Fiorini after F. Vanni, Saint Catherine of Sienna.
From *Legenda Maior*, 1597 (Paris, Bibliothèque nationale).

The Female Body
and Religious Practice in the
Later Middle Ages

Caroline Walker Bynum

Introduction

One night in the early fifteenth century, as she prayed to the Virgin Mary, the Franciscan reformer Colette of Corbie received a vision of Christ. The Christ who came to Colette was not the sweet-faced bridegroom nor the adorable baby familiar to us from medieval paintings and illuminations. Christ appeared to Colette as a dish completely filled with "carved-up flesh like that of a child," while the voice of God warned her that it was human sin that minced his son into such tiny pieces.[1]

A hundred years earlier, in the Rhineland, a Dominican friend of the nun Lukardis of Oberweimar received a vision of the Crucifixion. Yet the figures he saw were not the executed bodies of Christ and two thieves common in both art and visionary experience. Rather the friar saw his friend Lukardis and two others nailed to crosses, and the voice of God informed him that it was Lukardis who was to be identified with Christ because she suffered most.[2]

These visions startle the modern reader. Conditioned by classic accounts such as Johann Huizinga's and recent popularizations such as Barbara Tuchman's to see the late Middle Ages as violent in its daily practice, morbid, graphic and literal-minded in its images, we are nonetheless surprised to find Christ depicted as chopped meat or to read of a crucified body as female.[3] The images seem, if not disgusting, at least distasteful. Boundaries appear to be violated here — boundaries between spiritual and physical, male and female, self and matter. There is something profoundly alien to modern sensibilities about the role of body in medieval piety.

It is not my purpose in this essay to explore our modern discomfort with such boundary crossing, but rather to provide a context for understanding the ease with which medieval people mixed categories. Nonetheless, we do well to begin by recognizing the essential strangeness of medieval religious experience. The recent outpouring of work on the history of the body, especially the female body, has largely equated body with sexuality and understood discipline or control of body as the rejection of sex or of woman.[4] We must wipe away such assumptions before we come to medieval source material. Medieval images of the body have less to do with sexuality than with fertility and decay.[5] Control, discipline, even torture of the flesh is, in medieval devotion, not so much the rejection of physicality as the elevation of it – a horrible yet delicious elevation – into a means of access to the divine.[6]

In the discussion that follows, I wish first to illustrate the new religious significance body acquired in the period from 1200 to 1500, and second to argue that female spirituality in the same period was especially somatic – so much so that the emergence of certain bizarre miracles characteristic of women may actually mark a turning point in the history of the body in the West. Then I wish to explain briefly the ecclesiastical and social setting of women's somatic and visionary piety, before turning to an exploration of its context in two sets of medieval assumptions – assumptions about male/female and assumptions about soul/body. The final two sections of the essay discuss these assumptions at length in order to show that the very dualisms modern commentators have emphasized so much were far from absolute in the late Middle Ages. Not only did theology, natural philosophy and folk tradition mingle male and female in their understanding of human character and human physiology; theological and psychological discussion also sometimes mingled body and soul. The spirituality of medieval women owed its intense bodily quality in part to the association of the female with the fleshly made by philosophers and theologians alike. But its somatic quality also derived from the fact that by the thirteenth century the prevalent concept of person was of a psychosomatic unity, the orthodox position in eschatology required resurrection of body as well as soul at the end of time, and the philosophical, medical and folk understandings of body saw men and women as variations on a single physiological structure. Compared to other periods of Christian history and other world religions, medieval spirituality – especially female spirituality – was peculiarly bodily; this was so not only because medieval assumptions associated female with flesh, but also because theology and natural philosophy saw persons as in some real sense body as well as soul.[7]

The Body in Late Medieval Piety

One aspect of the medieval enthusiasm for body as means of religious access remains prominent in modern Catholic Europe. The cult of relics is well known. From the early Middle Ages down into modern times, pieces of dead holy people have been revered as the loci of the sacred. Medieval relics were jealously guarded, feared, fought for and sometimes even stolen from fellow Christians.[8] According to at least some learned and some popular opinion, relics were far more than mere aids to pious memory; they were the saints themselves, living already with God in the incorrupt and glorified bodies more ordinary mortals would attain only at the end of time.[9]

The cult of relics was only one of the ways in which late medieval piety emphasized body as the locus of the sacred. The graphic physical processes of living people were revered as well. Holy people spat or blew into the mouths of others to effect cures or convey grace.[10] The ill clamored for the bath water of would-be saints to drink or bathe in, and preferred it if these would-be saints themselves washed seldom and therefore left skin and lice floating in the water.[11] Following Francis of Assisi, who kissed lepers, several Italian saints ate pus or lice from poor or sick bodies, thus incorporating into themselves the illness and misfortune of others.[12] Holy virgins in the Low Countries lactated miraculously and cured their adherents with the breast milk they exuded.[13]

Medieval people, moreover, manipulated their own bodies for religious goals. Both male and female saints regularly engaged in what modern people call self-torture — jumping into ovens or icy ponds, driving knives, nails or nettles into their flesh, whipping or hanging themselves in elaborate pantomimes of Christ's Crucifixion.[14] Understood sometimes as chastening of sexual urges or as punishment for sin, such acts were more frequently described as union with the body of Jesus. The fourteenth-century Dominican Henry Suso, for example, said of ascetic practices:

> If suffering brought with it no other gain than that by our griefs and pains we grow in likeness to Christ, our prototype, it would still be a priceless benefit.... Even if God should choose to give the same eternal reward to those who suffer and to those who do not, we should nevertheless prefer afflictions as our earthly portion in order to resemble our leader.[15]

The ecstatic, even erotic, overtones of such union are often quite clear. Starving her body into submission, the Italian tertiary Angela of Foligno spoke of encounter with Jesus as "love and inestimable satiety, which, although it satiated, generated at the same time insatiable hunger, so that all her members were unstrung...."[16]

Pious folk in the later Middle Ages also gave extraordinary religious significance to the body of God. Not only did they believe that at the moment of consecration the bread on the altar became Christ; they also experienced miracles in which the bread turned into bloody flesh on the paten or in the mouth of the recipient.[17] Increasingly, therefore, eucharistic reception became symbolic cannibalism: devotees consumed and thus incorporated (as they are understood to do in other cannibal cultures, such as the Iroquois or Aztec) the power of the tortured god.[18] Moreover, pious practice came to revere the consecrated wafer as a physical remnant (or relic) of Christ — the only such relic that could exist on earth, Christ's body having been assumed into heaven. As the cult of the eucharistic host developed in the late twelfth century, consecrated wafers were reserved in reliquaries and honored with the sort of candles and lamps that burned before the relics of the saints.[19] Such an understanding of the host as relic is clearly illustrated by the story of Bishop Hugh of Lincoln, who chewed off a bit from the bone of Mary Magdalen preserved at Fécamp and defended himself to her outraged supporters by claiming that if he could touch Christ's body in the mass he could certainly chew the Magdalen's arm.[20]

Specific members of Christ's body were revered by the devout in ways that astonish and sometimes offend us. As Leo Steinberg has demonstrated, artists in the fifteenth century often called attention to the penis of the infant or the adult Christ.[21] And the cult of the holy foreskin was popular in the later Middle Ages. Although the hagiographer Raymond of Capua and the artists of early modern Europe depict Catherine of Siena as marrying Christ with a ring of gold and precious stones, Catherine herself says she married him with his circumcised flesh.[22] Birgitta of Sweden received a revelation from God saying where Christ's foreskin was preserved on earth; and the Viennese Beguine Agnes Blannbekin received the foreskin in her mouth in a vision and found it to taste as sweet as honey.[23]

The Female Body and Female Experience

Behavior in which bodiliness provides access to the sacred seems to have increased dramatically in frequency in the twelfth century and to have been more characteristic of women than of men. Although both men and women manipulated their bodies from the outside, so to speak, by flagellation and other forms of self-inflicted suffering, cases of psychosomatic manipulation (or manipulation from within) are almost exclusively female. I refer here to a number of phenomena that are sometimes called "paramystical" by modern scholars of religion and "hysterical" or "conversion phenomena" by modern psychologists.

Trances, levitations, catatonic seizures or other forms of bodily rigidity, miraculous elongation or enlargement of parts of the body, swellings of sweet mucus in the throat (sometimes known as the "globus hystericus") and ecstatic nosebleeds are seldom if at all reported of male saints but are quite common in the *vitae* of thirteenth- and fourteenth-century women. The inability to eat anything except the eucharistic host (which Rudolf Bell calls "holy anorexia") is reported only of women for most of the Middle Ages.[24] Although a few stories of fasting girls are told from Carolingian Europe, reports that see such inedia as a manifestation of sanctity begin to proliferate about 1200. These reports often include claims to other forms of miraculous bodily closure as well: women who do not eat are reputed neither to excrete nor to menstruate.

Despite the fame of Francis of Assisi's stigmata, he and the modern figure Padre Pio are the only males in history who have claimed all five visible wounds. There are, however, dozens of such claims for late medieval women. Francis (d.1226) may indeed have been the first case (although even this is uncertain); but stigmata rapidly became a female miracle, and only for women did the stigmatic wounds bleed periodically.[25] Miraculous lactation was, of course, female behavior, and it appears to have originated in the Low Countries in the early thirteenth century. Other kinds of holy exuding — particularly the exuding of sweet-smelling oil after death — seem more characteristic of women as well.[26] Bodily swelling understood as "mystical pregnancy" was usually (although not always) a female claim.[27] The most bizarre cases of pictures etched on hearts and discovered during preparation for burial are told of women.[28] Indeed, if we look outside the religious sphere, we find that writings by rather matter-of-fact fourteenth-century surgeons express an odd combination of reverence and almost prurient curiosity about what is contained inside women — that is, their "secrets."[29]

Although a number of blood prodigies are attributed to the bodies of male saints, female bodies provide a disproportionate percentage of the wonder-working relics in late medieval Europe.[30] As Claude Carozzi has argued, we can sometimes, in hagiographical accounts, see a woman turning into a relic even before her own death.[31] Moreover, incorruptibility either of the whole cadaver or of a part seems a virtual requirement for female sanctity by the early modern period. According to Thurston, incorruptibility (that is, remaining lifelike and supple for long years after death) has been claimed for all six of the female saints added to the universal Roman calendar between 1400 and 1900 (although it is mentioned for fewer than half of the male saints).[32] In short, women's bodies were more apt than men's to display unusual changes, closures, openings or exudings; such changes were either more common or much more frequently reported after 1200; religious significance was attached to such changes when they seemed to parallel either events in Christ's life or in the mass.

Another kind of bodily experience — illness or recurrent pain — was also more apt to be given religious significance in women's lives than in men's. In their statistical study of saints, Weinstein and Bell have pointed out that, although women were only seventeen and one-half percent of those canonized or revered as saints between 1000 and 1700, they were over fifty percent of those in whose lives patient suffering of illness was the major element of sanctity.[33] Ernst Benz, Richard Kieckhefer and Elizabeth Petroff have also pointed out the prominence of illness — as theme and as fact — in women's spirituality.[34] Some visionary women (such as Julian of Norwich) prayed for disease as a gift from God; some (such as Lidwina of Schiedam) at first desired to be cured. But, whatever the cause of disease or the saint's initial reaction to it, many medieval women — for example, Serafina of San Gimignano, Villana de' Botti, Margaret of Ypres, Dorothy of Montau, Gertrude of Helfta and Alpais of Cudot — made physical and mental anguish an opportunity for their own salvation and that of others.[35] Hagiographers fairly frequently described their female subjects as impelled to bodily frenzy by God's presence; Beatrice of Nazareth wondered whether it would be desirable to drive herself insane out of love for God.[36] Dauphine of Puimichel commented that if people knew how useful diseases were to the spirit, they would purchase them in the marketplace.[37] The leper Alice of Schaerbeke explained that illness could be offered for the redemption of one's neighbor:

> Dear sister, do not grieve [for me]; and do not think that I suffer for or expiate my own
> sins; I suffer rather for those who are already dead and in the place of penitence [i.e.,
> purgatory] and for the sins of the world....[38]

By 1500 there are extant women's *vitae*, such as Catherine of Genoa's, in which much of the account is devoted to physiological changes in the saint's dying body.

It is true that medieval writers, like modern ones, frequently saw disease as a condition to be avoided.[39] Indeed, cures of illness were the most common miracles performed by saints. But it is also true that sickness and suffering were sometimes seen by medieval people as conditions "to be endured" rather than "cured." Alpais of Cudot, for example, clearly indicated such an attitude when she saw the devil appear in a vision as a doctor. To Alpais, as to Elsbeth Achler and Catherine of Siena, the offer of cure was a temptation.[40] Indeed, a nun of the monastery of Töss composed a poem in which Christ said to her: "The sicker you are, the dearer you are to me."[41]

There is reason to believe that conditions that both we and medieval people would see as "illnesses" were given different meanings depending on whether they occurred in male or female bodies. Illness was more likely to be described as something "to be endured" when it happened to women. For example, in a ninth-century account of the posthumous miracles of Walburga, a man and a woman suffering from what we would term an "eating disorder" both present themselves before the saint's relics. The man is cured of his loathing for food when he is offered a chalice by three nuns; the woman, however, turns from voracious hunger to inability to eat – a condition of which she is not "cured." Rather, she is miraculously sustained for three years without eating.[42]

Statistics tell the same story. Sigal, in his recent study of miracles in eleventh- and twelfth-century France, finds that females account for only between eighteen and forty-two percent of recipients of miraculous cures. (The percentage varies with the disease cured.) Females are an even smaller percentage of the miraculous cures of children and adolescents, and of the cures that take place at shrines rather than at a distance. These facts cannot be accounted for by sex ratios in the population or by disproportionate percentages of men among those falling ill. Rather, they clearly indicate, as Sigal argues, that the society found it more valuable to cure one sex than the other. They also suggest that endurance of a condition of illness without supernatural amelioration was considered more appropriate to women, whether the endurance was a prelude to sanctity or not.[43]

The tendency of women to somatize religious experience and to give positive significance to bodily occurrences is related to what is generally recognized (for example, by scholars such as Dinzelbacher and Dronke) to be a more experiential quality in their mystical writing.[44] Male writers too, of course, use extremely physical and physiological language to speak of encounter with God. Indeed, the locus classicus for descriptions of eating God or being eaten by Him is Bernard of Clairvaux's sermons on the *Song of Songs*, later graphically echoed in John Tauler's sermons for Corpus Christi.[45] But men's writing often lacks the immediacy of women's; the male voice is impersonal. It is striking to note that, however fulsome or startling their imagery, men write of "*the* mystical experience," giving a general description which may be used as a theory or yardstick, whereas women write of "*my* mystical experience," speaking directly of something that may have occurred to them alone.[46] This is true even when, as in the case of Hildegard of Bingen or Julian of Norwich, a highly sophisticated theology is elaborated over many years as a gloss on visionary experiences.

Women regularly speak of tasting God, of kissing Him deeply, of going into His heart or entrails, of being covered by His blood. Their descriptions of themselves or of other women often, from a modern point of view, hopelessly blur the line between spiritual or psychological, on the one hand, and bodily or even sexual, on the other. Lidwina of Schiedam and Gertrude of Delft, for example, felt such maternal desire for the Christ child that milk flowed from their breasts; Beatrice of Nazareth experienced a joy in Christ that contorted her face and racked her with hysterical laughter; Lukardis of Oberweimar and Margaret of Faenza kissed their spiritual sisters with open mouths and grace flowed from one to the other with an ardor that left both women shaken. The thirteenth-century poet and mystic Hadewijch spoke of Christ penetrating her until she lost herself in the ecstasy of love. She wrote:

> After that he came himself to me, took me entirely in his arms and pressed me to him; and all my members felt his in full felicity, in accordance with the desire of my heart and my humanity. So I was outwardly satisfied and fully transported. Also then, for a short while, I had the strength to bear this; but soon, after a short time, I lost that manly beauty outwardly in the sight of his form. I saw him completely come to naught and so fade and all at once dissolve that I could no longer distinguish him within me. Then it was to me as if we were one without difference.[47]

Watching sisters sometimes saw the bodies of mystical women elongate or levitate or swoon in ecstatic trances; but the visionary women themselves often did not bother to make clear where the events happened – whether in body, heart or soul, whether in the eye of the mind or before the eyes of the body. Indeed, in the books of women's *Revelations*, which are really a new literary genre by the late fourteenth or early fifteenth century, the point is not to provide proof that one woman or a group of women received charismatic gifts so much as to communicate and share a piety in which spiritual-somatic experiences lie at the center.[48]

It would be wrong to draw an absolute contrast between male and female piety. Medieval men also saw visions, and their hagiographers described their affective experiences of God.[49] But those men (such as Bernard of Clairvaux, Francis of Assisi, Suso, Ruysbroeck or Richard Rolle) whose religiosity was most experiential and visionary often understood themselves in feminine images and learned their pious practices from women.[50] Moreover, whether they denigrated, admired or used the experiences of mystical women, men such as Albert the Great, Eckhart and Gerson spoke explicitly of somatic and visionary experiences as peculiarly female. David of Augsburg ridiculed them as "erotic ticklings." John Tauler wrote more sympathetically, but even he made it clear that he was a bit suspicious of such piety.[51]

Thus, if we speak phenomenologically, it seems clear that when "the other" breaks through into the lives of individuals, it often throws men into profound stillness. Male mystics write repeatedly of being at a core or ground or inner point (as Eckhart or Walter Hilton put it).[52] Women, on the other hand, are "switched on" by "the other," heightened into an affectivity or sensuality that goes beyond both the senses and our words for describing them. Even those female mystics, such as Hadewijch and Margaret Porete, who distrust or reject affectivity, speak with intimate knowledge of that which they wish to transmute or transcend.[53]

Women's sense that Christ is body, received and perceived by body, is vividly reflected in a vision given to the little-known French nun, Marguerite of Oingt (d. 1310). Marguerite saw herself as a withered tree which suddenly flowered when inundated by a great river of water (representing Christ). Marguerite then saw, written on the flowering branches of her self, the names of the five senses: sight, hearing, taste, smell and touch. It is hard to imagine a more pointed way of indicating that the effect of experiencing Christ is to "turn on," so to speak, the bodily senses of the receiving mystic.[54]

The Italian mystic Angela of Foligno (d. 1309), in words undoubtedly reworked by a scholastically educated redactor, expresses the same awareness when she says:

[The soul in this present life knows] the lesser in the greater and the greater in the lesser, for it discovers uncreated God and "humanated" God, that is divinity and humanity, in Christ, united and conjoined in one person.... And sometimes...the soul receives greater delight in the lesser.... For the soul is more conformed and adapted to the lesser which it sees in Christ the incarnate God, than it is to that which it sees in Christ the uncreated God; because the soul is a creature who is the life of the flesh and of all the members of its body. Thus it discovers both God "humanated" and God uncreated, Christ the creator and Christ the creature, and in that Christ it discovers soul with flesh and blood and with all the members of his most sacred body. And this is why, when the human intellect discovers, sees, and knows in this mystery Christ the man and Christ-God..., this intellect feels delight and expands in him, because it sees God "humanated" and God uncreated conformed and made like itself — because, that is, the human soul sees the soul of Christ, his eyes, his flesh, and his body. But while it looks..., it should not forget also to turn to the higher..., the divine....[55]

To Angela, the encounter with the body of Christ into which grace lifts her is beyond ordinary affectivity, for it is simultaneously a transport of pain and of delight. Even filtered through the screen provided by her confessor-redactor, the exuberance of Angela's enthusiasm contrasts sharply with the moderation and hesitation of a Tauler or an Eckhart. She says:

Once, when I was at Vespers and was contemplating the Crucifix...suddenly my soul was lifted into love, and all the members of my body felt a very great joy. And I saw and felt that Christ, within me, embraced my soul with that arm by which he was crucified...and I felt such great security that I could not doubt it was God.... So I rejoice when I see that hand which he holds out with the signs of the nails, saying to me: "Behold what I bore for you."

Now I can feel no sadness at the Passion...for all my joy is in that suffering God-Man. And it seems to my soul that it enters within that wound in the side of Christ and walks there with delight....[56]

In such piety, body is not so much a hindrance to the soul's ascent as the opportunity for it. Body is the instrument upon which the mystic rings changes of pain and of delight. It is from body — whether whipped into frenzy by the ascetic herself or gratified with an ecstasy given by God – that sweet melodies and aromas rise to the very throne of heaven.[57]

Thus, as many recent scholars have argued, the spiritualities of male and female mystics were different, and this difference has something to do with body.[58] Women were more apt to somatize religious experience and to write in intense bodily metaphors; women mystics were more likely than men to receive graphically physical visions of God; both men and women were inclined to attribute to women and encourage in them intense asceticisms and ecstasies. Moreover, the most bizarre bodily occurrences associated with women (e.g., stigmata, incorruptibility of the cadaver in death, mystical lactations and pregnancies, catatonic trances, ecstatic nosebleeds, miraculous inedia, eating and drinking pus, visions of bleeding hosts) either first appear in the twelfth and thirteenth centuries or increase significantly in frequency at that time. These facts suggest– hard as it is for sober modern historians to countenance such arguments – that the body itself may actually have a history. The body, and in particular the female body, seems to have begun to behave in new ways at a particular moment in the European past.[59] The question is: Why is this so?

The Ecclesiastical and Social Context

Many explanations can be proposed for the bodily quality of female spirituality in the later Middle Ages. I have written elsewhere about the importance of charismatic authorization for women at a time when clerical control increased in the Church, and it is customary now for scholars to emphasize women's mysticism as a form of female empowerment.[60] Since the Gregorian Reform of the late eleventh century, priest and layperson had been sharply separated in status and form of life; clerical dignity had become ever more elevated and awesome. Thus, one might argue that women *had* to stress the experience of Christ and manifest it outwardly in their flesh, because they did not have clerical office as an authorization for speaking. This argument must also recognize that the clergy themselves encouraged such female behavior both because female asceticism, eucharistic devotion and mystical trances brought women more closely under the supervision of spiritual directors, and because women's visions functioned for males too as means of learning the will of God. Moreover, theologians and prelates found women's experiential piety useful in the thirteenth-century fight against heresy. The increased emphasis on bodily miracles and indeed the appearance of new miracles of bodily transformation came at exactly the time of the campaign against Cathar dualism. Women whose bodies became one with the crucified man on the cross in stigmata, and visions in which the consecrated wafer suddenly turned into bleeding meat, were powerful evidence against the Cathar assertion that matter and flesh could not be the creations of a good God. Some of the earliest supporters of this bodily aspect of women's piety, James of Vitry and Thomas of Cantimpré, held it up explicitly as a reproach to the dualists.[61]

In addition, we must not forget the educational context. At least since the work of Grundmann in the 1930s, we have been aware of how much women's writing was shaped both by their lack of formal theological training and by the availability of the new vernacular languages with their characteristic literary genres.[62] In other words, part of the reason for the more open, experiential style of women's writings is the fact that women usually wrote not in the formal scholastic Latin taught in universities but in the vernaculars — that is, in the languages they grew up speaking. The major literary genres available in these languages were various kinds of love poetry and romantic stories: the vocabulary provided by such genres was therefore a vocabulary of feelings. A comparison of two women from much the same milieu, Mechtild of Hackeborn and Mechtild of Magdeburg, shows clearly that the one who wrote in Latin wrote more impersonally and to a much greater extent under the influence of the liturgy, whereas the vernacular poet wrote more experientially, with a greater sense both of personal vulnerability and of an immediate and special relationship to God.[63] Furthermore, women's works, especially their accounts of visions, were often dictated (that is, spoken) rather than penned — a fact that is clearly one of the explanations for women's more discursive, conversational, aggregative, tentative, empathetic and self-reflective style. As Elizabeth Petroff has recently pointed out, the prose of a female writer such as Julian of Norwich, which tends to circle around its point, evoking a state of being, displays exactly those traits Walter Ong has seen as characteristic of oral thought and expression.[64]

Social context also sheds light on the nature of women's piety. Secular society expected women to be intimately involved in caring for the bodies of others (especially the young, the sick and the dying). To some extent, women simply took these roles over into their most profound religious experiences. Not only did female mystics kiss, bathe and suckle babies in visions and grieve with Mary as she received

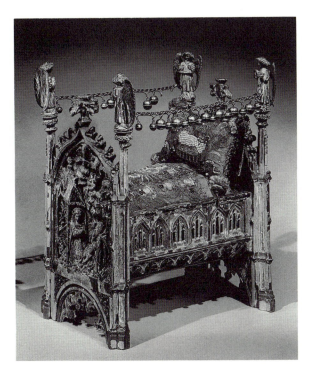

Figure 1: Liturgical cradle from the Grand Beguinage in Louvain, 15th century (New York, Metropolitan Museum of Art, New York).

her son's dead body for burial; they actually acted out maternal and nuptial roles in the liturgy, decorating lifesize statues of the Christ child for the Christmas crèche or dressing in bridal garb when going to receive their bridegroom in the Eucharist. Anyone who has stood before the lovely Beguine cradle on display in the Metropolitan Museum in New York and realized that it is a liturgical object must have thought, at least for a moment: "Why these nuns and Beguines were just little girls, playing with dolls!" (figure 1).[65]

It is possible that there is, in addition, a biological element in women's predisposition to certain kinds of bodily experiences. The fact that, in many cultures, women seem more given to spirit possession and more apt to somatize their inner emotional or spiritual states suggests a physiological explanation. In cultures as different as medieval Europe, medieval China and modern America, self-mutilation and self-starvation seem to be more characteristic of women than of men.[66] But we should be cautious about espousing biological explanations too hastily. Biology and culture are almost impossible to distinguish in these matters, because men and

173

women differ from each other consistently across societies in their social and psychological as well as their physiological experiences. The various cultures in which women are more inclined than men to fast, to mutilate themselves, to experience the gift of tongues and to somatize spiritual states are all societies that associate the female with self-sacrifice and service.

Intellectual Traditions: Dualism and Misogyny

Basic assumptions about body and about gender provide another context against which we must place the new miracles of bodily transformation and the graphic physiological visions of the later Middle Ages. There were intellectual traditions that conditioned women *and men* to certain expectations of women's bodies. Medieval thinkers associated *body* with *woman*; they therefore expected women's expressiveness to be more physical and physiological than men's. They also associated body with God, through the doctrine of the Incarnation, and eschewed sharp soul/body dichotomies more than did either patristic theologians or those of the early modern period. They could, therefore, give to the bodily experiences of members of both sexes a deeply spiritual significance.

It may appear odd to emphasize the bodiliness of God, or the bodiliness of women as a means of approaching God, in a discussion of the Middle Ages. Standard accounts of the period are much more inclined to emphasize its misogyny and dualism. And there is no denying these aspects of medieval attitudes. The practical dualism of medieval Christianity is well known. As Jacques Le Goff has pointed out, twelfth- and thirteenth-century literature presented the body not merely as dust but as rottenness, a garment masking the food of worms.[67] Ascetic theologians often wrote of spirit and flesh warring with each other. Both in Latin and in the emerging vernaculars, the genre of the debate between body and soul became popular. In one Latin version, so well-known it survives in at least 132 manuscripts, Soul describes herself as a noble creature blackened by Flesh, which must be overcome by hunger, thirst and beatings.[68] Indeed, chastity for men and virginity for women were almost preconditions for sanctity. Even in the later Middle Ages, when some married saints were added to the calendar, rejection of actual conjugal sex was taken as a major sign of the saint's growth toward holiness.[69]

It is also clear that theological, scientific and folk traditions associated women with body, lust, weakness and irrationality, men with spirit or reason or strength.[70] Patristic exegetes, for example, argued that woman (or Eve) represents the appetites, man (or Adam) represents soul or intellect.[71] As Weinstein and Bell have pointed out, hagiographers were inclined to see female sin as bodily or sexual, as arising from within the woman's body, whereas male sinners were depicted as tempted from without — often indeed as tempted by the proffered bodiliness of women.[72] In James of Voragine's *Golden Legend*, a collection of saints' lives retold for use by thirteenth-century preachers in edifying sermons, the major achievement of holy women is dying in defense of their virginity. Defense of chastity is an extremely infrequent theme in the male lives James tells. Resurrection from the dead is, however, a fairly common motif in accounts of holy men, and these men are raised in order to complete tasks or make reparation for deeds done on earth. This pattern suggests that women's lives can be complete only when death has assured perpetual virginity. In contrast, male lives are complete when virtue is won, evil defeated or restitution made. Whereas an early demise is advisable for women, assuring that their weak bodies can no longer be tempted or violated, death itself may be temporarily suspended to give men time to assert themselves and finish the job of winning salvation.[73]

As these examples demonstrate, medieval writers did associate body and flesh with woman, and they did sometimes draw from this dualist and misogynist conclusions. But what I would like to suggest here is that the impact of medieval conceptions of woman and of body was more complex than scholars have realized, because the concepts themselves were more complex. Medieval men and women did not take the equation of woman with body merely as the basis for misogyny. They also extrapolated from it to an association of woman with the body or the humanity of Christ. Indeed, they often went so far as to treat Christ's flesh as female, at least in certain of its salvific functions, especially its bleeding and nurturing. This fact helps us to understand why it was women more than men who imitated Christ bodily, especially in stigmata.

Moreover, if we look closely at the various traditions that associated woman with body or flesh, we find that neither medieval gender contrasts nor medieval notions of soul and body were as dichotomous as we have been led to think by projecting modern contrasts back onto them.[74] Thus, I would like to argue that we must consider not just the dichotomy but also the mixing or fusing of the genders implicit in medieval assumptions. Only in this way will we understand how mystical women could see themselves and be seen by men as especially apt to imitate and fuse with the male body of Christ. We must also consider the ways in which treatments of body and soul, particularly in the period after 1200, tended to mix rather than separate the two components of the person. Such background is necessary in order to comprehend how medieval people of both sexes could see the holy manifest in that same flesh which lured humans into lust and greed during their lives and, after death, putrefied in the grave.

Medieval traditions concerning male/female and body/soul are complex enough that I need to take them up separately and in some detail.

Woman Is to Man as Body Is to Soul

As all medievalists are by now aware, the body of Christ was sometimes depicted as female in medieval devotional texts – partly, of course, because *ecclesia*, Christ's body, was a female personification, partly because the tender, nurturing aspect of God's care for souls was regularly described as motherly. Both male and female mystics called Jesus "mother" in his eucharistic feeding of Christians with liquid exuded from his breast and in his bleeding on the Cross which gave birth to our hope of eternal life.[75] In the thirteenth century Margaret of Oingt described Jesus' pain on the Cross as birth pangs; Guerric of Igny in the twelfth century, and Catherine of Siena and the anonymous monk of Farne in the fourteenth, wrote of Christ nursing the soul at his breast; the fourteenth-century English mystic Julian of Norwich spoke of creation as a maternal act because God, in taking on our humanity in the Incarnation, gives himself to us as a mother gives herself to the fetus she bears.[76]

Iconography illustrates the same theme. In the moralized Bibles of the thirteenth and fourteenth centuries, artists depicted the Church being born from Christ's side, as Eve is born of Adam[77] (figure 2). Miniatures and panel paintings showed Christ exuding wine or blood into chalices or even into hungry mouths and drew visual parallels between his wound and Mary's breast offered to suckle sinners[78] (figures 3, 4, 5). We know that such traditions lie behind sixteenth-century depictions of Christ feeding Catherine of Siena from his side, because the various versions of Catherine's *vita* speak of Christ nursing her at his breast.[79] The motif of "Jesus as mother" may

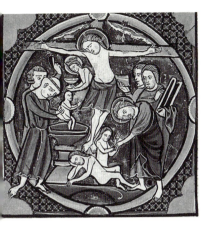

Figure 2: Eve made from the rib of Adam and the Church from the hip of Christ (Paris, Bibliothèque nationale).

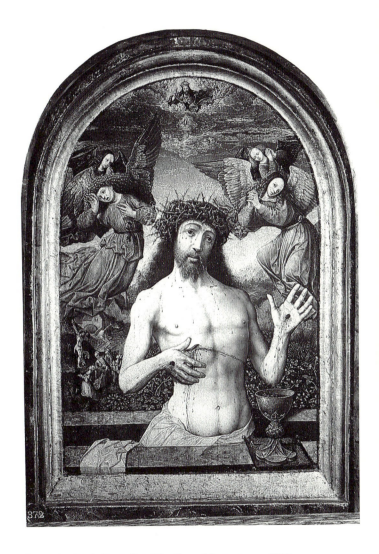

Figure 3: Jacob Cornelisz, The Man of Sorrows, ca. 1510 (Antwerp, Mayer van den Bergh Museum).

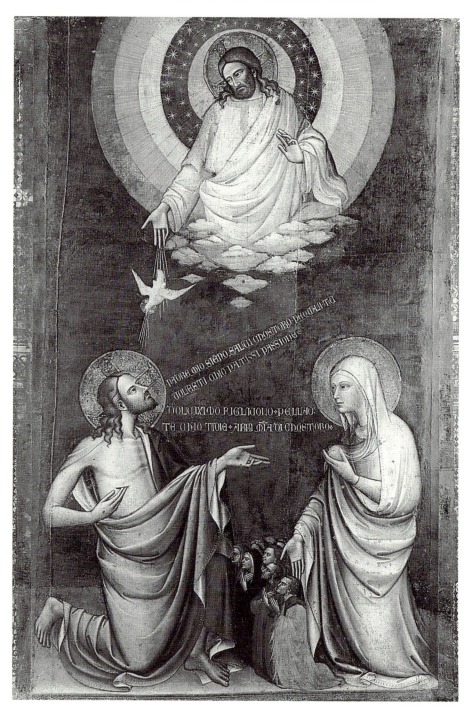

Figure 4: Unknown, The Intercession of Christ and the Virgin, ca. 1402
(New York, Metropolitan Museum of Art, Cloisters Collection).

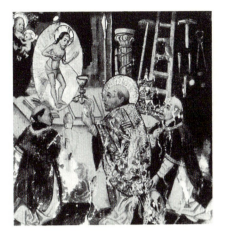

Figure 5: Mass of Saint Gregory,
Spanish altarpiece, end of the 15th century
(Spain, Parish Church of Villoldo).

also help explain the unusual northern Renaissance paintings by Jan Gossaert that depict the infant Christ with engorged breasts[80] (figure 6).

There were two separate strands on which medieval mystics drew in identifying woman with flesh and Christ's flesh with the female. Although it is easiest to cite these strands from treatises on theology, natural philosophy and medicine, recent work by French historians of medicine and anthropologists makes it abundantly clear that we have to deal here not merely with learned ideas but with assumptions widespread in the culture.[81] I have written about these elsewhere, but it seems advisable to repeat some of the material in order to make my argument clear.[82]

The first set of roots is theological. Medieval interpreters of the Bible regularly taught that "spirit is to flesh as male is to female" — that is, that the dichotomy male/female can serve as a symbol for the dichotomies strong/weak, rational/irrational, soul/body. This use of pairs of symbols led some medieval writers to see the male as symbol of Christ's divinity, the female as symbol of his humanity. Hildegard of Bingen, for example, argued that in Christ "divinity is to humanity as male is to female." Hildegard's association of women with Christ's humanity underlay her reiterated position that women were appropriately denied the priesthood because they had another way of joining with Christ. As Christ's brides in mystical union, women were the body of Christ, not merely his representatives. The analogy "male is to female as divinity is to humanity" also underlay Elisabeth of Schönau's vision — confusing even to its recipient — in which a female virgin, representing

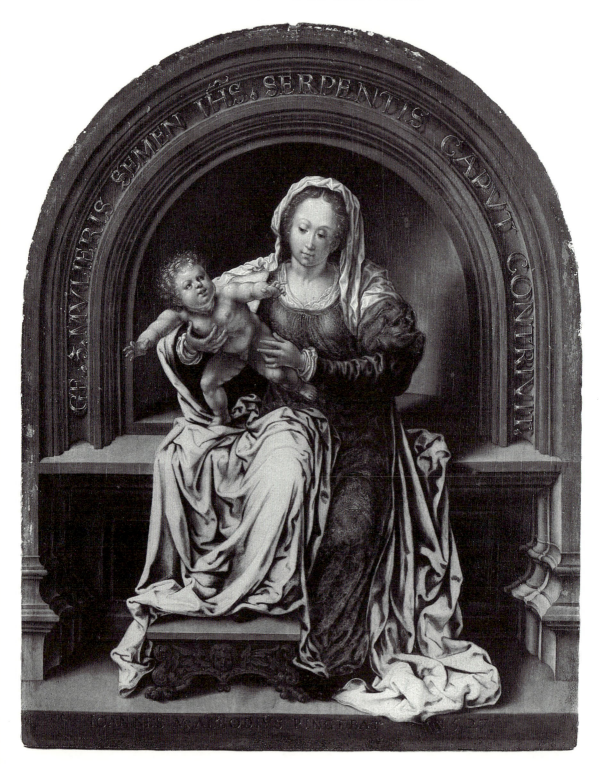

igure 6: Jan Gossaert, Madonna and Child, 1527
Munich, Staatsgemäldesammlungen).

Christ's humanity, appeared sitting on the sun (his divinity). The analogy is reflected in the many medieval texts that say that Christ married human nature as a man marries a woman, and it lies behind miniatures that depict not only *ecclesia* but also *humanitas* as female.

Such an association of Christ's humanity with the female and the fleshly was also supported by the theological doctrine of the Virgin Birth and the emerging notions of the Immaculate Conception and bodily Assumption. Because Christ had no human father, his body came entirely from Mary and was therefore closely associated with female flesh. As Thomas Aquinas put it:

> According to Aristotle, the male semen does not play the role of "matter" in the conception of animals. It is rather prime agent, so to speak, while the female alone supplies the matter. So even if male semen were lacking in Christ's conception it does not follow that the necessary matter was missing.
>
> ...it is not given to the blessed Virgin to be father of Christ but mother.... So it is to be held that in the actual conception of Christ, the blessed Virgin did not actively effect anything in the conceiving, but ministered the matter only. But she actively effected something before the conception by preparing the matter to be apt for conception.

Associating the flesh of Christ with Mary in another way, Bonaventure wrote:

> Indeed she [Mary] is raised above the hierarchy of the perfect [in heaven].... And thus it can be said that she is there corporeally, for she has a special sort of perfection in the celestial city.... The soul of Christ is not from her soul — since soul does not come by transmission [from the parents] — but his body is from her body. Therefore she will not be there [in heaven] in the mode of perfection unless she is there corporeally.[83]

Since some theologians increasingly stressed Mary's humanity as sinless from her conception, they were able to suggest that just as the Logos (the divinity of Christ separate from that of God) preexisted the Incarnation, so the humanity of Christ also preexisted the Incarnation in the sinless humanity of Mary. Such arguments could, of course, be carried to dubious theological lengths. But orthodox prayers and mass commentaries from the period also speak of Mary as the humanity of Christ, especially its bodily component or flesh. Catherine of Siena said that Christ's flesh was Mary's, sealed like hot wax by the Holy Spirit; Hildegard of Bingen wrote that Mary is the *tunica humanitatis* Christ puts on; Francis of Assisi called her Christ's robe or tabernacle. The notion is clearly depicted in eucharistic tabernacles which Mary surmounts as if she *were* the container, in monstrances made in her image (figure 7, a seventeenth-century example), and in the so-called "opening Virgins" — small statues of *Maria lactans* which open to show the Trinity inside (figure 8). As Carol Purtle and Barbara Lane have demonstrated, such a concept is also reflected in those late medieval paintings in which Mary takes on priestly characteristics (figure 9). Such images of Mary as priest have nothing to do with claiming sacerdotal functions for ordinary women. Mary is priest because it is she who offers to ordinary mortals the saving flesh of God, which comes most regularly and predictably in the mass.[84]

Scientific ideas — especially theories of conception or generation — were a second set of roots for the medieval tendency to associate flesh with female, and God's body with woman's body.[85] According to the Aristotelian theory of conception, held by some medieval scientists and theologians, the mother provides the matter of the fetus and the father its form or life or spirit. This theory clearly associates woman with the unformed physical stuff of which the fully human is made. According to the competing theory of conception available at the time — Galen's theory — two seeds were necessary, one from the father and one from the mother. This theory in a sense associates both father and mother with the physiological stuff. But even according to Galen the mother is the oven or vessel in which the fetus cooks, and her body feeds the growing child, providing its stuff as it matures.[86] Moreover, Giles of Rome in the thirteenth century, who rejected the Galenic theory as mediated by Avicenna and turned to Aristotle, argued against Galen that if woman provided both the menstrual matter and seed then she might impregnate herself and the male would have no role at all. Such an argument shows not only the tendency to associate matter with woman, but also a fear that this threatens the importance of the male contribution to life.[87]

Physiological theory associated matter, food and flesh with female in another sense. All medieval biologists thought the mother's blood fed the child in the womb and then, transmuted into breast milk, fed the baby outside the womb as well.[88] For example, a fourteenth-century surgeon wrote that milk is blood "twice cooked."[89] One of the Arab texts most frequently used by Western doctors argued: "Since the infant has just been nourished from menstrual blood [in the womb], it needs nurture whose nature is closest to menstrual blood, and the matter that has this quality is milk, because milk is formed from menstrual blood."[90] Thus, blood was the basic

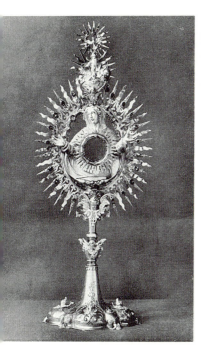

Figure 7: Monstrance from the Cloister
of Weyarn, Bavaria, 1652.

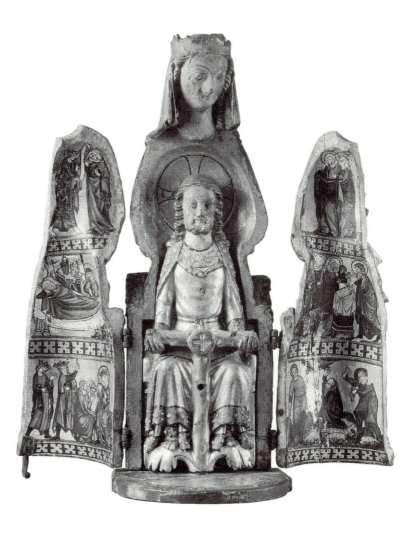

Figure 8: Shrine (Vierge Ouvrante): Virgin and Child, Middle Rhine
(New York, Metropolitan Museum of Art).

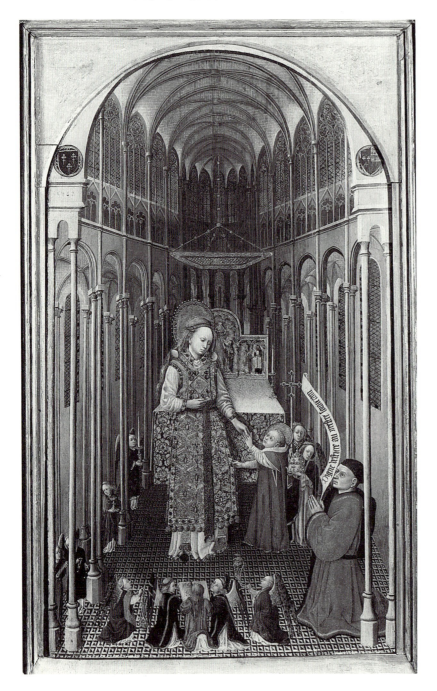

Figure 9: The Priesthood of the Virgin, French panel painting
commissioned for the Cathedral of Amiens, ca. 1437 (Paris, Louvre).

body fluid, and female blood was the fundamental support of human life. Medical theory also held that the shedding of blood purged or cleansed those who shed it.[91] Indeed, bleeding was held to be necessary for the washing away of superfluity, so much so that physiologists sometimes spoke of males as menstruating (presumably they meant hemorrhoidal bleeding) and recommended bleeding with leeches if they did not do so. Such medical conceptions of blood could lead to the association of Christ's bleeding on the Cross — which purges our sin in the Atonement and feeds our souls in the Eucharist — with female bleeding and feeding.

The sets of medieval assumptions just described associated female and flesh with the body of God. Not only was Christ enfleshed with flesh from a woman; his own flesh did womanly things: it bled, it bled food and it gave birth to new life. If certain key moments in the life of Christ were described by devotional writers as "female," it is no wonder that women's physiological processes were given religious significance. Such processes were especially open to religious interpretation when they were not just ordinary but also extraordinary — that is, when they were continuations of normal physiology yet miracles as well (as in the cases of virgin lactation or periodic stigmatic bleeding). Not surprisingly, women strove to experience such bodily moments, which recapitulated events in the life of Christ. And, not surprisingly, men (for whom such experiences were not in any sense "ordinary") both revered these women and suspected them of fraud or collusion with the devil.[92]

The analysis I have just given seems, however, to beg an important question. For the human Christ was, after all, male. And, as we all know from the many medieval discussions of women's incapacity for the priesthood, the inferior female body was in certain contexts and by certain theologians prohibited from representing God.[93] How then did it happen that medieval women came more frequently than medieval men to literal, bodily *imitatio Christi*, both in stigmata and in other forms of miraculous sufferings and exudings?

The answer lies in part in the fact that — for all their application of male/female contrasts to organize life symbolically — medieval thinkers used gender imagery fluidly, not literally. Medieval theologians and natural philosophers often mixed and fused the genders, treating not just the body of Christ but all bodies as both male and female.

From the patristic period on, those who saw the female as representing flesh, while the male symbolized spirit, wrote of real people as both. To say this is not to deny that men were seen as superior in rationality and strength. Clearly they were. But existing, particular human beings were understood as having both feminine and masculine characteristics.[94] Moreover, because of the emphasis on reversal that lay at the heart of the Christian tradition, devotional writers sometimes used the description "woman" or "weak woman" in order to attribute an inferiority that would — exactly because it was inferior — be made superior by God.[95] For example, male mystics such as Bernard of Clairvaux, Eckhart and John Gerson spoke of devout men as fecund mothers or weak women. The women writers about whom Peter Dronke has written so sensitively sometimes used "weak woman" as an ironic self-description in order to underline their special standing before God.[96]

This mixing of the genders is even more apparent in the scientific tradition, where in one sense it is not even clear that there were two sexes. As Thomas Laqueur and Marie-Christine Pouchelle have recently pointed out, medieval natural philosophers argued that men and women are really a superior and inferior version of the same physiology. Woman's reproductive system was just man's turned inside out. For example, the fourteenth-century surgeons Henri de Mondeville and Guy de Chauliac said: "The apparatus of generation in women is like the apparatus of generation in men, except that it is reversed"; "the womb is like a penis reversed or put inside." In the sixteenth century, Paré even suggested that women could turn into men if, owing to an accident, their internal organs were suddenly pushed outward.[97]

Medieval scientific ideas, especially in their Aristotelian version, made the male body paradigmatic. It was the form or pattern or definition of what we are as humans; what was particularly womanly was the unformedness, the "stuffness" or physicality of our humanness. Such a notion identified woman with breaches in boundaries, with lack of shape or definition, with openings and exudings and spillings forth.[98] But this conception also made men and women versions of the same thing. Men and women had the same sex organs; men's were just better arranged. These assumptions made the boundary between the sexes extremely permeable.

Permeability or interchangeability of the sexes is seen in a number of aspects of physiological theory. For example, all human exudings — menstruation, sweating, lactation, emission of semen, etc. — were seen as bleedings; and all bleedings — lactation, menstruation, nosebleeds, hemorrhoidal bleeding, etc. — were taken to be analogous. Thus, it was not far-fetched for a medical writer to refer to a man menstruating or lactating, or to a woman emitting seed.[99]

Because biological sex seemed so labile, the question of how to account for the observed sharpness of sexual difference — that is, for the fact that persons are distinctly male or female in gross anatomy — puzzled medieval writers. In discussions of generation, for example, natural philosophers held that the sex of the fetus resulted either from a combination of parts from both parents, or from the stronger or weaker impact of male seed on the menstruum, or from location of the fetus on the right or left side of the womb. Such explanations seem to put male and female along a continuum and leave it totally unclear why there are not at least as many hermaphrodites (midpoints on the spectrum) as there are males or females (endpoints on the spectrum).[100] Perhaps because of this uncertainty, the nature and cause of hermaphroditism, as of other embryological anomalies, was much discussed.[101]

Moreover, tales of pregnant men were fairly common in folklore and miracle stories from the twelfth to fifteenth centuries. These tales hardly suggest that doctors or ordinary folk actually thought males could become pregnant. Their purpose was either to ridicule the clergy (the pregnant male was often a cleric) or to warn against the dangers of unacceptable positions in sexual intercourse. Nonetheless, the popularity of the satiric notion that woman-on-top sex might drive the seed down into the man, impregnating him, suggests that those telling the tale have no good explanation why such things in fact do not happen.[102]

Medieval assumptions about maleness and femaleness associated body — particularly in its fleshly, oozing, unformed physicality — with woman. But such assumptions saw the physiological structure of the body as paradigmatically male. Thus, medieval thinkers put actual men and women on a continuum and saw their bodies as functioning in essentially the same ways. Such ideas made it easy for writers and artists to fuse or interchange the genders and, therefore, to use both genders symbolically to talk about self and God. As mystics and theologians in the thirteenth, fourteenth and fifteenth centuries increasingly emphasized the human body of Christ, that body was seen both as the paradigmatic male body of Aristotelian physiological theory and as the womanly, nurturing flesh that Christ's holy mother received from her female forebear.[103]

Female *imitatio Christi* mingled the genders in its most profound metaphors and its most profound experiences. Women could fuse with Christ's body because they *were* in some sense body, yet women never forgot the maleness of Christ. Indeed, exactly because maleness was humanly superior, the God who especially redeemed and loved the lowly stooped to marry *female* flesh. Hildegard of Bingen saw *ecclesia* as both Christ's bride and Christ's body. Julian of Norwich, who forged the most sophisticated theology of the motherhood of God, never ceased to refer to "Christ our mother" with the male pronoun. Some mystics, such as Hadewijch and Angela of Foligno, met Christ erotically as female to his maleness; others, such as Catherine of Siena or Margery Kempe, met him maternally, nursing him in their arms. But women mystics often simply became the flesh of Christ, because their flesh could do what his could do: bleed, feed, die and give life to others.[104]

The Body/Soul Relationship and the Significance of Body

Before concluding this examination of the religious significance of the female body, one conceptual boundary remains to be considered — that between body and soul. For the theological writing of the thirteenth and fourteenth centuries came to treat the relationship between body and soul as much tighter and more integral than it had earlier been understood to be. It seems reasonable to suppose that the extraordinary importance given to body, especially female body, in thirteenth- to fifteenth-century religion, and what appear to be the historical beginnings of certain somatic events (such as stigmata or miraculous lactation), owe something to the fact that theorists in the High Middle Ages did not see body primarily as the enemy of soul, the container of soul or the servant of soul; rather, they saw the person as a psychosomatic unity, as body and soul together.

Received wisdom has held that pious folk in the Middle Ages were practical dualists who hated and attacked the body.[105] Moreover, some feminist analysis has recently claimed that the Thomistic-Aristotelian association of form/matter with male/female laid the basis for modern theories of sex polarity and male supremacy, and for a certain denigration of the bodily or experiential as well.[106] There is truth in all this, of course. But when one reads medieval discussions, one is struck less by the polarities and dichotomies than by the muddle theologians and natural philosophers made of them, either by inserting entities between body and soul or by obscuring their differences. Those who wrote about body in the thirteenth and fourteenth centuries were in fact concerned to bridge the gap between material and spiritual and to give to body positive significance. Nor should we be surprised to find this so in a religion whose central tenet was the incarnation – the enfleshing – of its God.[107]

No scholastic theologian and no mystic (male or female) denied that the distinction between body and soul was in a technical, philosophical sense a real distinction. None rejected the Pauline idea that flesh (which, to Paul, means "sin" more than "body")[108] is a weight pulling spirit down. Nonetheless, theological speculation in the period of high scholasticism modified considerably the traditional platonic notion that the person is a soul, making use of a body.[109] A concept of person as soul *and* body (or, in modern parlance, a psychosomatic unity) undergirds scholastic discussions of such topics as bodily resurrection, miracles, embryology, asceticism, Christology and the Immaculate Conception. Indeed, it is because medieval thinkers felt it necessary to tie body and soul together, to bridge the gap between them while allowing body to retain a reality and significance of its own, that their writings in these areas are so extraordinarily difficult to understand. But, despite the obscurity of their theoretical writings, these theologians were in no way isolated from pious practice. They preached about miracles or trained others to preach; they inquired into accusations of heresy, claims for canonization and disputes over relics; they sometimes even supervised convents or advised others who did so. It thus seems likely that their attitudes toward the body shaped and reflected the environment within which holy women found it easy to experience bizarre bodily miracles and people of both sexes admired them.

The thirteenth and fourteenth centuries saw a proliferation of treatises and quodlibetal questions concerning various aspects of body.[110] (Quodlibetal disputations were debates by university students and masters on freely chosen rather than set topics; they are therefore an excellent index of which issues excited contemporary interest.) There was, for example, much discussion of the resurrection of the body;[111] and this fundamental tenet of Christian belief was treated not so much as a manifestation of divine power (as it had been in the patristic period) but as a consequence of human nature. Certain scholastic theologians (e.g., Peter of Capua) even questioned whether bodily resurrection after the Last Judgment might be natural – i.e., not a gift of divine grace but an implication of the fact that God created human

nature as a body/soul unity.[112] Most theorists answered that resurrection was supernatural. But in several papal and conciliar pronouncements, Christians were required
to hold that the damned as well as the saved rise bodily, nevermore to suffer corruption;[113] and moralists repeatedly explained this doctrine by arguing that body sinned
or gained merit alongside soul and must, therefore, also receive reward or punishment eternally.[114] Such arguments imply that persons *are* in some sense their bodies,
not merely souls temporarily inhabiting matter. As is well known, heretics of the
twelfth to fourteenth centuries were castigated for holding the obverse opinion.[115]
What most bothered orthodox polemicists about heretical opinions was not the moral
argument (i.e., the idea that flesh drags spirit down) but the ontological-cosmo-
logical one (i.e., the idea that matter and body cannot be included in the human).[116]

Scholastic treatises often combined theological with scientific (i.e., natural philosophical) interests. The attention devoted to Mary's virgin conception of Christ, and
the significantly larger amount of attention devoted to Mary's own Immaculate Conception and her bodily Assumption, suggest that religious writers were fascinated
by those Christian doctrines that forced an examination of bodily processes.[117] Some
even considered explicitly the physiological effects of religious practice. Albert the
Great, for example, asked whether cessation of eating and of menstruation in holy
women was damaging to their health.[118] A number of the major theologians of the
thirteenth century (e.g., Albert the Great, Giles of Rome, Richard of Middleton)
wrote both on embryology and on the resurrection of the body, and explicitly stated
that there was a connection between the topics, for both bore on the question of
the nature and identity of the human person.[119] A quick perusal of book 2, chapters 56 to 90, of the *Summa contra gentiles* convinces the reader that Aquinas assumed
that questions of psychology, embryology and eschatology must be solved together.
Moreover, a large section of Aquinas's long discussion of miracles in his *On the Power
of God* is concerned with whether demons or angels can make use of physical human
bodies and, if so, exactly how they might do it. Since this kind of miracle did not
loom large among those actually reported in Aquinas's day, one is tempted to attribute his interest in the question to the general fascination with which he and his
contemporaries viewed the body/soul nexus.[120] Hagiographers too combined an
interest in bodily miracles with exploration of medical lore, especially embryology.
For example, Thomas of Cantimpré, the hagiographer who showed the greatest

interest in collecting somatic miracles, especially female ones,[121] wrote on gynecology as well.[122]

In theological treatments of psychology and embryology we see a tendency to confuse the body/soul boundary. Thirteenth- to fifteenth-century explorations into psychology used the Aristotelian conception of soul – that is, the idea that soul is the principle of life. According to such theory, plants and animals as well as humans have souls. This idea made it difficult for those who wrote about the biological process of conception to say at what point the fetus was ensouled with the rational soul given by God, or indeed whether it had one or several souls as it developed. Moreover, under the influence of Avicenna, theologians and natural philosophers tried to work out a theory of "spirits" or "powers" located between soul and body as a sort of rarefied instrument to connect the two. Such discussions drew a sharper line between levels of soul than between soul and body.[123]

One of the reasons for the obscuring of the body/soul boundary in these treatments lay in Aristotle's theory itself, which actually worked less well to explain embryological development than the Galenic two-seed theory preferred by doctors.[124] As part of their general adoption of Aristotelian philosophy, theologians were drawn to the idea that the father provides the form for the fetus and the mother the matter (or menstrual material), but the concept proved difficult to use in detail. How does the father's seed, which is material, carry form or vital spirit? It is hard to follow Giles of Rome's explanation, in the *De formatione corporis humani in utero*, of how the father's body concocts a seed with vital spirits, which in some sense engenders spirits in the menstrual matter, which in turn form organs. But one thing is clear: the line between soul and body, form and matter, disappears in a complex apparatus that obscures the transition point from one to the other.[125]

In discussions of eschatology from the same period, we find the human person treated as a similarly tight and integral union of soul and body. Indeed, the doctrine of the resurrection of the body seemed to require a theory of the person in which body was integral. Accounts of the history of philosophy have long seen it as one of Aquinas's greatest achievements to utilize the Aristotelian form/matter dichotomy as a way of explaining that bodily resurrection after the Last Judgment is philosophically necessary.[126] According to Aquinas's use of hylomorphic analysis, the soul as a substantial form survives the death of the body, but the full person does not exist until body (matter) is restored to its form at the end of time. "The soul...is not the full man and my soul is not I [*anima...non est totus homo et anima mea non est ego*]."[127]

What historians of philosophy have not fully realized, however, is that Aquinas's conservative opponents, as much as Aquinas himself, gave positive significance to body. Theologians in the second half of the thirteenth century debated whether material continuity was necessary for bodily resurrection. Did God have to reassemble in the resurrected body the same bits of matter that had before been animated by a particular soul? They also debated whether the human person was to be explained by a plurality of forms or by a single form.[128] These debates are too complex to explain fully here, but what is important for our purposes is that both conservative theologians and those who followed Aquinas wanted to make body integral to person. Aquinas made body philosophically necessary, but in some sense telescoped body into form by holding both that soul is enough to account for individual continuity and that soul is the *forma corporeitatis*.[129] (In other words, it is soul that accounts for the "whatness" of body. Thus any matter that soul informs at the end of time will be *its* body.)[130] Those who opposed Thomas, following an older, platonic tradition, struggled to give body a greater substantial reality by positing a separate *forma corporeitatis* and arguing for material continuity in the resurrection. But to them too, the union of body and soul is necessary for personhood — and for happiness. Bonaventure wrote, in a sermon on the Assumption of the Virgin Mary:

> Her happiness would not be complete unless she [Mary] were there personally [i.e., bodily assumed into heaven]. The person is not the soul; it is a composite. Thus it is established that she must be there as a composite, that is, of soul and body. Otherwise she would not be there [in heaven] in perfect joy; for (as Augustine says) the minds of the saints [before their resurrections] are hindered, because of their natural inclination for their bodies, from being totally borne into God.[131]

Indeed, one can argue that those who differed with Aquinas, following a more Platonic, Augustinian or Franciscan tradition, gave even more importance to body than did the Thomists.[132] Henry of Ghent, for example, held to the theory of a separate *forma corporeitatis* so that the gifts of the glorified body could be understood as real changes *of that body*, not merely as a consequence of change in the soul.[133] In general, Franciscan thinkers emphasized the yearning of soul and body for each other after death. Richard of Middleton and Bonaventure actually saw this yearning as a motive for the saints in heaven: the blessed supposedly pray all the harder for us sinners because they will receive again their own deeply desired bodies only when the number of the elect is filled up and the Judgment comes.[134] More than a hundred years before Bonaventure, Bernard of Clairvaux (the great Cistercian who anticipated many aspects of Franciscan piety) spoke thus of the joys of bodily resurrection:

> Do not be surprised if the glorified body seems to give the spirit something, for it was a real help when man was sick and mortal. How true that text is which says that all things turn to the good of those who love God [Rom. 8.28]. The sick, dead and resurrected body is a help to the soul who loves God; the first for the fruits of penance, the second for repose and the third for consummation. Truly the soul does not want to be perfected, without that from whose good services it feels it has benefited...in every way.... Listen to the bridegroom in the Canticle inviting us to this triple progress: 'Eat, friends, and drink; be inebriated, dearest ones.' He calls to those working in the body to eat; he invites those who have set aside their bodies to drink; and he impels those who have resumed their bodies to inebriate themselves, calling them his dearest ones, as if they were filled with charity.... It is right to call them dearest who are drunk with love....[135]

Discussions of eschatology emphasized the fascination and value of body in other ways as well, sometimes even obscuring differences between body and soul. In some of their more adventuresome explorations of the future life, theologians elevated aspects of body into the spiritual realm. They wondered, for example, whether the blessed in their glorified bodies would truly taste and smell, as well as see, the pleasures of heaven.[136] At other moments in theological discussion, soul seems almost to spill over into body. The gifts (*dotes*) of subtlety, impassibility, clarity and agility that characterize the bodies of the saved were understood to be a flowing over of the beatific vision — perhaps even a way in which soul expresses itself as body.[137]

A number of the issues theologians raised enabled them to explore the nature of bodiliness at its very boundaries. For example, they debated whether we can open and close our eyes in the glorified body, how old we will be in heaven, whether we will rise in two sexes, whether the wounds of the martyrs will still be present in the glorified body, and how the damned in their restored bodies (which are incorruptible but not impassible) can cry without losing any bodily matter through the dissolution of tears.[138] In such discussion, jejune though it has seemed to most modern commentators, a very profound conception of body is adumbrated — one in which both innate and acquired physical differences between persons, including biological sex and even the marks of human suffering, *are* the person for eternity. Theologians agreed that human beings rise in two sexes and with the traces not only of martyrdom but of other particularities as well.[139] Although defects will be repaired in glory and woman's sex can, in Aristotelian terms, be seen as a defect, theologians nonetheless asserted that, for reasons they could not fully explain, God's creation was more perfect in two sexes than in one.[140] What is temporary or temporal, according to this view, is not physical distinctiveness or gender, but the change we call corruption (or decay or dissolution) of material being.[141] This conception of body as integral to person — indeed, of body as being the conveyor of personal specificity — helps us understand how relics could in this culture be treated as if they *were* the saints.[142]

Moreover, the idea that body as well as soul is rewarded (or punished) at the end of time — an idea reflected not just in theology but also in the literary genre of the debate between Body and Soul — seemed to give significance to physical rewards that might come *before* death or the Last Judgment. The catatonic trances and miraculous inedia of living holy women, like the incorrupt bodies they sometimes displayed beyond the grave, could easily be understood as having achieved in advance the final incorruption and impassibility of the glorified body in heaven. Indeed, Christ was understood to have assumed all general defects of body in the Incarnation because, as Thomas said, "we know human nature only as it is subject to defect," and all particular defects are caused by the general defects of corruption and passibility.[143] Thus, even the ugliness of disease and suffering can be not only lifted up into the curative pangs of purgatory but also transmuted, through Christ's wondrous yet fully human body, into the beauty of heaven. (Presumably, stigmatics will still bear their marks before the throne of God, although the wounds will no longer bleed periodically.)[144]

By the 1330s the faithful were required to believe that the beatific vision could come to the blessed before the end of time; and theologians held, although in different ways, that the gifts of the glorified body were in some sense a consequence of the soul's vision of God.[145] Indeed, some theologians argued that a special miracle had been necessary to block the manifestation of God's glory in the human body of his son Jesus; the body Jesus displayed at the Transfiguration was, they held, his normal body, manifesting the beatific vision he constantly possessed.[146] Theologians were, of course, cautious about stating that any specific person had actually received the beatific vision. But in the context of such opinion, it is not surprising that hagiographers made extravagant claims, describing their holy subjects as rosy and beautiful despite (perhaps even because of) flagellation and self-starvation, excruciating disease and death itself.[147] Aquinas wrote that the martyrs were enabled to bear up under pain exactly because the beatific vision flows over naturally into the body.[148]

The widely shared assumption that bodies not only reflect the glory their souls receive in God's presence but are also the place where persons are rewarded or punished in their specificity underlies the many hagiographical stories and *exempla* from this period in which incorruption or other miraculous marks touch only part of a body. Caesarius of Heisterbach, for example, told of a master who copied many books; after death, his right hand was found undecayed although the rest of his body had turned to dust.[149] In another tale from Caesarius's collection, a pious man who said his prayers as he walked returned after death in a vision with the words *Ave Maria* written on his boots; God, says Caesarius, puts "the mark of glory most of all on those members by which it is earned."[150] Given the tremendous emphasis on female virginity as an avenue to sanctity, it is hardly surprising that the bodies of many female saints were found wholly intact many years after burial.[151] As Caesarius might have put it, God marked their unviolated bodies with permanent inviolability.

It is, moreover, hardly surprising that, as the doctrine of purgatory was elaborated, the experiences of souls there were imagined as bodily events, even though theologians taught that souls in this state subsisted without their bodies. Bodily metaphors for spiritual states are used in many societies. But more seems to be involved in these Christian ideas than mere convenience of metaphor. In technical theology as in popular miracle stories, pain was understood to be the experience of a psychosomatic unit. Aquinas said about the suffering of Christ's soul: "soul and body are one being. So when body is disturbed by some corporeal suffering, soul is of necessity disturbed indirectly as a result [*per accidens*]...."[152] More generally in the culture, the reverse was assumed as well: when soul is disturbed, body is disturbed. Pain and imperviousness to it happen to a personal entity that is body and soul together.[153] So many forces in the religious life of the period conspired to suggest that persons *are* their bodies that preachers found it almost impossible to speak of immortal souls without clothing them in their quite particular flesh. The many tales of temporary resurrections of the dead, of corpses bleeding to accuse their murderers or sitting up to revere the Eucharist, of cadavers growing or smelling sweet or even exuding food after death, point to a widespread cultural assumption that person is body as well as soul, body integrally bound with soul.[154]

Conclusion

About the topics I have discussed above, much more could be said. But I have explained and explored enough to make it quite clear that the extraordinary bodily quality of women's piety between 1200 and 1500 must be understood in the context of attitudes toward woman and toward body peculiar to the later Middle Ages. Because preachers, confessors and spiritual directors assumed the person to be a psychosomatic unity, they not only read unusual bodily events as expressions of soul, but also expected body itself to offer a means of access to the divine. Because they worshiped a God who became incarnate and died for the sins of others, they viewed all bodily events – the hideous wounds of martyrs or stigmatics as well as the rosy-faced beauty of virgins – as possible manifestations of grace. Because they associated the female with the fleshly, they expected somatic expressions to characterize women's spirituality.

We must never forget the pain and frustration, the isolation and feelings of helplessness, that accompanied the quest of religious women. For all her charismatic empowerment, woman was inferior to man in the Middle Ages; her voice was often silenced, even more frequently ignored. Not every use of the phrase "weak woman" by a female writer was ironic; women clearly internalized the negative value placed on them by the culture in which they lived. Moreover, for all its expressiveness and lability, body was inferior to soul. The locus of fertility and of mystical encounter, it was also the locus of temptation and decomposition. Whereas soul was immortal, body rose again only after decay and as a result of the grace of Christ's Resurrection. Body was not always a friend or a tool or a gateway to heaven. Nonetheless, one of the most striking characteristics of this period in Western religious history is the extent to which female bodily experience was understood to be union with God.

The thirteenth-century Flemish Saint Christina the Astonishing, whose body lac-

196

tated and levitated in mystical encounter, supposedly spoke of her own asceticism in a little dialogue that has many literary antecedents:

> Then wailing bitterly she began to beat her breast and her body…"O miserable and wretched body! How long will you torment me…? Why do you delay me from seeing the face of Christ? When will you abandon me so that my soul can return freely to its Creator?"…[T]hen, taking the part of the body, she would say…"O miserable soul! Why are you tormenting me in this way? What is keeping you in me and what is it that you love in me? Why do you not allow me to return to the earth from where I was taken and why do you not let me be at rest until I am restored to you on the Last Day of Judgment?"… [S]he would then rest a little in silence.… Then, taking her feet with both hands, she would kiss the soles of her feet with greatest affection and would say, "O most beloved body! Why have I beaten you? Why have I reviled you? Did you not obey me in every good deed I undertook to do with God's help? You have endured the torment and hardships most generously and most patiently which the spirit placed on you.… Now, O best and sweetest body…is an end of your hardship, now you will rest in the dust and will sleep for a little and then, at last, when the trumpet blows, you will rise again purified of all corruptibility and you will be joined in eternal happiness with the soul you have had as a companion in the present sadness."[155]

Christina's words express much of what a thirteenth-century woman and her hagiographer assumed about female body. Source of temptation and torment, body is also a beloved companion and helpmeet; delay and hindrance on earth, it is essential to the person herself and will be perfected and glorified in heaven.

Christina's words can be supplemented by a later and more gruesome dialogue, which is nonetheless descended from the genre in which Thomas of Cantimpré, her hagiographer, wrote. In the fifteenth-century *Disputacion Betwyx the Body and Wormes*, the anonymous author modifies the traditional debate between Body and Soul to dramatize death and decay.[156] Here a female body, so misled about the significance of flesh that she actually boasts of her descent from Eve, is forced to hear the message of Worms, who will strip the body of its stinking flesh, scouring the bones (figure 10). Nonetheless, the poem does not end with the feast of Worms, nor with the triumph of devils carrying Body off to hell. The poet argues for victory over death, not by denying the horrors of decay, but by identifying corruption with the suffering of Christ on the Cross.[157] As Christina says in Thomas's quite similar account: Body

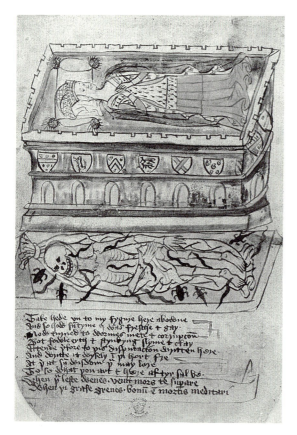

Figure 10: *A Disputacion Betwyx e Body and Wormes*,
15th-century English poem (London, British Library).

itself will rise again. Welcoming the "kys" of Worms and agreeing to "dwell to gedyr"
with them in "luf" until Judgment Day as "neghbors" and "frendes," Body arms herself with "gode sufferaunce" and anticipates the coming "blis of heuen" through
the "mene and mediacione" of "our blissed Lord, our verry patrone."[158]

In such a dialogue, the modern reader glimpses the startling significance attributed to body, and especially female body, in the later Middle Ages. Clothing of decay
and potential food for worms, female flesh was also an integral component of female
person. Created and redeemed by God, it was a means of encounter with Him.
Healed and elevated by grace, it was destined for glory at the Last Judgment. And
in that Judgment it rose as female. Although medieval theologians did not fully
understand why, they were convinced that God's creation was more perfect in two
sexes than in one.

NOTES

1. Peter of Vaux, "Life of Colette of Corbie," trans. Stephen Juliacus, ch. 10, par. 84, in *Acta sanctorum* (hereafter AASS), March, vol. 1 (Paris, 1865), p. 558. See Caroline Walker Bynum, *Holy Feast and Holy Fast: The Religious Significance of Food to Medieval Women* (hereafter HFHF) (Berkeley: University of California Press, 1987), p. 67.

2. Life of Lukardis, ch. 55, *Analecta Bollandiana* 18 (1899), p. 340.

3. Johann Huizinga, *The Waning of the Middle Ages: A Study of Forms of Life, Thought and Art in France and the Netherlands in the XIVth and XVth Centuries* (1924), trans. F. Hopman (Pbk reprint: Garden City: Doubleday, 1956); Barbara W. Tuchman, *A Distant Mirror: The Calamitous Fourteenth Century* (New York: Knopf, 1978).

4. For discussion of the modern period, see Catherine Gallagher and Thomas Laqueur, eds., *The Making of the Modern Body: Sexuality and Society in the Nineteenth Century* (Berkeley: University of California Press, 1987). For discussion of the Middle Ages, see Danielle Jacquart and Claude Thomasset, *Sexualité et savoir médical au Moyen Age* (Paris: Presses universitaires de France, 1985); Jacques Le Goff, "Corps et idéologie dans l'Occident médiéval: La révolution corporelle," in *L'Imaginaire médiéval: Essais* (Paris: Gallimard, 1985), pp. 123-27; and Michel Sot, "Mépris du monde et résistance des corps aux XIe et XIIe siècles," and Jacques Dalarun, "Eve, Marie ou Madeleine? La dignité du corps féminin dans hagiographie médiévale," in *Médiévales* 8 (1985), *Le souci du corps*, pp. 6-32.

5. A close reading of the evidence Le Goff presents in "Corps et idéologie" makes this clear. In the twelfth- and thirteenth-century literature he cites, disease and deformity are symbols of sin or of the corruption of society (not primarily of sex); the disgust displayed toward body is ultimately a disgust toward the putrefaction that will be manifest most clearly in the grave.

6. I have discussed this in "Women Mystics and Eucharistic Devotion in the Thirteenth Century," *Women's Studies* 11 (1984), pp. 179-214; in "Fast, Feast and Flesh: The Religious Significance of Food to Medieval Women," *Representations* 11 (Summer 1985), pp. 1-25; and in HFHF. The point is also made by Peter Dinzelbacher, "Europäische Frauenmystik des Mittelalters: Ein Überblick," in *Frauenmystik im Mittelalter*, ed. P. Dinzelbacher and D. Bauer, Wissenschaftliche Studientagung der Akademie der Diozese Rottenburg-Stuttgart 22-25. Februar 1984, in Weingarten (Ostfildern: Schwabenverlag, 1985), pp. 11-23; by Peter Brown, *The Cult of the Saints: Its Rise and Function in Latin Christianity* (Chicago: University of Chicago Press, 1981); by Jacques Gelis and Odile Redon, Preface, and Michel Bouvier, "De l'incorruptibilité des corps saints," in *Les miracles miroirs des corps*, eds. Gelis and Redon (Paris: Presses et publications de l'université de Paris VIII, 1983), pp. 9-20, 193-221; by Marie-Christine Pouchelle, "Représentations du corps dans la *Legende dorée*," *Ethnologie française* 6

(1976), pp. 293-308; by Dominique de Courcelles, "Les corps des saints dans les cantiques catalans de la fin du moyen âge," *Médiévales* 8 (1985): *Le souci du corps*, pp. 43-56; and, in a different way, by Herbert Thurston, *The Physical Phenomena of Mysticism* (hereafter PP) (Chicago: Henry Regnery, 1952).

7. I have treated some of the material that follows in HFHF, although from a somewhat different point of view. I should, however, point out here that the material in the final two sections of this essay is new and goes considerably beyond anything touched on in HFHF.

8. P. Séjourné, "Reliques," *Dictionnaire de théologie catholique* (hereafter DTC) (Paris: Letouzey et Ané, 1903-72), vol. 13, pt. 2, cols. 2330-65; Patrick J. Geary, *Furta Sacra: Thefts of Relics in the Central Middle Ages* (Princeton, 1978), esp. pp. 152-54; and E.A.R. Brown, "Death and the Human Body in the Later Middle Ages: The Legislation of Boniface VIII on the Division of the Corpse," *Viator* 12 (1981), pp. 221-70, esp. pp. 223-24.

9. See Peter the Venerable, Sermon 4, *Patrologia latina*, ed. J.-P. Migne (hereafter PL), vol. 189 (Paris: 1890), cols. 1001-03; reedited by Giles Constable, "Petri Venerabilis Sermones Tres," *Revue Bénédictine* 64 (1954), pp. 269-70. See also Caesarius of Heisterbach, *Dialogus miraculorum*, ed. Joseph Strange, 2 vols. (Cologne: Heberle, 1851), bk. 8, ch. 87, vol. 2, pp. 145-46.

10. See, for example, the case of Lukardis, HFHF, pp.113-14. See also, "Life of Lutgard of Aywières," bk. 1, chs. 1-2, and bk. 2, ch. 1, AASS, June, vol. 4 (Paris and Rome, 1867), pp. 192-94; and "Life of Benevenuta of Bojano," ch. 10, par. 82, AASS, October, vol. 13 (1883), p. 172.

11. Nicole Hermann-Mascard, *Les Reliques des saints: Formation coutumière d'un droit*, Société d'Histoire du Droit: collection d'histoire institutionnelle et sociale 6 (Paris: Edition Klincksieck, 1975), p. 274, n.21. As examples, see the process of canonization of 1276 for Margaret of Hungary, in Vilmos Fraknói, *Monumenta romana episcopatus vesprimiensis (1103-1526)*, vol. 1 (Budapest: Collegium Historicorum Hungarorum Romanum, 1896), pp. 237-38, 266, 267, 288; and the case of Lidwina of Schiedam, "Fast, Feast and Flesh," p. 5.

12. Angela of Foligno, *Le Livre de l'expérience des vrais fidèles: texte latin publié d'après le manuscrit d'Assise*, eds. and trans. M.-J. Ferré and L. Baudry (Paris: Editions E. Droz, 1927), par. 53, p. 106 (cf., *ibid.*, par. 80, p. 166); Raymond of Capua, *Legenda maior* of Catherine of Siena, AASS, April, vol. 3 (1866), pt. 2, ch. 4, pars. 155 and 162-63, and pt. 3, ch. 7, pars. 412 and 414, pp. 901-03, 963; Catherine of Genoa, *Il dialogo spirituale* and *Vita*, ch. 12, ed. Umile Bonzi da Genova, *S. Caterina Fieschi Adorno*, vol. 2, *Edizione critica dei manoscritti Cateriniani* (Turin: Marietti, 1962), pp. 422-27, 140-41. And see Thomas of Celano, "First Life of Francis of Assisi," bk. 1, ch. 7, par. 17, in *Analecta Franciscana* 10 (Quaracchi: Collegium S. Bonaventurae, 1941), p. 16; Celano, "Second Life," bk. 1, ch. 5, par. 9, in *ibid.*, pp. 135-63; Bonaventure, *Legenda maior* of Francis, pt. 1, ch. 1, pars. 5-6, in *ibid.*, pp. 562-63;

and Bonaventure, *Legenda minor*, ch. 1, eighth lesson, in *ibid.*, pp. 657-58.

13. HFHF, pp. 122-23, 126, 211, 273-75.

14. Giles Constable, *Attitudes Toward Self-Inflicted Suffering in the Middle Ages,* The Ninth Stephen J. Brademas Sr. Lecture (Brookline, Mass.: Hellenic College Press, 1982); Richard Kieckhefer, *Unquiet Souls: Fourteenth-Century Saints and Their Religious Milieu* (Chicago: University of Chicago Press, 1984), chs. 3-5; Brenda Bolton, "*Mulieres sanctae*," *Studies in Church History* 10: *Sanctity and Secularity: The Church and the World*, ed. D. Baker (1973), pp. 77-93, and *idem*, "*Vitae Matrum*: A Further Aspect of the *Frauenfrage*," *Medieval Women: Dedicated and Presented to Professor Rosalind M.T. Hill...*, ed. D. Baker, Studies in Church History: Subsidia 1 (Oxford, 1970), pp. 253-73.

15. "Life of Suso," ch. 31, in Henry Suso, *Deutsche Schriften im Auftrag der Württembergischen Kommission für Landesgeschichte*, ed. Karl Bihlmeyer (Stuttgart: Kohlhammer, 1907), pp. 91-92; trans. M. Ann Edwards, *The Exemplar: Life and Writings of Blessed Henry Suso, O.P.*, ed. Nicholas Heller, 2 vols. (Dubuque: Priory Press, 1962), vol. 1, pp. 87-88.

16. Angela of Foligno, *Le Livre*, par. 75, pp. 156-58.

17. Peter Browe, *Die Eucharistischen Wunder des Mittelalters*, Breslauer Studien zur historischen Theologie NF 4 (Breslau: Müller and Seiffert, 1938).

18. Peggy Reeves Sanday, *Divine Hunger: Cannibalism as a Cultural System* (New York: Cambridge University Press, 1986), and Louis-Vincent Thomas, *Le Cadavre: De la biologie à l'anthropologie* (Brussels: Editions complexe, 1980), pp. 159-69.

19. Ronald C. Finucane, *Miracles and Pilgrims: Popular Beliefs in Medieval England* (Totowa, N.J.: Rowan and Littlefield, 1977), pp. 197-98: Benedicta Ward, *Miracles and the Medieval Mind: Record and Event, 1000-1215* (Philadelphia: University of Pennsylvania Press, 1982), pp. 15-18; Gary Macy, *The Theologies of the Eucharist in the Early Scholastic Period: A Study of the Salvific Function of the Sacrament According to the Theologians, c.1080–c.1220* (Oxford: Oxford University Press, 1984), pp. 87-95; HFHF, p. 255.

20. Adam of Eynsham, *Life of Hugh of Lincoln*, eds. D. Douie and H. Farmer, 2 vols. (London: Thomas Nelson and Sons, 1961), bk. 5, ch. 15, vol. 2, p. 170.

21. Leo Steinberg, *The Sexuality of Christ in Renaissance Art and in Modern Oblivion* (New York, Pantheon, 1983).

22. See Louis Canet in Robert Fawtier and Louis Canet, *La double expérience de Catherine Benincasa (Sainte Catherine de Siene)* (Paris: Gallimard, 1948), pp. 245-46.

23. Peter Dinzelbacher, "Die 'Vita et Revelationes' der Wiener Begine Agnes Blannbekin (+1315) im Rahmen der Viten-und Offenbarungsliteratur ihrer Zeit," in Dinzelbacher and Bauer, eds., *Frauen-*

mystik, pp. 152-177.

24. See Thurston, PP; Dinzelbacher, "Überblick"; *idem, Vision und Visionsliteratur im Mittelalter* (Stuttgart: Hiersemann, 1981); Rudolph M. Bell, *Holy Anorexia* (Chicago: University of Chicago Press, 1985); and HFHF. As all four of the important recent books on saints make clear, these phenomena are particularly documented for Low Country women in the thirteenth century, for women in the Rhineland in the late thirteenth and early fourteenth centuries, and for north Italian women in the fourteenth to fifteenth centuries: see André Vauchez, *La sainteté en Occident aux derniers siècles du moyen âge d'après les procès de canonisation et les documents hagiographiques*, Bibliothèque des Études Françaises d'Athènes et de Rome 241 (Rome: Ecole française de Rome, 1981); Donald Weinstein and Rudolph M. Bell, *Saints and Society: The Two Worlds of Western Christendom, 1000–1700* (hereafter SS) (Chicago: University of Chicago Press, 1982); Michael Goodich, *Vita Perfecta: The Ideal of Sainthood in the Thirteenth Century*, Monographien zur Geschichte des Mittelalters 25 (Stuttgart: Hiersemann, 1982); and Kieckhefer, *Unquiet Souls*.

25. Thurston, PP, esp. pp. 69, 95-99, 123; Antoine Imbert-Gourbeyre, *La Stigmatisation: L'Extase divine et les miracles de Lourdes: Réponse aux libres-penseurs*, 2 vols. (Clermont-Ferrand, 1894), which must be used with caution; Pierre Debongnie, "Essai critique sur l'histoire des stigmatisations au Moyen Age," *Etudes carmélitaines* 21.2 (1936), pp. 22-59; E. Amann, "Stigmatisation," DTC, vol. 14, pt. 1, cols. 2617-19.

26. J.-K. Huysmans, *Sainte Lydwine de Schiedam* (Paris, 1901), pp. 288-91, which, however, contains no documentation; Thurston, PP, pp. 268-70; Hermann-Mascard, *Les Reliques*, pp. 68-69; Charles W. Jones, *Saint Nicolas of Myra, Bari and Manhattan: Biography of a Legend* (Chicago: University of Chicago Press, 1978), pp. 144-53; and Bynum, "Fast, Feast and Flesh," nn. 22, 81, 82, 85. Women also account for most of the cases of exuding sweet odors: see Thurston, PP, pp. 222-32.

27. HFHF, pp. 203-04, 257, 268-69; Bynum, "Women Mystics," p. 202.

28. Clare of Montefalco's spiritual sisters tore out her heart after her death and found the insignia of the Passion incised upon it; see Vauchez, *La sainteté*, p. 408. Three precious stones, with images of the Holy Family on them, were supposedly found in the heart of Margaret of Città di Castello; see "Life of Margaret," ch. 8, *Analecta Bollandiana* 19 (1900), pp. 27-28. On mystical espousal rings and miraculous bodily elongation, see Thurston, PP, pp. 139 and 200.

29. The point is Pouchelle's; see Marie-Christine Pouchelle, *Corps et chirurgie à l'apogée du Moyen Age* (Paris: Flammarion, 1983), pp. 132-36. She claims that the earliest official dissections (in 1315) were dissections of female bodies. The dissections to which she refers were clearly not the first dissections or autopsies of any sort. Dissections arising out of embalming or for the purpose of deter-

mining the cause of death in legal cases were practiced at least from the early thirteenth century; dissections of the human body for teaching purposes were practiced at Bologna about 1300. See Walter Artelt, *Die ältesten Nachrichten über die Sektion menschlicher Leichen im mittelalterlichen Abendland*, Abhandlungen zur Geschichte der Medizin und der Naturwissenschaften 34 (Berlin: Ebering, 1940), pp. 3-25; Mary Niven Alston, "The Attitude of the Church Towards Dissection Before 1500," *Bulletin of the History of Medicine* 16 (1944), pp. 221-38; Ynez Viole O'Neill, "Innocent III and the Evolution of Anatomy," *Medical History* 20.4 (1976), pp. 429-33; Nancy G. Siraisi, "The Medical Learning of Albertus Magnus," in James A. Weisheipl, ed., *Albertus Magnus and the Sciences: Commemorative Essays, 1980* (Toronto: Pontifical Institute of Medieval Studies, 1980), p. 395; and Jacquart and Thomasset, *Sexualité*, p. 49.

30. According to the tables in Weinstein and Bell, SS, women provide twenty-seven percent of the wonder-working relics, although only seventeen and one-half percent of the saints. On blood prodigies, see Thurston, PP, pp. 283-93.

31. Claude Carozzi, "Douceline et les autres," in *La religion populaire en Languedoc du XIIIe siècle à la moitié du XIVe siècle*, Cahiers de Fanjeaux 11 (Toulouse, 1967), pp. 251-67; and see de Courcelles, "Les corps des saints," esp. p. 51.

32. Thurston, PP, pp. 233-82, esp. pp. 246-52. Of the forty-two saints living between 1400 and 1900 whose feasts are kept by the universal church, there are claims of incorruption in twenty-two cases, and in seven more there are reports of odd phenomena which imply non-decay. Seventeen of the incorrupt are male, but of the six females among the forty-two, five are incorrupt and for the sixth (Jane Frances de Chantal), who was embalmed, there appears to be a claim for extraordinary survival. There are thus more incorrupt male bodies, but all the female bodies are claimed to be incorrupt. On incorruption, see also Bouvier, "De l'incorruptibilité"; João de Pina-Cabral, *Sons of Adam, Daughters of Eve: The Peasant World of the Alto Minho* (Oxford, 1986), pp. 230-38; and Bynum, "Holy Anorexia in Modern Portugal," in *Culture, Medicine and Psychiatry* 12 (1988), pp. 259-68. For examples of miraculous bodily closure in women saints, see Bynum, "Fast, Feast and Flesh," n.54.

33. Weinstein and Bell, SS, pp. 234-35.

34. Ernst Benz, *Die Vision: Erfahrungsformen und Bilderwelt* (Stuttgart: Ernst Klett, 1969), pp. 17-34; Kieckhefer, *Unquiet Souls*, pp. 57-58; and Elizabeth A. Petroff, *Medieval Women's Visionary Literature* (Oxford; Oxford University Press, 1986), pp. 37-44.

35. Julian of Norwich, *A Book of Showings*, long text, chs. 2-4, eds. E. Colledge and J. Walsh, 2 vols., P.I.M.S. Studies and Texts 35 (Toronto: Pontifical Institute of Medieval Studies, 1978), vol. 2, pp. 285-98; "Life of Villana de' Botti," ch. 1, pars. 11-12, AASS, August, vol. 5 (1868), pp. 866-67;

z o n e

Caroline Walker Bynum, *Jesus as Mother: Studies in the Spirituality of the High Middle Ages* (Berkeley: University of California Press, 1982), pp. 192 and 253 n.295; L. Reypens, ed., *Vita Beatricis: De autobiografie van de Z. Beatrijs van Tienen O. Cist. 1200-1268* (Antwerp: Ruusbroec-Genootschap, 1964), p. 64; G.G. Meersseman, ed., "Life of Margaret of Ypres," in "Frères prêcheurs et mouvement dévot en Flandre au XIIIe siècle," *Archivum fratrum praedicatorum* 18 (1948), pp. 125-26; Bynum, "Fast, Feast and Flesh," pp. 4-8; Kieckhefer, *Unquiet Souls*, pp. 22-33; "Life of Alpais of Cudot," AASS, November, vol. 2.1 (1894), pp. 167-209; "Life of Serafina of San Gimignano," AASS, March, vol. 2 (1865), pp. 232-38.

36. *Vita Beatricis*, ed. Reypens, bk. 3, ch. 6, pp. 134-36. See also pp. 45-49, 63, 99, 154-55. The poet Hadewijch also speaks of ecstasy as "insanity"; see poem 15, Poems in Couplets, in Hadewijch, *The Complete Works*, trans. C. Hart (New York: Paulist Press, 1980), pp. 350-52. Philip of Clairvaux in his "Life of Elisabeth of Spalbeek" calls her ecstasy *imbecillitas*; see *Catalogus codicum hagiographicorum Bibliothecae regiae Bruxellensis*, Subsidia hagiographica 1, vol. 1.1 (Brussels, 1886), p. 364.

37. Process of canonization, art. 33, in Jacques Cambell, ed., *Enquête pour le procès de canonisation de Dauphine de Puimichel, comtesse d'Ariano (+26-xi-1360)* (Turin: Erasmo, 1978), p. 52.

38. "Life of Alice," ch. 3, para. 26, AASS, June, vol. 2 (1867), p. 476. And see "Life of Lutgard of Aywières," bk. 3, ch. 1, AASS, p. 204. The emphasis on service is important. Even those women who languished alone in illness thought of themselves as saving others through their suffering. Although all recent works on saints (Vauchez, *La sainteté*, Weinsten and Bell, SS, Goodich, *Vita Perfecta* and Kieckhefer, *Unquiet Souls*) have contrasted contemplative women with active ones and have seen the active form of life to be more characteristic of Italian women, I take issue with this dichotomy; see HFHF, chs. 1 and 4.

39. See Jerome Kroll and Bernard Bachrach, "Sin and the Etiology of Disease in Pre-Crusade Europe," *Journal of the History of Medicine and Allied Sciences* 41 (1986), pp. 395-414; Alain Saint-Denis, "Soins du corps et médecine contre la souffrance à l'Hôtel-Dieu de Laon au XIIIe siècle," *Médiévales* 8 (1985): *Le souci du corps*, pp. 33-42; Katharine Park, "Medicine and Society in Medieval Europe, 500-1500," in Andrew Wear, ed., *Medicine in Society* (Cambridge: Cambridge University Press), ch. 2, forthcoming.

40. "Life of Alpais," bk. 3, ch. 4, and bk. 4, ch. 1, AASS, pp.196-97 and 198. For Elsbeth Achler, see Bihlmeyer, ed., "Die Schwäbische Mystikerin Elsbeth Achler von Reute († 1420)...," *Festgabe Philipp Strauch zum 80. Geburtstag am 23. September 1932*, ed. G. Bäsecke and F. J. Schneider (Halle: Niemeyer, 1932), pp. 88-109. On Catherine, see Raymond of Capua, *Legenda maior*, pt. 2, ch. 5, par. 167, AASS, p. 904.

41. Elsbet Stagel, *Das Leben der Schwestern zu Töss beschrieben von Elsbet Stagel*, ed. Ferdinand Vetter, Deutsche Texte des Mittelalters 6 (Berlin: Weidmann, 1906), p. 37.

42. "Life of Walburga" (d. 779) by Wolfhard of Eichstadt, in AASS, February, vol. 3 (Antwerp, 1658), pp. 528 and 540-42.

43. Pierre-André Sigal, *L'homme et les miracles dans la France médiévale (XI–XIIe siècle)*, (Paris: Editions du Cerf, 1985), esp. pp. 259-61.

44. Dinzelbacher, "Überblick"; and Peter Dronke, *Women Writers of the Middle Ages: A Critical Study of Texts from Perpetua († 203) to Marguerite Porete († 1310)* (Cambridge: Cambridge University Press, 1984), pp. x-xi.

45. See, for example, Bernard of Clairvaux, *Sermones super Cantica Canticorum*, sermon 71, *Sancti Bernardi opera*, ed. J. Leclercq, C.H. Talbot and H.M. Rochais (Rome: Editiones Cistercienses, 1958), vol. 2, pp. 214-24; John Tauler, sermon 31, in *Die Predigten Taulers*, ed. Ferdinand Vetter (Berlin: Wiedman, 1910), p. 310. See also Huizinga, *Waning*, pp. 197-200.

46. This point is made in a number of the papers in Dinzelbacher and Bauer, eds., *Frauenmystik*. See esp. Franz Wöhrer, "Aspekte der englischen Frauenmystik im späten 14. und beginnenden 15. Jahrhundert," pp. 314-40.

47. See above nn.10, 13, 26, 27, 36; and Hadewijch, vision 7, in *Complete Works*, trans. C. Hart, pp. 280-81.

48. See Siegfried Ringler, "Die Rezeption mittelalterlicher Frauenmystik als wissenschaftliches Problem, dargestellt am Werk der Christine Ebner," and Dinzelbacher, "Agnes Blannbekin," in Dinzelbacher and Bauer, eds., *Frauenmystik*, pp. 178-200 and 152-77; and Bynum, "Women Mystics," pp. 185-92. Miraculous elements tend to be more or less stressed in accounts of visions depending on the audience for which they are composed; see Simone Roisin, *L'Hagiographie Cistercienne dans le diocèse de Liège au XIIIe siècle* (Louvain, 1947).

49. For a comparison of male and female visions, see Dinzelbacher, *Vision*, pp. 151-55 and 226-28; Kieckhefer, *Unquiet Souls*, p. 172; Bynum, "Women Mystics," pp. 181-84.

50. Bynum, *Jesus as Mother*, pp. 110-69; HFHF, ch. 3; and Hester G. Gelber, "A Theatre of Virtue: The Exemplary World of St. Francis of Assisi," *Saints and Virtues*, ed. J.S. Hawley (Berkeley: University of California Press, 1987), pp.15-35.

51. Browe, *Die Wunder*, pp. 110-11; Tauler, sermon 31, *Die Predigten*, pp. 310-11.

52. Wöhrer, "Aspekte der englischen Frauenmystik."

53. For Hadewijch, see *Complete Works*, trans. C. Hart. For Marguerite Porete, see Romana Guarnieri, ed., "Il 'Miroir des simples âmes' di Margherita Porete," *Archivio Italiano per la storia della*

pietà 4 (1965), pp. 501-635, and Dronke, *Women Writers*, pp. 202-28.

54. Marguerite of Oingt, *Les oeuvres de Marguerite d'Oingt*, ed. and trans. Antonin Duraffour, Pierre Gardette and P. Durdilly (Paris: Société d'édition 'Les belles lettres,' 1965), p. 147.

55. Angela of Foligno, *Le livre*, par. 167, pp. 382-84.

56. *Ibid.*, pars. 66 and 151, pp. 138-40 and 326. For the contrast between Eckhart and women mystics, see Otto Langer, "Zur dominikanischen Frauenmystik im spätmittelalterlichen Deutschland," in Dinzelbacher and Bauer, eds., *Frauenmystik*, pp. 341-46.

57. See HFHF, p. 210.

58. This difference cuts across differences of class or region. The few female saints we know of from poorer groups in society are remarkably similar in their pious practices to the saintly princesses and noblewomen of the period; see Weinstein and Bell, SS, pp. 216 and 220-38. On regional differences, see n.38 above.

59. For helpful remarks on this topic, see Barbara Duden, "A Repertory of Body History," *Zone* 5 (1989).

60. *Jesus as Mother*, pp. 9-21 and 170-262; and "Women Mystics," pp. 192-96. The argument is implied in the title of a recent collection, *Women of Spirit: Female Leadership in the Jewish and Christian Traditions*, eds. Rosemary Reuther and Eleanor McLaughlin (New York: Simon and Schuster, 1979). Petroff, *Women's Visionary Literature*, p. 27, argues that writing itself was considered a male acitivity; therefore women needed direct divine inspiration to call a writing and speaking voice into existence.

61. HFHF, pp. 76-77, 229, 253. Eucharistic visions, especially visions of the bleeding host, occurred to women more frequently than to men; see Browe, *Die Wunder*.

62. Herbert Grundmann, "Die Frauen und die Literatur im Mittelalter: Ein Beitrag zur Frage nach der Entstehung des Schrifttums in der Volksprache," *Archiv für Kulturgeschichte* 26 (1936), pp. 129-61.

63. Margot Schmidt, "Elemente der Schau bei Mechtild von Magdeburg und Mechtild von Hackeborn: Zur Bedeutung der geistlichen Sinne," in Dinzelbacher and Bauer, eds., *Frauenmystik*, pp. 123-151.

64. Petroff, *Women's Visionary Literature*, pp. 28-32.

65. For Hildegard of Bingen dressing her nuns as brides to receive communion, see "Letter of Abbess T[engswich] of Andernach to Hildegard," epistle 116, PL 197, col. 336c. For examples of cradles and baby Christ figures used by women in the liturgy, see Elisabeth Vavra, "Bildmotiv und Frauenmystik – Funktion und Rezeption," in Dinzelbacher and Bauer, eds., *Frauenmystik*, pp. 201-30; Ursula Schlegel, "The Christchild as Devotional Image in Medieval Italian Sculpture: A Contribution to Ambrogio Lorenzetti Studies," *The Art Bulletin* 52.1 (March 1970), pp. 1-10; and Petroff, *Wom-*

en's Visionary Literature, p. 54, n.22. The crib in the Metropolitan Museum is fifteenth century and from the Grand Beguinage in Louvain.

66. Thurston, PP; I.M. Lewis, *Ecstatic Religion: An Anthropological Study of Spirit Possession and Shamanism* (Harmondsworth: Penguin, 1971); Bynum, "Holy Anorexia in Modern Portugal"; Katherine Carlitz, "Private Suffering as a Public Statement: Biographies of Virtuous Women in Sixteenth-Century China," paper delivered at the Seventh Berkshire Conference on the History of Women, June 1987; Robert McClory, "Cutters: Mutilation: The New Wave in Female Self-Abuse," *Reader: Chicago's Free Weekly* 15.48 (September 5, 1986), pp. 29-38.

67. Le Goff, "Corps et idéologie," pp. 123-25.

68. Robert W. Ackerman, "*The Debate of the Body and the Soul* and Parochial Christianity," *Speculum* 37 (1962), pp. 541-65, esp. pp. 552-53. In the dialogue, Flesh does try to retaliate by suggesting that sin lies rather in the will — i.e., that it should really be charged to Soul's account.

69. Clarissa Atkinson, "Precious Balsam in a Fragile Glass: The Ideology of Virginity in the Later Middle Ages," *Journal of Family History* 8.2 (Summer 1982), pp. 131-43; Marc Glasser, "Marriage in Medieval Hagiography," *Studies in Medieval and Renaissance History* n.s. 4 (1981), pp. 3-34.

70. Kari Elisabeth Børresen, *Subordination et équivalence: Nature et rôle de la femme d'après Augustin et Thomas d'Aquin* (Oslo, 1968); Vern L. Bullough, "Medieval Medical and Scientific Views of Women," *Viator* 4 (1973), pp. 487-93; Eleanor McLaughlin, "Equality of Souls, Inequality of Sexes: Women in Medieval Theology," *Religion and Sexism: Images of Women in the Jewish and Christian Traditions*, eds. Reuther and McLaughlin (New York: Simon and Schuster, 1974), pp. 213-66; Marie-Thérèse d'Alverny, "Comment les théologiens et les philosophes voient la femme?" *La femme dans les civilisations des Xe–XIIIe siècles: Actes du colloque tenu à Poitiers les 23-25 Septembre 1976, Cahiers de civilisation médiévale* 20 (1977), pp. 105-29; Natalie Z. Davis, *Society and Culture in Early Modern France* (Stanford: Stanford University Press, 1975), pp. 124-31.

71. Medieval theologians sometimes carried the dichotomy further, suggesting that the mother was responsible for the nurture of the child's body but the father was charged with its *educatio* — that is, the nourishing of its soul. See John T. Noonan, Jr., *Contraception: A History of Its Treatment by the Catholic Theologians and Canonists*, enlarged ed. (Cambridge, Mass.: Harvard University Press, 1986), p. 280. Female theologians agreed with male ones about the dichotomy but sometimes used it in unusual ways. See, for example, the discussion of Hildegard of Bingen in Prudence Allen, *The Concept of Woman: The Aristotelian Revolution 750 B.C. — A.D. 1250* (Montreal and London: Eden Press, 1985), p. 297, and the works on Hildegard cited in n.104 below.

72. Weinstein and Bell, SS, pp. 234-36; Dalarun, "Eve, Marie ou Madeleine?"

73. James of Voragine, *Legenda aurea vulgo historia lombardica dicta*, ed. T. Graesse (Dresden and Leipzig: Libraria Arnoldiana, 1846). According to my very rough count, twenty-three of twenty-four female martyrs defend their virginity. (Twelve die.) There are only six cases of male saints whose virginity is threatened. (Only one dies.) In contrast, there are forty-eight temporary resurrections of men, only nine of women. Such an emphasis on the inviolability of the living female body should be placed against the background of the culture's similar emphasis on the incorruptibility of the female dead and in the context also of various miraculous body closures; see above n.32 and below n.98. On the extraordinary popularity and diffusion of the Golden Legend, see Brenda Dunn-Lardeau, ed., *Legenda aurea: Sept siècles de diffusion* (Montreal and Paris: Bellarmin and J. Vrin, 1986).

74. For an influential article that projects back into the earlier Western tradition the modern nature/culture contrast, see Sherry Ortner, "Is Female to Male as Nature Is to Culture?" in Michelle Z. Rosaldo and Louise Lamphere, eds., *Women, Culture and Society* (Stanford: Stanford University Press, 1974), pp. 67-86. For criticisms of Ortner's approach, on these and other grounds, see Eleanor Leacock and June Nash, "Ideologies of Sex: Archetypes and Stereotypes," *Issues in Cross-Cultural Research* 285 (New York: New York Academy of Sciences, 1977), pp. 618-45; and Carol P. MacCormack and M. Strathern, eds., *Nature, Culture and Gender* (Cambridge: Cambridge University Press, 1980). The point about the mixing of genders has been nicely made by Eleanor McLaughlin, " 'Christ My Mother': Feminine Naming and Metaphor in Medieval Spirituality," *Nashota Review* 15 (1975).

75. See Valerie Lagorio, "Variations on the Theme of God's Motherhood in Medieval English Mystical and Devotional Writings," *Studia mystica* 8 (1985), pp. 15-37, which gives citations to earlier literature on the subject.

76. HFHF, pp. 266-67.

77. Gertrud Schiller, *Ikonographie der christlichen Kunst*, vol. 4, pt. 1: *Die Kirche* (Gütersloh: Gerd Mohn, 1976), plates 217-19; and Robert Zapperi, *L'Homme enceint: L'Homme, la femme et le pouvoir*, trans. M.-A.M. Vigueur (Paris: Presses Universitaires de France, 1983), pp. 19-46.

78. For Christ bleeding into the chalice (either in the so-called "Mass of St. Gregory" or the "Eucharistic Man of Sorrows"), see Gertrud Schiller, *Iconography of Christian Art*, trans. J. Seligman, vol. 2, *The Passion of Jesus Christ* (London: Humphries, 1972), plates 707, 708, 710, 806; and Ewald M. Vetter, "Mulier amicta sole und mater salvatoris," *Münchner Jahrbuch der bildenden Kunst*, ser. 3, vols. 9 and 10 (1958-59), pp. 32-71, esp. p. 51. For the so-called "Double Intercession," in which Christ's wound is made parallel to Mary's lactating breast, see Schiller, *Iconography*, vol. 2, *Passion*, pls. 798 and 802; Barbara G. Lane, *The Altar and the Altarpiece: Sacramental Themes in Early Netherlandish Painting* (New York: Harper & Row, 1984), pp. 7-8; and A. Monballieu, "Het Antonius

Tsgrootentriptiekje (1507) uit Tongerloo van Goosen van der Weyden," *Jaarboek van het Koninklijk Museum voor Schone Kunsten Antwerpen* (1967), pp. 13-36. I am grateful to Stephen Wight and James Marrow for help with this point and with the material in the next two notes.

79. HFHF, pp. 165-80. By the sixteenth century, artists often showed Catherine drinking from Christ's side while he lifted the open wound toward her mouth with his fingers in the same gesture *Maria lactans* usually employs to present her nipple to her baby son. See engravings by M. Florini (1597) and Pieter de Jode (1600 or 1606), after Francisco Vanni; W. Pleister, "Katharina von Siena," *Lexikon der christlichen Ikonographie*, ed. W. Braunfels (Vienna: Herder, 1974), vol. 7, col. 305, pl. 4; and "Peeter de Jode I," *Wurzbuch Niederländisches Kunstler Lexikon* (Leipzig: Halm und Goldmann, 1906), vol. 1, p. 759, item 12. See also the painting of Catherine's vision by Ludovico Gimignani (1643-97) reproduced in Jean-Noël Vuarnet, *Extases féminines* (Paris: Artaud, 1980), n.p., and the eighteenth-century painting of the same scene by Gaetano Lapis reproduced in Giuliana Zandri, "Documenti per Santa Caterina da Siena in Via Giulia," *Commentari* 22 (1971), p. 242, fig. 2.

80. The picture reproduced in figure 6 exists in at least four versions; the best (signed and dated to 1527) is in Munich. See *Le siècle de Bruegel: La peinture en Belgique au XVIe siècle*, 2nd ed. (Brussels: Musées Royaux des Beaux-Arts de Belgique, 1963), pp. 106-07, item 115; and Max J. Friedländer, *Early Netherlandish Painting*, vol. 8, *Jan Gossart and Bernart van Orley*, notes by Pauwels and Herzog, trans. H. Norden (Leyden: Sijhoff, 1972), pl. 29. Several other depictions of the Virgin and child by Gossart show a similar enlarging of the child's breasts: see Friedländer, *Jan Gossart*, pl. 31, no. 30, pl. 36, nos. 38a and b; and Larry Silver, "*Figure nude, historie e poesie*: Jan Gossaert and the Renaissance Nude in the Netherlands," *Nederlands kunsthistorisch Jaarboek* 36 (1986), pp. 25-28. One of these uses the two-fingered lifting gesture by which the Virgin calls attention to the child's nipple: Friedländer, *Jan Gossart*, pl. 31, no. 30. Gossart also draws attention to the Virgin's breast, especially by having the child lean on it, stroke it or cuddle against it as he sleeps; see *ibid.*, pls. 33, 36, 38; and Silver, "*Figure nude*," p. 28, pl. 45. It is possible that one should not seek a Christological explanation for this iconographic emphasis, since Gossart appears in at least one place to represent *putti* with engorged breasts; see the *putti* on the base of the columns depicted on shutters now in the Toledo Museum; Friedländer, *Jan Gossart*, pl. 17. Gossart shared the late medieval–Renaissance fascination with hermaphrodites; he drew the famous statue of the *Resting Apollo* or *Hermaphrodite* on his trip to Rome in 1508 and illustrated the story of Hermaphroditus and Salmacis: see Max Friedländer, *Early Netherlandish Painting: From Van Eyck to Bruegel*, trans. Marguerite Kay (New York: Phaidon, 1965), p. 96 and pl. 210; and Silver, "*Figure nude*," p. 17. His hermaphroditic infants may reflect this interest or may indeed simply be Mannerist efforts to shock. Critical discussion of Gossart always emphasizes

the "massive," "heavy," "carnal" quality of the bodies he depicts; his attention to the breast and especially to the engorged male breast has not been commented on.

81. Pouchelle, *Corps*, pp. 157-60. It is a truism that medical and theological opinion were not, in the Middle Ages, fully compatible; this was especially true of opinion about sexual practice and abstinence. See Joan Cadden, "Medieval Scientific and Medical Views of Sexuality: Questions of Propriety," *Medievalia et Humanistica* n.s. 14 (1986), pp. 157-71; and Jacquart and Thomasset, *Sexualité*, p. 265ff. Nonetheless, in the ideas about gender which I discuss here, medical, theological and folk conceptions were quite often compatible and similar. See also Park, "Medicine and Society in Medieval Europe."

82. See HFHF and Bynum, "The Body of Christ in the Later Middle Ages: A Reply to Leo Steinberg," *Renaissance Quarterly* 39.3 (1986), pp. 399-439. In what follows, I shall not, for the most part, repeat documentation given in those two studies.

83. Thomas Aquinas, *Summa theologiae*, Blackfriars ed., 61 vols. (New York: McGraw-Hill, 1964-81), pt. 3a, q. 28, art. 1, vol. 51, p. 41, and 3a, q. 32, art. 4, vol. 52, p. 55. Bonaventure, *De assumptione B. Virginis Mariae*, sermon 1, sec. 2, in *S. Bonaventurae opera omnia*, ed. Collegium S. Bonaventurae (Quarrachi: Collegium S. Bonaventurae, 1901), vol. 9, p. 690.

84. Lane, *Altar*, pp. 71-72; Carol J. Purtle, *The Marian Paintings of Jan van Eyck* (Princeton, 1982), pp. 13-15, 27-29 and passim; Vetter, "Mulier amicta sole und mater salvatoris"; and Bynum, "Reply to Steinberg," pl. 8.

85. Erna Lesky, *Die Zeugungs- und Vererbungslehren der Antike und ihr Nachwirken* (Mainz, 1950); Joseph Needham, *A History of Embryology*, 2nd ed. (Cambridge: Cambridge University Press, 1959), pp. 37-74; Anthony Preus, "Galen's Criticism of Aristotle's Conception Theory," *Journal of the History of Biology* 10 (1977), pp. 65-85; Thomas Laqueur, "Orgasm, Generation and the Politics of Reproductive Biology," in *The Making of the Modern Body*, eds. Gallagher and Laqueur; *idem*, *The Female Orgasm and the Body Politic*, work in progress; and Pouchelle, *Corps*. Galen's two-seed theory holds that both male and female contribute to the matter of the fetus; Galen is unclear, however, on what the female seed is — i.e., on whether it is the menstruum or a female lubricant; see Preus, "Galen's Criticism." The situation in the Middle Ages was further complicated by the fact that Galen was known partly in spurious texts; see Luke Demaitre and Anthony A. Travill, "Human Embryology and Development in the Works of Albertus Magnus," in *Albertus Magnus and the Sciences*, ed. Weisheipl, pp. 414-16. The account of Galen and his influence in Allen, *Concept of Woman*, is oversimplified.

86. Pouchelle, *Corps*, p. 234 and passim.

87. M. Anthony Hewson, *Giles of Rome and the Medieval Theory of Conception: A Study of the* De

formatione corporis humani in utero (London: University of London, Athlone Press, 1975); and Jacquart and Thomasset, *Sexualité*, pp. 87-92.

88. See Mary McLaughlin, "Survivors and Surrogates: Children and Parents from the Ninth to the Thirteenth Centuries," *The History of Childhood*, ed. L. DeMause (New York: Psychohistory Press, 1974), pp. 115-18; Charles T. Wood, "The Doctors' Dilemma: Sin, Salvation and the Menstrual Cycle in Medieval Thought," *Speculum* 56 (1981), pp. 710-27, esp. p. 719; Pouchelle, *Corps*, pp. 263-66. The Aristotelian idea that blood is the basic fluid, concocted into milk, semen, etc., is a partial departure from the earlier theory of the four humors and not fully compatible with it; see Preus, "Galen's Criticism," pp. 76-78.

89. Pouchelle, *Corps*, p. 264. Some anatomists actually held that the womb and breasts were connected by a blood vessel; see Jacquart and Thomasset, *Sexualité*, pp. 59-60, 71-72.

90. *Ibid.*, p. 100.

91. Blood was a highly ambiguous symbol. But exactly because the culture held it to be in some ways impure, the shedding of blood, either naturally or through cauterization or leeching, was purgative. Thus, although menstrual blood was taboo, menstruation was a necessary and positive function. See Pouchelle, *Corps*, pp. 115-23; Jacquart and Thomasset, *Sexualité*, pp. 99-108; Kroll and Bachrach, "Sin and...Disease," esp. p. 409; and L. Gougaud, "La pratique de la phlébotomie dans les cloîtres," *Revue Mabillon* 53 (1924), pp. 1-13.

92. Male suspicion of women's visionary and charismatic experiences, like male distrust of the female body, was never absent. It seems to have increased in the later fourteenth, fifteenth and sixteenth centuries. See Vauchez, *La Sainteté*, pp. 439-48; Weinstein and Bell, SS, pp. 228-32; and Edouard Dumoutet, *Corpus Domini: Aux sources de la pieté eucharistique médiévale* (Paris, 1942), p. 125. The increase in witchcraft accusations in the same period is an aspect of this mistrust.

93. Francine Cardman, "The Medieval Question of Women and Orders," *The Thomist* 42 (October 1978), pp. 582-99.

94. For examples of hagiographers who praise women as "virile," see "Life of Ida of Louvain," AASS, April, vol. 2 (1865), p. 159; and "Life of Ida of Léau," AASS, October, vol. 13 (1883), p. 112. The compliment could, of course, cut both ways.

95. According to Christ and Paul, the first shall be last, the meek shall inherit the earth, and the foolishness of men is wisdom before God. See Bynum, *Jesus as Mother*, pp. 127-28, and *idem*, "Women's Stories, Women's Symbols: A Critique of Victor Turner's Theory of Liminality," *Anthropology and the Study of Religion*, ed. F. Reynolds and R. Moore (Chicago: Center for the Scientific Study of Religion, 1984), pp. 105-24.

96. Bynum, *Jesus as Mother*, pp. 110-69; HFHF, pp. 80 and 281; Vauchez, *La Sainteté*, p. 446 n.511; Dronke, *Women Writers*.

97. Laqueur, *Female Orgasm*; Pouchelle, *Corps*, pp. 223-27, 307-10, 323-25; Jacquart and Thomasset, *Sexualité*, pp. 50-52; Claude Thomasset, "La réprésentation de la sexualité et de la génération dans la pensée scientifique médiévale," in *Love and Marriage in the Twelfth Century*, eds. Willy Van Hoecke and A. Welkenhuysen, Mediaevalia Lovaniensia, ser. 1, studia 8 (Louvain: The University Press, 1981), pp. 1-17, esp. pp. 7-8.

98. In discussing women's right to drink wine in the monastery, Abelard claims that women are rarely inebriated because their bodies are humid and pierced with many holes. See Allen, *Concept of Woman*, p. 281. See also Pouchelle, *Corps*, pp. 310 and 323-27, and Jacquart and Thomasset, *Sexualité*, p. 66, on the general sense in the culture that the female body is full of openings. Such assumptions are part of the background to the emphasis in saints' lives on miraculous closure; see above nn.29 and 32, and Pouchelle, *Corps*, pp. 224-28. To religious writers, the good female body is closed and intact; the bad woman's body is open, windy and breachable. At the same time, the closed, secret and virgin body of a woman is fascinating and threatening, inviting investigation.

99. See above n.85.

100. There is much about this in Allen, *Concept of Woman* (although the individual accounts are not always correct). See also Jacquart and Thomasset, *Sexualité*, pp. 193-95; and Thomasset, "La réprésentation."

101. See Demaitre and Travill, "Albertus Magnus," pp. 432-34; Thomasset, "La réprésentation," pp. 5-7; J.M. Thijssen, "Twins as Monsters: Albertus Magnus's Theory of the Generation of Twins and Its Philosophical Context," *Bulletin of the History of Medicine* 61 (1967), pp. 237-46; and André Pecker, *Hygiène et maladie de la femme au cours des siècles* (Paris: Dacosta, 1961), c. 5 – a quasi-popular account that nonetheless makes the interest in hermaphrodites quite clear. Stories of bearded women were also popular at the close of the Middle Ages.

102. Zapperi, *L'Homme enceint*; and Pouchelle, *Corps*, pp. 142 and 223.

103. On the increased attention to the physicality of Christ in the later Middle Ages, see Kieckhefer, *Unquiet Souls*, pp. 89-121. On the increasingly positive sense of body generally, see Alan E. Bernstein, "Political Anatomy," *University Publishing* (Winter 1978), pp. 8-9.

104. On Hildegard, see Barbara Newman, *Sister of Wisdom: St. Hildegard's Theology of the Feminine* (Berkeley: University of California Press, 1987); and Elisabeth Gössmann, "Das Menschenbild der Hildegard von Bingen und Elisabeth von Schoenau vor dem Hintergrund der frühscholastischen Anthropologie," in Dinzelbacher and Bauer, eds., *Frauenmystik*, pp. 24-47. On Julian, see E. McLaugh-

lin, " 'Christ Our Mother.' " On Margery Kempe, see Clarissa W. Atkinson, *Mystic and Pilgrim: The Book and the World of Margery Kempe* (Ithaca: Cornell University Press, 1983).

105. See above nn. 4, 5, 67-73.

106. Allen, *Concept of Woman*. See also Maryanne Cline Horowitz, "Aristotle and Women," *Journal of the History of Biology* 9 (1976), pp. 186-213.

107. A recent nonscholarly book that argues this position is Frank Bottomley, *Attitudes Toward the Body in Western Christendom* (London: Lepus Books, 1979).

108. See Oscar Cullman, "Immortality of the Soul or Resurrection of the Dead? The Witness of the New Testament," in Terence Penelhum, ed., *Immortality* (Belmont, Cal.: Wadsworth, 1973), pp. 53-84.

109. Richard Heinzmann, *Die Unsterblichkeit der Seele und die Auferstehung des Leibes: Eine problemgeschichtliche Untersuchung der frühscholastischen Sentenzen- und Summenliteratur von Anselm von Laon bis Wilhelm von Auxerre*, Beiträge zur Geschichte der Philosophie und Theologie des Mittelalters: Texte und Untersuchungen 40.3 (Münster: Aschendorff, 1965); and Hermann J. Weber, *Die Lehre von der Auferstehung der Toten in den Haupttraktaten der scholastischen Theologie von Alexander von Hales zu Duns Skotus*, Freiburger Theologische Studien (Freiburg: Herder, 1973). Thomas Aquinas, *Quaestiones disputatae de potentia Dei absolute*, q. 5, art. 10, ed. P.M. Pession, in Thomas Aquinas, *Quaestiones disputatae*, vol. 2, ed. P. Bazzi et al., 8th ed. (Rome: Marietti, 1949), pp. 43-44, says explicitly that Porphyry's idea that the soul is happiest without the body, and Plato's idea that the body is a tool of the soul, are wrong; the soul is more like God when it is united to the body than when it is separated, because it is then more perfect.

110. Hewson, *Giles of Rome*, p. 56, n.21.

111. See the works cited in n.109 above.

112. Weber, *Auferstehung*, pp. 80-106.

113. A. Michel, "Résurrection des morts," DTC 13, pt. 2, cols. 2501-03. Benedict XII, in the bull *Benedictus Deus*, cited the profession of faith of Michael Paleologus at the Second Council of Lyon of 1274 which asserted that *omnes homines* appear before the tribunal of Christ in the Last Judgment *cum suis corporibus*. See below n.144.

114. Michel, "Résurrection des morts," cols. 2501-71. And see Aquinas, *On the Truth of the Catholic Faith: Summa contra gentiles*, trans. Anton Pegis et al., 4 vols. in 5 (New York: Image Books, 1955-57), 4, ch. 85, par. 4, vol. 4, pp. 323-24; and Wilhelm Kübel, "Die Lehre von der Auferstehung der Toten nach Albertus Magnus," *Studia Albertina: Festschrift für Bernhard Geyer zum 70. Geburtstage*, ed. H. Ostlender, Beiträge zur Geschichte der Philosophie und Theologie der Mittelalters, Supplementband 4 (Münster: Aschendorff, 1952), pp. 279-318. For the position that *all* must rise and that *body* must

be rewarded or punished for good or evil deeds, theologians regularly cited 2 Cor.5.10.

115. See, for example, Moneta of Cremona, *Adversus Catharos et Valdenses libri quinque* (Rome, 1743. Reprint: Ridgewood, N.J.: Gregg Press, 1964), bk. 4, chs. 8-12, pp. 346-88; and on Moneta, Georg Schmitz-Valckenberg, *Grundlehren katharischer Sekten des 13. Jahrhunderts: Eine theologische Untersuchung mit besonderer Berücksichtigung von Adversus Catharos et Valdenses des Moneta von Cremona*, Münchener Universitäts-Schriften: Kath. Theologische Fakultät: Veröffentlichungen des Grabmann-Institutes zur Erforschung der mittelalterlichen Theologie und Philosophie, NF 11 (Munich: Schöningh, 1971), pp. 196-207.

116. Many of the extant sources on the Cathar position (both anti-Cathar polemic and Cathar material itself) suggest that the dualists' insistence on "spiritual body" and their denial of any resurrection of physical body was based on their abhorrence of matter — its tangibility, putrefiability, dissolvability. One has the sense that, to the Cathars (at least as they appeared to orthodox eyes), the paradigmatic body was the cadaver. See Walter L. Wakefield and Austin P. Evans, eds., *Heresies of the High Middle Ages: Selected Sources Translated and Annotated*, Record of Civilization 81 (New York: Columbia University Press, 1969), pp. 167, 231, 238-39, 297, 311-13, 321-23, 337, 339-42, 343-45, 353, 357, 361, 380. See also M.D. Lambert, "The Motives of the Cathars: Some Reflections...," *Religious Motivation: Biographical and Sociological Problems for the Church Historian*, Studies in Church History 15 (1978), pp. 49-59.

117. Wood, "Doctors' Dilemma"; *idem*, "Gynecological Aspects of the Annunciation," to appear in *Actes du colloque l'Annonciation à la Renaissance* (Florence: Casa Usher); Edward D. O'Connor, ed., *The Dogma of the Immaculate Conception: History and Significance* (Notre Dame, Ind.: University of Notre Dame Press, 1958).

118. Albert the Great, *De animalibus libri XXVI nach der Cölner Urschrift*, vol. 1, Beiträge zur Geschichte der Philosophie des Mittelalters: Texte und Untersuchungen 15 (Münster: Aschendorff, 1916), bk. 9, tract. 1, ch. 2, p. 682.

119. Weber, *Auferstehung*, pp. 13-41 and 235-36; Hewson, *Giles of Rome*, pp. 38-58; Kübel, "Die Lehre...nach Albertus," esp. p. 299.

120. Aquinas, *De potentia Dei*, q. 6, arts. 5-10, pp. 49-54. Aquinas argues (art. 8) that Christ willed to eat after the Resurrection to show the reality of his body; angels cannot, however, really eat and speak (i.e., move the organs and the air or divide food and send it throughout the body). The analysis makes it quite clear that the human body/soul nexus is far closer than that suggested by any model of a spirit using a material object (as the angels do). See esp. art. 8, reply to obj. 8, where Aquinas explains why Christ's eating after the Resurrection is different from the angels' eating, even though in

neither case can food be changed into flesh and blood.

121. Thomas wrote, probably in the following order, four lives of women saints, all of which are characterized by somatic miracles and highly experiential piety: a supplement to James of Vitry's "Life of Mary of Oignies," AASS, June, vol. 5 (1867), pp. 572-81; a "Life of Christina the Astonishing" (which contains the most remarkable somatic miracles of any thirteenth-century woman's *vita*) AASS, July, vol. 5 (1868), pp. 637-60; a "Life of Margaret of Ypres" (see above n.35); and a "Life of Lutgard of Aywières" (which he composed in order to obtain her finger as a relic), AASS, June, vol. 4, pp. 187-210. He also composed a *vita* of John, first abbot of Cantimpré. His *Bonum universale de apibus*, ed. Georges Colvener (Douai, 1627), is a collection of miracle stories, many of which display a concern for body. On this, see Henri Platelle, "Le recueil des miracles de Thomas de Cantimpré et la vie religieuse dans les Pays-Bas et le nord de la France au XIIIe siècle, " in *Assistance et assistés jusqu'à 1610*, Actes du 97e Congrès National des Sociétés Savantes, Nantes, 1972 (Paris: Bibliothèque Nationale, 1979), pp. 469-98; and Alexander Murray, "Confession as a Historical Source in the Thirteenth Century," in *The Writing of History in the Middle Ages: Essays Presented to Richard William Southern* (Oxford: Clarendon Press, 1981), pp. 275-322, especially pp. 286-305.

122. *Die Gynäkologie des Thomas von Brabant: Ein Beitrag zur Kenntnis der mittelalterlichen Gynäkologie und ihrer Quellen*, ed. C. Ferckel (Munich: Carl Kuhn, 1912), an edition of part of bk.1 of Thomas of Cantimpré's *De naturis rerum*; there is a new ed. by Helmut Boese, *Liber de natura rerum: Editio princeps secundum codices manuscriptos*, vol. 1, *Text* (New York and Berlin: De Gruyter, 1973). On Thomas's encyclopedia, see Pierre Michaud-Quantin, "Les petites encyclopédies du XIIIe siècle," *Cahiers d'histoire mondiale* 9.2 (1966), *Encyclopédies et civilisations*, pp. 580-95; G.J.J. Walstra "Thomas de Cantimpré, *De naturis rerum*: Etat de la question," *Vivarium* 5 (1967), pp. 146-71, and 6 (1968), pp. 46-61; and Helmut Boese, "Zur Textüberlieferung von Thomas Cantimpratensis' *Liber de natura rerum*," *Archivum fratrum praedicatorum* 39 (1969), pp. 53-68.

123. See Katherine Park and Eckhart Kessler, "The Concept of Psychology," and K. Park, "The Organic Soul," in Charles B. Schmitt, ed., *The Cambridge History of Renaissance Philosophy* (Cambridge: Cambridge University Press) chs. 13 and 14, forthcoming; and E. Ruth Harvey, *The Inward Wits: Psychological Theory in the Middle Ages and the Renaissance*, Warburg Institute Surveys 6 (London: Warburg Institute, 1975).

124. See Preus, "Galen's Criticism." See also Michael Boylan, "The Galenic and Hippocratic Challenges to Aristotle's Conception Theory," *Journal of the History of Biology* 17 (1984), pp. 83-112.

125. See Hewson, *Giles of Rome*.

126. See the works cited in n.109 above, and Michel, "Résurrection des morts." For a modern

position on the survival question that agrees with Thomas, see Peter Geach, "Immortality," in Penelhum, *Immortality*, p. 11ff.

127. Aquinas, Commentary on 1 Cor. 15, lect. 2, quoted in Emile Mersch and Robert Brunet, "Corps mystique et spiritualité," *Dictionnaire de spiritualité, ascétique et mystique: doctrine et histoire*, vol. 2, pt. 2 (Paris: Beauchesne, 1953), col. 2352.

128. In general, see Heinzmann, *Unsterblichkeit*, pt. 2 passim, and Weber, *Auferstehung*, passim, esp. pp. 125-57 and 217-54. On the question of the necessity of material continuity for numerical continuity, answers ranged from William of Auxerre (in the early thirteenth century), who argued that the ashes of Paul must rise as the body of Paul (Heinzmann, *Unsterblichkeit*, p. 243, n.11), to Durandus (in the early fourteenth century) who held that God can make the body of Peter out of dust that was once the body of Paul (Weber, *Auferstehung*, p. 228ff., especially p. 241, n.400).

129. Because of this telescoping of body into soul, some recent interpreters have debated how important body is to Thomas. Does it really add anything to the capacities of soul? See Norbert Luyten, "The Significance of the Body in a Thomistic Anthropology," *Philosophy Today* 7 (1963), pp. 175-93; J. Giles Milhaven, "Physical Experience: Contrasting Appraisals by Male Theologians and Women Mystics in the Middle Ages," paper given at the Holy Cross Symposium "The Word Becomes Flesh," November 9, 1985; Richard Swinburne, *The Evolution of the Soul* (Oxford: Clarendon Press, 1986), pp. 299-306, esp. n.9; and the article by Bazan cited in n.130 below. Nonetheless, Aquinas did argue that, without body, the soul in heaven before the end of time would in a certain sense lack memory and other passions; see *Summa contra gentiles* 2, ch. 81, pars. 12, 14-15, vol. 2, pp. 264-66.

130. *Summa contra gentiles* 4, ch. 81, par. 7, vol. 4, p. 303: "Corporeity, however, can be taken in two ways. In one way, it can be taken as the substantial form of a body.... Therefore, coporeity, as the substantial form in man, cannot be other than the rational soul...." See Bernardo C. Bazan, "La corporalité selon saint Thomas," *Revue philosophique de Louvain* 81, ser. 4.49 (1983), pp. 369-409, esp. pp. 407-08. Bazan says that, according to Thomas, "Notre corporalité est toute pénétrée de spiritualité, car sa source est l'âme rationnelle."

131. Bonaventure, *De assumptione B. Virginis Mariae*, sermon 1, sec. 2, p. 690. See also Aquinas, *Summa contra gentiles* 4, ch. 79, par. 11, vol. 4, p. 299; and the passage from *De potentia Dei*, cited in n.109 above.

132. Heinzmann, *Unsterblichkeit*, p. 188, quotes a passage from the *Summa called Breves dies hominis* in which Plato is represented as supporting the position that resurrection is natural because of the longing of soul for body. This suggests that contemporaries were aware that a Platonic position tends in some ways to give more weight to body than an Aristotelian one (and not necessarily negative weight).

133. Weber, *Auferstehung*, p. 326. The doctrine of the plurality of forms seems to lurk behind much of Franciscan teaching on the gifts (*dotes*) of the glorified body, for thinkers such as Bonaventure and Richard of Middleton hold that body is in some way predisposed for the flowing over of glory into it before it receives the *dotes*; see *ibid.*, p. 314ff. Such a position tends to give substantial reality to body.

134. Weber, *Auferstehung*, p. 304, n.197; and see *ibid.*, pp. 266 and 135-36.

135. Bernard, *De diligendo Deo*, sec. 11, pars. 30-33, in *Tractatus et opuscula, Sancti Bernardi opera*, vol. 3 (1963), pp. 145-47; trans. Robert Walton, *The Works of Bernard of Clairvaux*, vol. 5, *Treatises*, vol. 2, Cistercian Fathers Series 13 (Washington D.C.: Cistercian Publications, 1974), pp. 122-24.

136. Weber, *Auferstehung*, pp. 255-63. Thomas held that risen bodies will have the capacity for touch; see *Summa contra gentiles* 4, ch. 84, par. 14, vol. 4, pp. 322-23. Risen bodies will not, however, eat: see *Summa contra gentiles* 4, ch. 83, vol. 4, pp. 311-20.

137. Nikolaus Wicki, *Die Lehre von der himmlischen Seligkeit in der mittelalterlichen Scholastik von Petrus Lombardus bis Thomas von Aquinas*, Studia Friburgensia NF 9 (Freiburg: Universitätsverlag, 1954); Joseph Göring, "The *De Dotibus* of Robert Grosseteste," *Mediaeval Studies* 44 (1982), pp. 83-109; and Weber, *Auferstehung*, pp. 314-42.

138. See, for example, Hugh of St. Victor, *De sacramentis* 2, pt. 18, ch. 18; PL 176 (1854), col. 616A; Peter Lombard, *Sententiae in IV libris distinctae*, vol. 2, 3rd ed., Spicilegium Bonaventurianum 5 (Grottaferrata: Collegium Bonaventurae ad Claras Aquas, 1981), bk. 4, distinctio 44, pp. 510-22; and *Summa contra gentiles* 4, ch. 90, par. 9, vol. 4, p. 334.

139. See, for example, *Summa contra gentiles* 4, ch. 88, vol. 4, pp. 328-30; and *Summa theologiae* 3a, q. 54, art. 4, vol. 55, pp. 30-35. See also Supplement to *Summa theologiae* 3, q. 96, art. 10, on whether the scars of the martyrs are an *aureole*; *Supplementum*, comp. and ed. by the Brothers of the Order, in *Sancti Thomae Aquinatis opera omnia*, vol. 12 (Rome: S.C. de Propaganda Fide, 1906), p. 238. In general, thirteenth-century theologians drew on Augustine's *City of God*, bk. 22, ch. 17 ("vitia detrahentur, natura servabitur") on this matter; see Weber, *Auferstehung*, p. 79, n.194.

140. Allen, *Concept of Woman*; Weber, *Auferstehung*, pp. 256-59. Weber quotes Augustinus Triumphus, writing on the resurrection, to the effect that, if persons were to rise in the opposite sex, they would not be the same persons: "Non omnes resurgentes eundem sexum habebunt, nam masculinus sexus et femininus, quamvis non sint differentiae formales facientes differentiam in specie, sunt tamen differentiae materiales facientes differentiam in numero. Et quia in resurrectione quilibet resurget non solum quantum ad id quod est de identitate specifica, secundum habet esse in specie humana, verum etiam resurget quantum ad id, quod est de identitate numerali, secundum quam

habet esse in tali individuo. Ideo oportet unumquodque cum sexu proprio et cum aliis pertinentibus ad integritatem suae individualis naturae resurgere, propter quod femina resurget cum sexu femineo et homo cum masculino, remota omni libidine et omni vitiositate naturae." Moneta of Cremona, writing against the Cathars, argued that God created sex difference: see Moneta, *Adversus Catharos*, bk. 1, ch. 2, sec. 4, and bk. 4, ch. 7, sec. 1, pp. 121 and 315.

141. The resurrected bodies of the damned will be incapable of corruption (i.e., of dissolution or of loss of their matter) but not incapable of suffering. See n.144 below.

142. Theologians were aware that some of the particular issues they raised in debates over eschatology had implications for the cult of relics – particularly the issue of whether the cadaver of John is still the body of John and whether its specific matter must rise in John at the Last Judgment. See Weber, *Auferstehung*, pp. 76-78, 150-53, 239, and n.128 above.

143. *Summa theologiae* 3a, q. 14, arts. 1-4, vol. 49, pp. 170-87, esp. p. 174.

144. Indeed, scholastic theologians held that the damned also receive their bodies *whole* after the resurrection, because only the permanence (i.e., the perfect balance or wholeness) of these bodies ensures that their punishment will be permanent and perpetual; see Kübel, "Die Lehre...nach Albertus," pp. 316-17.

145. After fierce debate, the issue was finally settled by Benedict XII in the bull *Benedictus Deus* of January 29, 1336; see Henry Denzinger, *Enchiridion symbolorum: Definitionum et declarationum de rebus fidei et morum*, 31st ed., ed. C. Rahner (Freiburg: Herder, 1957), pp. 229-30. For a brief overview, see M.J. Redle, "Beatific Vision," *New Catholic Encyclopedia* (Washington D.C.: Catholic University of America, 1967), vol. 2, pp. 186-93.

146. A. Challet, "Corps glorieux," DTC 3, cols. 1879-1906.

147. See, for example, the cases of Jane Mary of Maillé and Columba of Rieti, in HFHF, pp. 131-134, 148.

148. *Summa theologiae* 3a, q. 15, art. 5, obj. 3 and reply, vol. 49, pp. 204-07; and see also *ibid.*, 3a, q. 14, art. 1, obj. 2 and reply, pp. 170-75. Bernard of Clairvaux expresses the same opinion in *De diligendo Deo*, sec. 10, par. 29, *Tractatus et opuscula*, p. 144.

149. Caesarius, *Dialogus*, bk. 12, ch. 47, vol. 2, p. 354.

150. *Ibid.*, ch. 50, vol. 2, pp. 355-56; see also *ibid.*, ch. 54, p. 358. For the importance of marks of healing visible on the body, see Judith-Danielle Jacquet, "Le Miracle de la jambe noire," in Gelis and Redon, eds., *Les miracles miroirs des corps*, pp. 23-52.

151. See above, n.32. A related issue concerning incorruptibility, which I do not have space to treat here, is the incorruptibility of the bodies of great sinners; see Thomas, *Le cadavre*, pp. 39-43,

who however underestimates the importance of incorruptibility for sanctity.

152. *Summa theologiae* 3a, q. 15, art. 4, vol. 49, p. 202 (my translation).

153. Doctors showed their own awareness of such psychosomatic unity. For example, Henri de Mondeville, skeptical about miraculous cures, explained their apparent success thus: "If the human spirit believes that a thing is useful (which in itself is of no help), it may happen that by the imagination alone this thing aids the body." See Pouchelle, *Corps*, p. 107. Mondeville shows by many examples how "in acting on the soul one acts on the body" (*ibid.*, p. 108).

154. Henri Platelle, "La Voix du sang: Le cadavre qui saigne en presence de son meutrier," *La piété populaire au moyen age*, Actes du 99e Congrès National des Sociétés Savantes, Besançon 1974 (Paris: Bibliothèque Nationale, 1977), pp. 161-79; Finucane, *Miracles and Pilgrims*, pp. 73-75; Bouvier, "De l'incorruptibilité"; Philippe Aries, *The Hour of Our Death*, trans. Weaver (New York: Knopf, 1981), pp. 261-68 and 353ff.; Jacques Gelis, "De la mort à la vie: Les 'sanctuaires à réprit,'" *Ethnologie française* 11 (1981), pp. 211-24.

155. "Life of Christina Mirabilis," ch. 5, no. 36, par. 47-48, AASS, July, vol. 5, pp. 658-59; trans. Margot H. King, *The Life of Christina Mirabilis*, Matrologia latina 2 (Saskatoon: Peregrina, 1986), pp. 27-28. This little dialogue was supposedly witnessed by Thomas, abbot of St. Trond; see ch. 5, no. 36, par. 47, p. 658. See also, Petroff, *Women's Visionary Literature*, p. 36; and Ackerman, "*Debate of the Body and Soul* and Parochial Christianity."

156. For the text, see Karl Brunner, "Mittelenglische Todesgedichte," *Archiv für das Studium der neueren Sprachen* 167, n.s. 67 (1935), pp. 30-35. See also, Marjorie M. Malvern, "An Earnest 'Monyscyon' and 'thinge Delectabyll' Realized Verbally and Visually in 'A Disputacion Betwyx the Body and Wormes,' A Middle English Poem Inspired by Tomb Art and Northern Spirituality," *Viator* 13 (1982), pp. 415-43.

157. See Malvern, " 'Monyscyon'," pp. 427 and 432ff.

158. Stanzas 24, 28-29 in Brunner, "Mittelenglische Todesgedichte," p. 34.

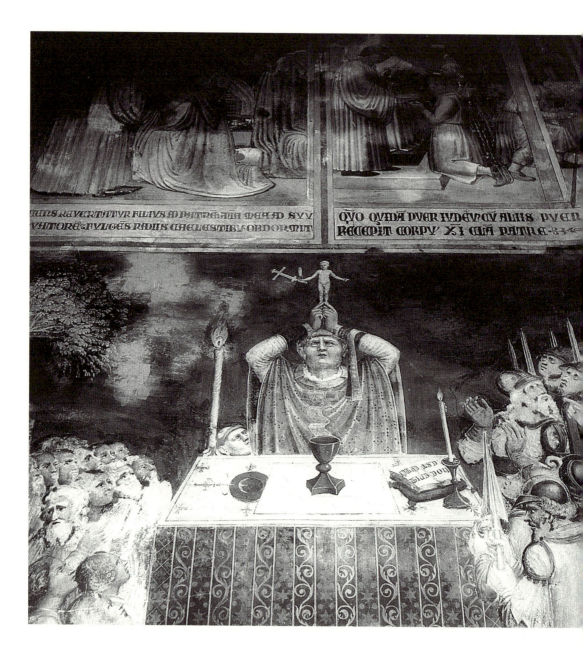

The Host started to bleed in the hands of a priest who doubted the Transubstantiation. Fresco depicting the Miracle of Bolsena, 1263 (Orvieto, Italy).

The Consecrated Host:
A Wondrous Excess

Piero Camporesi

The Mysterious Food

The divine flesh, transmitter of abstract, impalpable powers that put the soul into communication with the ineffable, was also widely perceived as a mysterious, super-human nourishment, a sort of divine marrow that would mete out both health and salvation (the two are indistinguishable in the single, ambiguous term *salus*). It was seen as a heavenly manna and balsam, a supernatural *pharmakon* — the "salubrious *elixir vitae* of His blood " (Giacomo Correglia, *Pratica del confessionario*). "It is with reason that Saint Ambrose called the divine sacrifice "*tutamen et salus animae et corporis*," tutelage and salvation of soul and body and remedy of all spiritual and cor-poreal ills.[1] Christ was the great therapist. By touching the "pulse of the soul," he drew out of it all the ills that lay at the roots of corporeal diseases. He was "the doctor who could heal all infirmities" through confession, the Eucharist and extreme unction. "Doctors acknowledge that a dead man's parts and members can be put to the same parts and members of incurable patients, head to head, mouth to mouth, hand to hand, and will have the power to heal them.... Now, if the body of a dead man can possess such virtue, how much more powerful the body of a God who is all virtue."[2] *Medicina sacramentalis*, the "cordial wafer... composed of the rarest pow-der" had to be taken "at least an hour before the meal." (Thus ran Saint Francis of Sales's spiritual recipe.) This exceptional tonic, *malorum omnium antidotum*, porten-tous reconstituent, the "very divine and very precious viand," the "sacred powder," had the inexplicable power of restoring lost energies.[3]

Even more miraculously and despite natural laws and the most fundamental prin-ciples of existence, the sacramental food could nourish bodies without painful, daily dependence on food. The blessed Gerardo Maiella, a lay brother of the Congre-

221

gazione de Redentore founded by Saint Alphonse de Liguori, could "restore all lost corporeal strength" with the "bread of angels," "so much sweeter and filling" than any earthly repast.[4] The effects of this supersubstantial bread were felt not only by saints and blessed souls but also by simple men and women of intense faith. This "vital food" (*cibus vitalis*) concealed a "manifold strength, not only for the soul, but also for the body [*multiplex fortitudo, non solum animae, sed et corporis*]."[5]

Among various other prodigies, Caesarius of Heisterbach tells us of a very pious woman who received Holy Communion every Sunday and felt absolutely no need to eat for the rest of the week.[6] Unable to believe the reasons for her unusual fasting, her bishop decided to test her and asked her confessor to give her Communion with a nonconsecrated wafer. Unaware of this trick, the following Sunday after Communion, the woman returned home and was suddenly seized by such hunger that she felt she would die unless she ate something as soon as possible. Fearing that this sudden, ferocious hunger was a sign of her sins, she ran to her confessor and told him of the terrible condition into which she had lapsed, all the time lamenting that she could be thoroughly bereft of divine grace. Having duly thanked the Omnipotent, who alone could have worked such a "great wonder" (*mirabilia magna*), the confessor immediately gave her the real body of Christ whose miraculous power immediately halted her terrible hunger and restored the grace of which the bishop — a tempter in reverse — had cheated her.

This exemplum, a rough, medieval parable, lent substantial drama to the occult and "infinite powers" of the consecrated Host, a "mysterious food" whose "sweetness makes all creatures lose their appetite" by sating hunger with "taste and pleasure." Even in modern times, the "effects of the Holy Sacrament in the body," its "admirable flavors" and "penetrating delights," were highly appreciated.[7] Jean-Baptiste Saint-Jure (1588-1657), one of the most authoritative Jesuits of the seventeenth century, noted that both body and soul were deeply affected by them:

> The institution of the Holy Sacrament was meant to provide nourishment to the soul, and indeed it is in the spirit that it mainly and primarily produces its salutary effects, and yet it is certain, in the opinion of both Holy Fathers and Doctors, that these effects also extend to the body, which also benefits by its virtue and vigor.... The same thing is true of the soul that duly receives Our Lord for, just as a well-groomed and perfumed man, upon visiting a friend, hugging him, caressing him and generally spending time

with him, leaves his scent in the room and on his friend after he has gone so that the friend cannot help but remember him even though he is no longer in sight, so does Our Lord, when He passes through the soul which receives Him corporeally, leave in it a kind of balsam and very agreeable scents, certain signs that He was there.[8]

The presence and memory of the divine visit manifested themselves aromatically; they spoke in a language of scent. The soothing and inebriating flesh of Christ, with its penetrating delights, drugged the spiritual flesh of the "human heart," and brought it "marvelous rest and peace." The heavenly physician came to earth to produce an aromatic ecstasy and "purify our flesh with His sacred touch." Just as salt possesses the "virtue of preserving dead flesh, which would otherwise putrefy and teem with worms," so the "infinitely holy and infinitely chaste" flesh transforms man's flesh with its divine aroma like "the flesh of some birds in the East Indies, which never rots because it is fed with aromatic flowers and plants."[9]

The bread of angels "surpasses the flavors of the tastiest things, and exceeds all the sweets that can flatter our senses." To the point that "he, in whom the Paschal Lamb dwells, feels admirable things, sees yet greater things, and speaks of unheard-of wonders," while the "strength of the mysterious wine he has imbibed fills his soul with inexplicable joy."[10]

As a "miracle of miracles," the "divine Sacrament" produced "holy and marvelous effects" which, as well as the internal effects it had on the soul, showed itself "in external signs and miracles": the possessed were exorcised, the lame were healed, incurable infirmities disappeared, "prisoners" were freed from their chains and warriors and duelists drew from it additional energy for their battle.[11]

"Before entering the battlefield with his army," Archduke Leopold of Austria "would order a solemn procession in which the divine Sacrament was carried around to beseech the help and protection of the God of victories; and he [the Archduke] would fortify himself and his soldiers with what the Scriptures refer to as *panis fortium*."[12]

As a rule, the magic particle infused those who ate it with "happiness, sweetness and spiritual pleasure," but at times instead of "pleasure," some experienced "tedium, sadness and bitterness."[13] Inexplicably, for them the "sweetness" and flavor of manna and honey exuded from the body of Christ was a bitter morsel. The opposing effects were clearly the work of an obscurely ambivalent power. Some of the longest fasts, therefore, were seen as the product of the Tempter's subtle skills. Martino Del Rio tells of a young woman whose throat was blocked by the devil and who, as a result, could neither eat nor drink for almost seventy days. And yet, surprisingly enough, after fasting so long, and then for fifteen additional days in the monastery where she had gone for help, the young woman was as fresh and buxom as ever. She did not look thinner and was neither tired nor sick. With the help of the Eucharist,[14] the demon was finally expelled.

These persons who, unlike most mortals, did not lead "the life of animals," who could live "beyond the usual limits of nature," who ate only the food of angels, who achieved "the monstrous and excessive feat" of living without eating, moved in a sphere of supernatural "excess and awe."[15] With angels and demons who also do not eat, they shared a startlingly ambiguous realm where holiness and abjection shifted roles, where the sacred was only a mask for the perverse face of the sacrilegious. In the late fifteenth century, a perplexed chronicler from Cesena records a rumor, originating in Umbria, that concerned the portentous fasts of a Dominican nun who had been repeatedly able to spend the forty days of Lent eating only divine flesh:

> Sister Columba, of the Dominican order, currently (1493) residing in Perosa, never drinks wine or eats cooked food, and has repeatedly spent the entire period of Lent without eating anything aside from what she receives at her daily Communion, the *corpus domini.* This is a great and miraculous thing, which could be either divine or demonic.[16]

The uncertain boundary between the divine and the demonic often extended into the shadowy realm of imposture: the simulation of sanctity, ecstasy or verbal contact with the angels, the affectation of ambiguous "sanctimonia," or even simply the vainglory of imagining oneself holy, as in the case of "a young woman of lowly origins," who, tricked by the devil, did her best to lend "credence and support to her vain claims of sanctity by duplicitous and false means."[17]

Any infraction, however involuntary, in the rigorous ritual of the consecration of bread and wine was seen as particularly serious. The delicate moment of transubstantiation — the transformation of nutritional substances into the blood and body of Christ — had to involve a faithful replica and precise repetition of both liturgical formulas and ceremonial prescriptions. The Eucharist, the sacrifice of the altar, a moment of the highest magico-liturgical tension, *grande mysterium*, the culmination of the entire Mass, the dramatic apex of divine participation and supernatural presence, could also become a stage for *mutationes, apparitiones, miracula*. Everything was possible in the arcane atmosphere of transubstantiation, in the prodigious alchemic balance of divine permutations: the heavenly and the demonic could explode into a war of conflicting powers.

Apparitiones et illusiones: the former were divine, the latter satanic. But it was not always easy to distinguish which was which. "Or do apparitions always emanate from God even when they are illusions [*An apparitiones praedictae semper a Deo procedant vel quandoque sint illusiones*]?" Often even apparitions fluctuated in an ambiguous atmosphere: "apparitions of this kind can be caused either by divine art, in which case they are miracles from God, or by demonic art and illusion [*posse apparitiones huiusmodi causari, vel divina arte, seu miraculosae a Deo, vel arte et illusione Daemonis*]."[18]

In the absence of apparitions, the altar nonetheless remained the disquieting space where the "visible priest" was to assume the awesome responsibility of representing the "invisible priest" and realizing "a sacrifice of infinite excellence." In other words, he was to represent and relive the ancient *mactatio* as perpetrated by "a priest of infinite perfection such as Christ" who, through the officiant, would perform "for the sake of his ministry [*causa ministerialis*]" the extraordinary transformation and immolation of himself.[19]

"Many priests are made exceedingly anxious [*Valde anxiatur nonnulli sacerdotes*]...." The "miracle of miracles" brought with it tension, restlessness and anxiety. The miracle of transubstantiation at the "mysterious and holy altar"[20] made the officiant feel like the executor of a supernatural act of occult violence. On the one hand, he was to perform a bloodless sacrifice ("altar sacrifices are performed every day by the hand of the priest... where adorable victims come as if in a state of death"). On the other hand, he had to turn into a necromantic mediator and transform "two inanimate substances," bread and wine, into supernatural food, thus bringing back to life "the body and the blood of Jesus Christ... in the guise of the body and the blood of a slaughtered lamb; whereby, at this point in every Mass, the Redeemer dies again mystically without really dying, at once alive and as if murdered."[21] Because, among the "amazing prodigies" and the "great and extraordinary miracles flashing in this mystery," "the ultimate one is that all these miracles and prodigies, which nature can only contemplate with dread, are worked by means of three or four little words emitted from the mouth of a man."[22]

If, with the words of His priest, God "annihilates the substances of bread and wine in the Mass, he does so in order to reproduce, through an infinitely greater miracle, the body of Jesus Christ in their place."[23] But, inexplicable wonder, by altering "the established causal order" and subverting its laws, with the words of the consecration the priest also severs

> the natural connection between the substances of bread and wine and their nonessential qualities, whereby the substance perishes while its accidents survive without any support. And this is all the more admirable in that the destruction of a substance, and the survival and endurance of its accidents without their natural support, has never before been witnessed in nature. An angel can support a huge machine in the air, but he cannot support the taste of wine, a color or an odor without substance. And though he can destroy the substance of bread, he cannot reduce it to nothing. These extraordinary prodigies happen daily during the Holy Mass, and they remind us of God's dominion over everything and everybody, that He is the Lord of life and death, and that, because of His infinite perfection, He deserves that creatures be consumed in His honor, and, finally, that just as He annihilates those substances, so can He annihilate us.[24]

The awesomeness of the sacrifice caused the dislocation of natural laws. It violated them through a series of impossible alchemic reactions that upset the relationship between substances and their accidents. Color, odor, flavor survived the annihilation of the substances that expressed them. By turning into flesh and blood, the primary substances — bread and wine — changed radically in essence, but their physical attributes survived their metamorphosis. The sacrifice turned the inanimate into the animate. The life of the heavenly enzyme, the Incorruptible, fermented out of unleavened bread. Vital, vivifying, beatifying food was born out of dead food. God had introduced himself into a balsamic "mysterious food"[25] in order to modify and remold those who ate and digested it, without being modified Himself. This extraordinary food belied both the laws of nutrition and the principles of digestion, according to which all food is altered and modified by its swallower:

> And as if in order to come to us, He punctually obeys a man's voice, He lowers Himself, makes Himself smaller, lives a hidden life, with eyes that do not see, ears that do not

hear. In a general mortification of the senses, He upsets the laws of nature, breaks apart the most united things, and fortifies the weakest things to produce effects that far surpass their virtues...[26]

These are the prodigies of the hypostatic union: "He is in us and we are in Him," "we become as one" (*unum quid efficimur*). Heavenly bread, divine flesh, incorruptible body, "dish of His table" that the pious receive directly from Heaven in the guise of bread and wine, the Omnipotent gives Himself

to us as food. Since nothing merges with us more intimately than food which, by means of natural heat, transforms itself into our own substance, and becomes one with us.... "He who eats of my flesh and drinks of my blood shall remain in me and I in him [*Qui manducat meam carnem et bibit meum sanguinem, in me manet, et ego in eo*]." But there is a difference between other food and this one: whereas the former transforms itself into us and becomes our own substance, the latter transforms us into itself.[27]

The "sacramental" food which, "in a morsel," contains "the quintessence of all good and the antidote to all evil," "incorruptible and immortal,"[28] does not change; rather, it changes us.

Balsamic moderator and sedative of the flesh, manna of the soul, inextricably joined to the flesh which, resurrected and embalmed to last forever, has been trusted to the incorruptible and aromatic eternity of the paradise of the blessed. The consecrated host is a pledge of unimaginable ecstasies, unseizable delights, a sure viaticum toward "immortal and incomprehensible light," toward "invisible light."[29] In its plenitude of sense and spirit it regenerates both soul and body:

Just as honey lends its own incorruptibility to the fruit that is dipped in it, so does the body of the Savior, in joining ours, lend us some of the seeds of immortality He deserved, and the special right to live forever.[30]

As an elixir and the "sweetest medicine," the Omnipotent "humiliates Himself by becoming our food," and in that food, He dies "mystically, morally and truly," following the ineluctable route to degradation of all substances that enter the carnal labyrinth of the human belly. The divine body must be absorbed by the "infamous body." The pure must fuse with the impure "in order to nourish our souls and our bodies with immortal life."[31]

Once the body has become "alive...at once tomb and temple," the "new sacramental life" acquired by the Host through Consecration slowly melts in the folds of the ventricular *antrum*, while the arcane powers of the magical words fade away in the relentless physiological functions which alter, transform and reshape everything.

In the Pit of the Stomach

Most likely, the introduction of the Host into the worshiper's mouth created a real trauma. As he swallowed it, all the terrifying images connected with this act — the body of the purest lamb entering the filth of the digestive apparatus, the divine flesh polluted by contact with mucous membranes, the juices of the corruptible flesh and the rot of the bowels — must have returned to his mind and seized him with vertiginous horror.

The stomach occupies a crucial place in all theological meditations on the Eucharist. This organ, and all the physiological processes connected to it, becomes the focus of close attention, of minute and thoughtful exploration, because this fleshy bag is the organic terminus where the ultimate and definitive prodigy of the supernatural metamorphosis occurs. With concern and anxiety, theologians follow the descent of Christ's body into the *antrum*, the damp and smelly bowels.

The journey of the Host from the mouth to the "road of the stomach" must be preceded by a complex ritual of purification. The fast, which must be rigorously observed, at least from midnight on, is described in minute detail. Omissions and inattention, which may often amount to sacrilege, are enough to invalidate the assumption of the particle. In those times when oral hygiene was still primitive and toothbrushes were unknown, even the involuntary retention of small bits of food between the teeth constituted a serious theological problem. Saint Thomas, who readily admitted being "greedy for sacraments,"[32] considered the issue in his *Summa* (3, q. 80, art. 8), and decided that "the remains of food" (*reliquiae cibi*) between the teeth, if casually swallowed, did not impede the reception of the Sacrament: "nevertheless, if the remains of food lingering in the mouth are by chance swallowed, they will not impede the taking of this Sacrament [*reliquiae tamen cibi remanentis in ore, si casualiter deglutiantur, non impediunt sumptionem huius sacramenti*]."[33] On the basis of this authority, theologians established that "neither saliva, nor blood, nor any other humor descending from the head and swallowed, nor the remains of food between teeth, if swallowed after midnight as saliva, would break the natural fast, since they were not absorbed as food."[34]

228

When sniffing tobacco became fashionable in Europe (in 1779, the pope himself opened a factory in Rome, thus hushing up, once and for all, the widespread suspicion that the "Indian" herb might be diabolical), those who could not help but indulge their *rapé*, or who were unable to abstain from the "fetid delights of Indian tobaccoes,"[35] were allowed to abandon themselves to their vice without fear, because its aromatic powder, free from the taint of Satan, was fully assimilated (at least insofar as sinning was concerned) into innocent saliva:

> The same thing can be said of tobacco. It is absorbed through the nostrils in the form of powder which is clearly not taken as food, since the latter is absorbed through the mouth and not through the nostrils; so that if it is swallowed, it goes down as saliva.[36]

When all the rules concerning the purity of the itinerary had been observed, the Host, made of the purest wheat flour, could begin its descent into the obscure intestinal meanders, into man's inner flesh, in *fundo ventriculi*, where the man-God, "swallowed into his chest,"[37] would eventually come to rest. Alone among all the Sacraments, which never went any farther than the surface of the body, the Eucharist penetrated all the way into man's bowels. Through this intimate, direct contact:

> We become living limbs which are truly joined to Christ, our Head. Indeed, in a way, we become one with Him: we became the limbs of His body, of His flesh, of His bones...by eating His divine flesh with His bones, we become, through this conjuction, even more specifically the limbs of His divine body...All the other Sacraments remain external to us since they are administered by means of unctions, baths, words uttered and heard and other exterior matters: but the Eucharist, having assumed the shape of food and drink, is received internally, and, as such, brings Jesus Himself inside our chest.[38]

The *manducatio*, the swallowing, ingestion and digestion of the consecrated bread was to take place according to the most perfect physiological rhythm, like the finest and most complete assimilation of natural food. In order to achieve the ideal fullness of grace, it was necessary that the natural warmth of the stomach carry out its action to the best of its ability and in absolute accordance with the mechanisms of digestion. The warmth of grace would then stimulate the gastric walls, thereby activating from inside the mechanism of perfect mutation by means of an impeccable assimilation of the natural species. The ventricle became the delicate locus of transubstantiation, the prodigious metamorphosis that leads, first of all, to the assimilation of the divine into the human, and then to the passage and the fusion of the human into the divine – the crucible where the swallowed food becomes one with the swallower. There is, however, one fundamental difference: "corporeal food becomes one with its swallower by transforming itself into the person who has absorbed it. The opposite occurs in the Eucharist, where it is not the food that turns into the person who has received it but rather the person who spiritually turns into the received food."[39]

Nevertheless, the receiver's supernatural transformation occurred according to the ways and times of human physiology. All natural matters had to submit to the normal rhythm of the digestive process. Divine grace could manifest itself only after the eucharistic food, having reached the warm bag of the stomach, had been melted into mush by the warmth of this natural oven. The mere introduction of the wafer into the oral cavity was irrelevant to the outcome of a perfect reception of the consecrated bread, since the prodigies of the *corpus mysticum*, the miracles of total *communio*, the absolute fusion of divine and human flesh, the release of "grace's action," could only occur in the stomach.

This is part of the reason why the sick could not receive the Host. "They cannot swallow, but they should be cured as soon as possible so that they may also absorb the Host: since the Eucharist confers no grace when taken only by the tongue or the palate, nor when it is kept in the mouth; it is necessary that it should proceed down the throat [*deglutire non possunt, sed sollicite curari solet, ut hostiam traiiciant: non ergo eucharistia gratiam confert statim: ac linguam vel palatum attingit, vel quamdiu in ore retinetur; sed requiritur et expectatur trajectia per guttur*]."[40]

The analogy between the spiritual and the material, between the beneficial effects of a good digestion and the fruition of the supernatural benefits conferred by the Host, was complete. Just as the natural warmth of the stomach alone could guarantee the proper consumption of both food and drink, so only the spiritual warmth of the ingested Sacrament could produce the full effect of charismatic effusion, and to such an extent that some theologians refused to acknowledge the action of the Host when a person died with it still in his or her mouth.

Spiritual nourishment could not spread out in all its fullness except through bodily nourishment, even if "after the Eucharist has been taken and remains in the stomach, the digestive processes may cease physically, but morally it continues, as is its nature [*transacta sumptione et quando eucharistia durat in stomacho, non perseveret manducatio sacramenti physice, adhuc tamen moraliter perseverat ratione dispositionis*]."[41] Such premises gave rise to the issue of the time of grace, the complex *quaestio* of the duration of the supernatural effects and of Christ's permanence in the Host, and the amount of time necessary for a full assimilation of the natural elements. Generally speaking, it was believed that the transformation of the species took about an hour, though the length of time varied according to the character and temperature of each individual stomach. According to the Roman doctors consulted by Cardinal De Lugo, the assimilation of the species took about one quarter of an hour for priests and about one minute less for laymen. But others believed that the entire digestive process took a layman five Pater Nosters and Ave Marias, while in a priest it would only occur after he removed his sacred vestments. However, Cardinal De Lugo, himself a theologian, was of the opinion that even in a priest, the corruption of the Host was complete a quarter of an hour after Communion.

This is how theology answered the question "How long does Christ remain in the Eucharist [*Quamdiu Christus manet in eucharistia*]?" Answers to the question "When is grace received [*Quando recipiatur gratia*]?" were not nearly as homogeneous. According to some, the effects of grace started the moment all fragments (of the Host) reached the pit of the stomach, whereas others thought that it happened the moment that a single piece of the Host (and not all of them) completed the journey.[42]

The most important thing for all good Christians was to be filled with grace. Some asked to receive Communion in the same way priests did, in two different forms (*sub utraque specie*), bread and wine, assuming that "more grace is contained in both forms than in one [*plus gratiae dari sub utraque, quam sub una*]." Thus, it did not seem right to deny wine to the worshiper who wished to receive a double portion of grace.[43]

At this point, it is important to mention a singular tendency which can be easily explained in light of the analogy between the digestion of sacred food and the digestion of profane food. I am referring to the widespread conviction that the greater and more consistent the divine nourishment chewed and ingested, the greater and more lasting were the grace and other benefits emanating from it. Therefore, the worshipers who wanted it were given an unusually large Host or even several Hosts at one time.

The charge of grace contained in a Host was such that even if its natural components were accidentally vomited, provided they retained something of bread and

wine, they still deserved to be adored; and if they were reintroduced into the stomach, they still released their beatifying fermentation.[44]

The "very great and extraordinary miracles" that occurred on the "holy and mysterious table," and the "great wonder" of the consecrated Host that turned the eucharistic act into a terrible mystery, were objects of profound "admiration and awe."[45]

The stomach became a hidden altar where occult and incomprehensible acts took
place, a zone of liturgical mediation between Heaven and earth, the divine and the
beastly, where an unimaginable rite of transformation occurred:

> O sovereign and incomprehensible Majesty, is it really possible that, though You are in
> Heaven, I can see You in my stomach, where You have come after making so many mira-
> cles and turning nature upside down? I tremble all over and am seized with awe when-
> ever I think of this infinite favor.... I believe, without the slightest doubt, that You are,
> soul and body, inside my stomach.[46]

The moment of separation, the end of that extraordinary contact, and the disappearance of that terrible and yet elating presence was most delicate and painful:

> When, after having thus kept Our Lord, the species are digested and He ceases to be
> with us corporeally, we must pray for Him not to leave us.... But since You have decided
> to go away corporeally, and that I be thus mortified, I submit to Your holy and divine
> will and accept this, however bitter, separation.[47]

The final destiny of the material "accidents," that is to say of bread and wine,
and the mysterious events that accompanied their putrefaction, constituted the last
stage in a series of "miracles and prodigies that nature can only contemplate with
dread." For, as G.B. Sangiure explains:

> When these accidents rot, and their putrefaction generates worms, then some theolo-
> gians believe that God creates again some primary matter, and very probably the very
> bread that has been destroyed; and in it, and through it, he produces the substantial forms
> of those insects. According to Angelico, who teaches us yet a stranger thing, God would
> make the bulk of the consecrated Host serve the function of primary matter, and would
> draw from it the forms of these animals. The ultimate [wonder] is that all these miracles
> and prodigies that nature can only contemplate with dread are worked by means of three
> or four little words emitted from the mouth of a man. And this is indeed a marvelous
> thing, incomparably more so than when Joshua's voice halted the sun in the middle of
> its course, which was and will remain an object of awe for all the centuries to come.[48]

The "awesome sacrifice" seemed so enormous that not all Christians could accept it in its inhuman atrocity, and preferred to see it as a symbol or trope. This was the case for an "ancient hermit" who "though of great fame and life, erred because he was an idiot or a simpleton." According to this old devotee, "the body of Christ was not really in the consecrated Host, but, as he went around saying, it was only represented by it."[49] He and two other "ancient" hermits who, after having prayed to God for an entire week to draw their friend away from error, were attending the Sunday Mass with him, had a revelation the moment the bread was placed on the altar for consecration:

> All three saw a young child on the altar, and when the priest started breaking the Host, it seemed to them that an angel came down from Heaven and divided the child in two with a knife, and collected his blood in the chalice. And when the priest divided the Host into several parts to give Communion to the people, they saw that the angel was also dividing the child into several small parts. And when, at the end of the Mass, the hermit went to receive Communion, it seemed to him that he alone was given a part of the bloodied flesh of that child. Seeing this, he was filled with such dread that he screamed and said: "My Lord, now I really believe that the bread which is consecrated on the altar is Your holy body and the chalice, that is to say the wine, is Your blood." And immediately it seemed to him that the flesh had turned again into bread and he received Communion. Then, the other two hermits told him: "God, knowing that to eat raw flesh horrifies human nature, ordered that this sacrament assume the guise of bread and wine...."[50]

Believers, particularly in earlier centuries, confusedly understood God's sacrifice as a prodigy of abominable grandeur, and were quite conscious of the bloody fragments of divine flesh that descended into their stomachs in the guise of the Host. To their horror of the anthropophagous act, in itself nefarious, was added their sacred dismay at the thought of introducing illicit portions of an incommensurable food — global fragments of heavenly flesh into their infamous bowels.

The child slaughtered by the angel, his flesh cut up into small bloody bits — in the vision reported by Domenico Cavalca — reflects this profound attraction-repulsion toward the sacrificial mystery (the *mactatio*, the "mystical slaughter"), a fact emphasized further by the mention of the irrepressible disgust which the idea of digesting provokes in the deepest recesses of the self. Both the sensibility of believers and ecclesiastic doctrine (*incruente immolatur*, according to the Tridentine canon) have over time nearly obliterated this bloody offering, anesthetizing and reducing it to little more than a symbolic act. They have edulcorated and disincarnated it, reinterpreted it merely as a trope. In other words, they have unconsciously rejected the awesome notion of transubstantiation, and have refused its intolerable weight. But the image and feeling of a bloody totemic rite during which unworthy sons swallow the raw flesh of their Father (of a Father who, most perfect and pure victim – the only one worthy of his glory –has already immolated himself before his Creator) weighed on the conscience, at least until the eighteenth century, of all those who received Communion.

And in the middle of the eighteenth century, the bishop of Saint Agata dei Goti (as well as several other clergymen) did not hesitate to repropose that archaic form of the sacrificial meal and of the sacrifice of the King:

> What a refined expression of love, Saint Francis of Sales says, would we see in the act of a prince who, seated at his table, sent a portion of his meal to a pauper? And what if he sent him his entire meal? And what if he sent him his own arm to eat? In the Holy Communion, Jesus not only gives us part of his meal to eat, or part of his body, but his entire body....[51]

NOTES

1. C.G. Rosignoli, *Maraviglie di Dio nel Divinissimo Sacramento e nel Santissimo Sacrificio* (Turin: G.B. Zappata, 1704), p. 220.

2. P. Clemente Simoncelli, *Guida de morabundi* (Naples: Tomasi, 1962), p. 120.

3. Francis of Sales, *Lettere spirituali*, trans. French to Italian by a devotee (Padua: Stamperia del Seminario, 1728), pt. 1, p. 283.

4. C. Berruti, *Vita del venerabile servo di Dio Gerardo Maiella* (Naples: Miranda, 1847), p. 35.

5. Cesarius of Heisterbach, *Dialogus miraculorum*, ed. J. Strange (Cologne, Bonn, Brussels, 1851), vol. 2, p. 202.

6. *Ibid.*

7. Giovanni Battista Sangiure, S.J., *Erario della vita Cristiana e religiosa: Overo l'arte di conoscere Cristo Gesù, e di amarlo. Dove si tratta delle Virtù, e de' Punti più importanti della vita spirituale*. Trans. French back to Italian (Venice: N. Pezzana, 1711), pt. 3, respectively p. 228 ("possanza infinita," "cibo

misterioso"), p. 330 ("dolcezza fa perdere l'appetito di tutte le creature"), p. 238 ("con gusto e piacere"), p. 239 ("ammirabili gusti" and "penetranti delizie").

8. *Ibid.*, pp. 241 and 332.

9. *Ibid.*, p. 239 ("penetranti delizie," "cuore umano," "in un riposo e in una tranquillità meravigliosa"), p. 244 ("co'l suo sacro tocco, la carne nostra pura"), p. 243 ("virtù di conservare intera la carne morta, la quale altrimenti si putrefarrebbe e diventerebbe una scaturigine di vermi," "Infinitamente santa, infinitamente casta," "carni di alcuni uccelli dell'Indie orientali [che] non si corrompono giammai perchè si pascono di fiori e d'erbe aromatiche").

10. *Ibid.*, p. 240 ("sormonta tutti i sapori che contengono le cose gustose ed eccede tutte le dolcezze dalle quali possono i nostri sensi essere lusingati," "colui, in cui l'Agnelo Pasquale dimora, sente cose ammirabili, ne vede di grandi, ne dice di inaudite," "la forza del misterioso vino, che ha bevuto, gli riempie l'anima di una gioia inesplicabile").

11. Emerio de Bonis, S.J., *Trattata del Santissimo Sacramento dell'altare et del modo di riceverlo fruttuosamente. Con un altro trattata della Santissima Messa & del moda di udirla con frutta* (Brescia: P.M. Marchetti, 1598), p. 85.

12. C.G. Rosignoli, S.J., *Verità eterne, esposte in lettioni, ordinate principalmente per li giorni degli Esercizi Spirituali* (Milan: C. A. Malatesta, 1688), p. 364.

13. De Bonis, *Trattato del Santissimo Sacramento*, p. 60.

14. Martino Del Rio, *Disquisitionum magicarum libri sex* (Venice: apud Ioan. Antonium et Iacobum de Franciscis, 1606), vol. 3, p. 179.

15. Imperiali, *Le notti beriche Overo de' quesiti, e discorsi fisici, medici, politici, historici, e sacri libri* (Venice: Paulo Baglioni, 1655) 5: p. 67 ("vita d'animali," "oltre il costume solito della natura"), p. 62 ("mostruoso e trabocchevole effetto"), p. 67 ("stupori ed eccessi").

16. Giuliano Fantaguzzi, *"Caos." Cronache cesenati del sec. XV*, published for the first time with notes by Dino Bazzocchi (Cesena: Tipografia Bettini, 1915), p. 47.

17. Francis of Sales, *Lettere spirituali*, p. 177.

18. *Rubricae missalis Romani commentariis illustratae* (Rome: sumptibus Felicis Caesaretti, sub Signo Reginae, 1674), p. 362. The form *ly* or *li*, characteristic of theological texts of the late Middle Ages, was derived from a misunderstanding of the sign *h* with a dot on it which, if fact, means *hoc* (*nomen* or *verbum*). Bruno Nardi (Padua: Saggi sulla cultura veneta del Quattro e Cinquecento, 1971), pp. 124-29; cf. *lyhoma*, in Folengo's *Baldus* 25.492. (My thanks to Augusto Campana and Italo Mariotti for their help on this note.)

19. Giovanni Pietro Pinamonti, *L'albero della vita: Pregi, e frutti della S. Messa. Con la maniera di*

parteciparne copiosamente, in *Opere* (Venice: N. Pezzana, 1719), p. 425 ("sacerdote invisibile," "sagrifizio d'infinita Eccellenza," "un sacerdote d'infinita perfezione come Cristo").

20. Sangiure, S.J., *Erario della vita Cristiana*, pt. 3, p. 295.

21. Pinamonti, *L'albero della vita*, p. 426.

22. Sangiure, *Erario della vita Cristiana*, pp. 290 and 292.

23. Pinamonti, *L'albero della vita*, p. 427.

24. *Ibid.*, p. 426.

25. Sangiure, *Erario della vita Cristiana*, p. 228.

26. *Ibid.*, p. 308.

27. Alessandro Diotallevi, S.J., *La beneficenza di Dio verso gl'uomini e l'ingratitudine degli uomini versa Dio considerazioni* (Venice: A. Poletti, 1716), pp. 253 and 258.

28. *Ibid.*, pp. 259 and 274.

29. Sant'Aurelio Agostino, "I soliloqui," in *Le divote meditazioni* (Venice: Erede di Niccolò Pezzana, 1775), p. 209.

30. P. Segneri, *Il Cristiano istruito nella sua legge: Ragionamenti morali* (Venice: Baglioni, 1773), pt. 3, p. 74.

31. *Ibid.*, pp. 71 and 74.

32. Giacomo Lubrani, S.J., "I tre Cieli: Panegirico vii di S. Tommaso d'Aquino," in *Il Cielo domenicano. Col primo mobile della predicazione, con più Pianeti di Santita. Panegirici sacri* (Naples: Raillard, 1691), vol. 1, p. 124.

33. Fulgenzio Cuniliati, O.P., *Il catechista in pulpito* (Venice: T. Bettinelli, 1768), p. 218.

34. *Ibid.*

35. Emanuele Tesauro, *La filosofia morale derivata dall'alto fonte del grande Aristotele Stagirita* (Venice: N. Pezzana, 1712), p. 286.

36. Cuniliati, *Il catechista*, p. 218. For a more rigorous account (*an sumptio tabachi communionem impediat*), cf. Paolo Maria Quarti, *Rubricae missalis Romani, commentariis illustratae*, p. 458.

37. *Ibid.*, p. 225.

38. *Ibid.*, p. 232.

39. *Ibid.*, pp. 232-33.

40. Bartholomaeus Mastrius de Meldula, O.M.C., *Theologia moralis ad mentem DD: Seraphici et subtilis concinnata* (Venice: apud Antonium Moram, 1723), p. 433.

41. *Ibid.*

42. Alphonse de Liguori, *Theologia moralis*, vol. 2, p. 129.

43. *Ibid.*

44. *Ibid.*

45. Sangiure, *Erario della vita Cristiana*, pt. 3, pp. 290, 295, 324.

46. *Ibid.*, pp. 324-25.

47. *Ibid.*, pp. 330-31.

48. *Ibid.*, pp. 291-92. For the "various phases of the dispute over the Eucharist," cf. John Gregory Bourke, *Scatalogic Rites of All Nations* (Washington: W.H. Lowdwermilk & Co., 1891).

49. Domenico Cavalca, *Le vite dei SS. Padri* (Milan: Istituto Editoriale Italiano, 1915), vol. 2, p. 69.

50. *Ibid.*, pp. 69-71.

51. Alfonse de Liguori, *Apparecchio alla morte, cioe considerazioni sulle massime eterne* (Bassano: Remondini, 1767), p. 390. Cf. C.G. Jung, *Transformation Symbolism in the Mass* (Princeton, 1979).

From *La casa dell'eternità*, Milan, Garzanti, 1987.
Translated by Anna Cancogne.

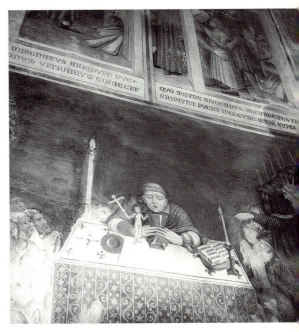

Fresco depicting the Miracle of Bolsena, 1263 (Orvieto, Italy).

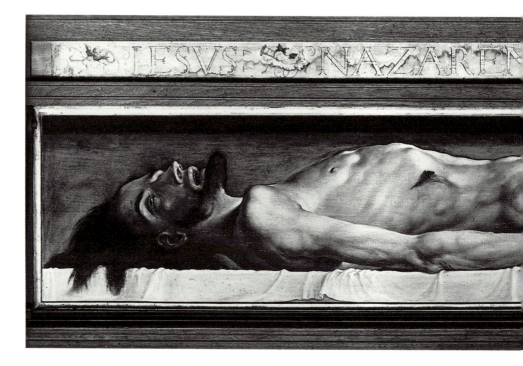

Hans Holbein the Younger, The Body of the Dead Christ in the Tomb, 1522
(Bâle, Musée des Beaux Arts).

Holbein's Dead Christ

Julia Kristeva

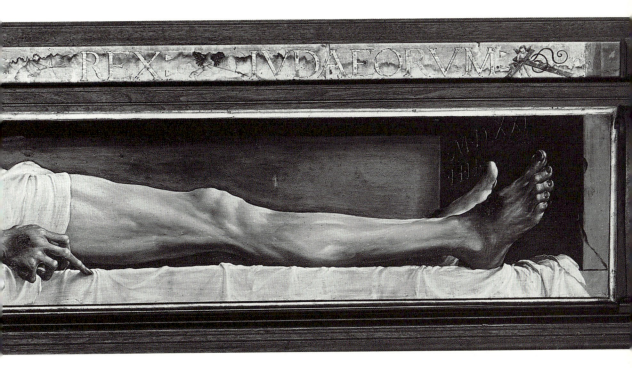

"Some May Lose Their Faith"

In 1522 (the underlying coat bears the date 1521) Hans Holbein the Younger (1497-1543) painted a disturbing picture, the *Body of the Dead Christ in the Tomb*, which may be seen at the Basel museum. The painting apparently made a tremendous impression on Dostoyevsky. At the very outset of *The Idiot*, Prince Myshkin attempted to speak of it, but to no avail; only through a new polyphonic twist of the plot did he see a reproduction of it at Rogozhin's house and, "struck by a sudden thought," he exclaimed: "That picture...that picture! Why, some people may *lose their faith* by looking at that picture?"[1] A little later, Ippolit, a peripheral character who nevertheless seems, in many respects, to be the narrator's and Myshkin's double, gave a striking account of it: "The picture depicted Christ, who has just been taken from the Cross. I believe that painters are usually in the habit of portraying Christ, whether on the Cross or taken down from the Cross, as still retaining a shade of extraordinary beauty on His face; that beauty they strive to preserve even in His moments of greatest agony. In Rogozhin's picture there was no trace of beauty. It was a faithful representation of the dead body of a man who had undergone unbearable torments before the Crucifixion, been wounded, tortured, beaten by the guards, beaten by the people, when He carried the Cross and fell under its weight, and, at last, had suffered the agony of crucifixion, lasting for six hours (according to my calculation, at least). It is true, it is the face of a man who had only *just* been taken from the Cross — that is, still retaining a great deal of warmth and life; rigor mortis had not yet set in, so that there is still a look of suffering on the face of the dead man, as though He were still feeling it (that has been well caught by the artist); on the other hand, the face has not been spared in the least; it is nature itself, and, indeed, any man's corpse would look like that after such suffering. I know that the Christian church laid it down in the first few centuries of its existence that Christ really did suffer and that the Passion was not symbolic. His body on the Cross was therefore fully and entirely subject to the laws of nature. In the picture the face is terribly smashed with blows, swollen, covered with terrible, swollen and bloodstained bruises, the eyes open and squinting; the large, open whites of the eyes have a sort of dead and glassy glint. But, strange to say, as one looks at the dead body of this tortured man, one cannot help asking oneself the peculiar, and interesting question: if such a corpse (and it must have been just like that) was seen by all His disciples, by His future chief apostles, by the women who followed Him and stood by the Cross, by all who believed in Him and worshiped Him, then how could they possibly have believed, as they looked at the corpse, that that martyr would rise again? Here one cannot help being struck with the idea that if death is so horrible and if the laws of nature are so powerful, then how can they be overcome? How can they be overcome when even He did not conquer them, He who overcame nature during His lifetime and whom nature obeyed, who said *Talitha cumi!* and the damsel arose, who cried, *Lazarus come forth!* and the dead man came forth? Looking at that picture, you get the impression of nature as some enormous, implacable and dumb beast, or to put it more correctly, much more correctly, though it may seem strange, as some huge engine of the latest design, *which has senselessly seized, cut to pieces and swallowed up — impassively and unfeelingly — a great and priceless Being*, a Being worth the whole of nature and all its laws, worth the entire earth, which was perhaps created solely for the coming of that Being! The picture seems to give expression to the idea of a dark, insolent and senselessly eternal power, to which everything is subordinated, and this idea is suggested to you unconsciously. The people surrounding the dead man, none of whom is shown in the picture, must have been overwhelmed by a feeling of terrible anguish and dismay on that evening *which had shattered all their hopes and almost all their beliefs in one fell blow*. They must have parted in a state of the most dreadful terror, though each of them carried away within him a mighty thought which could never be wrested from him. And if, on the eve of the Crucifixion, the Master could have seen what He would look like when taken from the Cross, would He have mounted the Cross and died as He did? This question, too, you can't help asking yourself as you look at the picture."[2]

The Man of Sorrows

Holbein's painting represents a corpse stretched out by itself on a slab covered with a cloth that is hardly draped.[3] Life-size, the painted corpse is seen from the side, its head slightly turned toward the viewer, the hair spread out on the sheet. The right arm is in full view, resting alongside the emaciated, tortured body, and the hand protrudes slightly from the slab. The rounded chest suggests a triangle within the very low, elongated rectangle of the recess that constitutes the painting's frame. The chest bears the bloody mark of a spear, and the hand shows the stigmata of the Crucifixion, which stiffen the outstretched middle finger. Imprints of nails mark Christ's feet. The martyr's face bears the expression of hopeless grief; the empty stare, the sharp-lined profile, the dull blue-green complexion are those of a man who is truly dead, of Christ forsaken by the Father ("My God, my God, why hast thou forsaken me?") and without the promise of Resurrection.

The unadorned representation of human death, the well-nigh anatomical stripping of the corpse conveys to viewers an unbearable anguish before the death of God, which here is mingled with our own death because there isn't the slightest suggestion of transcendency. What is more, Hans Holbein has given up all architectural or compositional fancy. The tombstone weighs down on the upper portion of the painting, which is merely twelve inches high, and intensifies the feeling of permanent death: this corpse will never rise again.[4] The pall itself, reduced to a minimum of folds, emphasizes, through that economy of motion, the feeling of stiffness and stony cold.

The viewer's gaze penetrates this closed-in coffin from below and, following the painting from left to right, stops at the stone set against the corpse's feet, sloping at a wide angle toward the spectators.

What was the purpose of a painting with such peculiar dimensions? Does the *Dead Christ* belong to the altar that Holbein did for Hans Oberried in 1520-21, in which the two outside wings depicted the Passion and the center was saved for the Nativity and the Adoration?[5] There is nothing to support such a hypothesis, which, however, is not implausible when one takes into account a few features it shares with the outside wings of the altar that was partially destroyed during iconoclastic outbursts in Basel.

Among the various interpretations given by critics, one stands out and seems today the most plausible. The painting was done for a predella that remained independent and was to be positioned above the visitors as they filed in, from the side and the left (for instance from the church's central nave toward the southern aisle). In the Upper Rhine region, there are churches that contain funerary recesses where *sculpted* Christly bodies are displayed. Might Holbein's work be a painterly transposition of such recumbent statues? According to one hypothesis, this *Dead Christ* was the covering for a sacred tomb open only on Good Friday and closed the rest of the year. Finally, relying on X rays of the painting, Fridtjof Zschokke has shown that the *Dead Christ* was initially located in a semicircular recess, like the section of a tube. That location corresponds to the date inscribed next to the right foot and the signature: H. H. DXXI. One year later, Holbein substituted the arched recess with a rectangular one and signed above the feet: MDXXII H. H.[6]

The biographical and professional context of the *Dead Christ* is also worth recalling. Holbein painted a series of Madonnas (between 1520 and 1522), among them the very fine *Enthroned Virgin and Child* known as the "Solothurn Madonna." In 1521, his first son, Philip, was born. This is also the time of a strong friendship with Erasmus, whose portrait Holbein did in 1523.

There is the birth of a child — and the threat of death weighing down on it. But above all, death weighs on the painter as a father whom the coming generation would one day displace. Then there is the friendship with Erasmus and the renunciation not only of fanaticism but also, with some humanists, of faith itself. A small diptych of the same period, gothic in style and painted mostly in shades of brown, portrays *Christ as the Man of Sorrows*, and the *Virgin as the Mater Dolorosa* (Basel, 1519-20). The body of the man of sorrows, strangely athletic, brawny and tensed, is shown seated under a colonnade; the right hand, curled up in front of the sexual organ, seems spastic; the head alone, wearing a crown of thorns, with its aching face and gaping mouth, expresses a morbid suffering beyond vague eroticism. From what passion did such pain arise? Would the man-God be distressed, that is, haunted by death, *because* he is sexual, and prey to a sexual passion?

A Composition in Loneliness

Italian iconography embellishes, or at least ennobles, Christ's face during the Passion; but above all, it surrounds Christ with figures that are plunged not only in grief but also in the certainty of the Resurrection, as if to suggest the attitude we too should adopt when facing the Passion. Holbein, on the contrary, leaves the corpse strangely alone. It is perhaps this isolation — *an act of composition* — that endows the painting with its major melancholy burden, more so than its delineation and coloring. To be sure, Christ's suffering is expressed through three components inherent in line and color: the head bent backward, the contortion of the right hand bearing the stigmata, the position of the feet — the whole being bonded by means of a dark palette of grays, greens and browns. Nevertheless, such realism, harrowing on account of its very parsimony, is emphasized to the utmost through the painting's composition and location: a body stretched out alone, situated above the viewers and separated from them.

Cut off from us by its base but without any possibility for the gaze to extend to Heaven because the ceiling in the recess comes down low, Holbein's *Dead Christ* is inaccessible, distant and without a beyond. It is a way of looking at mankind from afar, even in death. Just as Erasmus saw folly from a distance. It is a vision that opens out not onto glory but onto endurance. Another, a new, morality resides in this painting.

Christ's dereliction is here at its worst: forsaken by the Father, He is apart from all of us. Unless Holbein, whose mind, pungent as it was, doesn't appear to have led him across the threshold of atheism, wanted to include us personally, humans, aliens, spectators that we are, in this crucial moment of Christ's life. With no intermediary, suggestion or indoctrination, whether pictorial or theological, other than our ability to imagine death, we are led to collapse in the horror of the caesura that is death or to dream of an invisible beyond. Does Holbein forsake us, as Christ, for an instant, had imagined Himself forsaken? Or does he, on the contrary, invite us to change the Christly tomb into a living tomb, to participate in the painted death and thus include it in our own life? In order to live with it and make it live, for if the living body in opposition to the rigid corpse is a dancing body, doesn't our life, through identification with death, become a "danse macabre," in keeping with Holbein's other well-known vision?

This enclosed recess, this well-isolated coffin simultaneously rejects us and invites us. Indeed, the corpse fills the entire field of the painting, without any labored reference to the Passion. Our gaze follows the slightest physical detail: it is, as it were, nailed, crucified and riveted to the hand placed at the center of the composition. Should we attempt to avert our gaze, it is quickly stopped, locked in on the distressed face or the feet propped against the black stone. And yet this walling-in allows for two prospects.

On the one hand, there is the insertion of date and signature, MDXXII H. H., at Christ's feet. Placing the painter's name, to which was often added that of the donor, in that position was common at the time. It is nevertheless possible that in abiding by that code Holbein inserted himself into the drama of the dead body. A sign of humility: the artist throwing himself at God's feet? Or a sign of equality? The painter's name is not lower than Christ's body – they are both at the same level, jammed into the recess, united in man's death, in death as the essential sign of mankind, of which the only surviving evidence is the ephemeral creation of a picture drawn here and now in 1521 and 1522!

We have, on the other hand, this hair and this hand that extend beyond the base as if they might slide over toward us, as if the frame could not hold back the corpse. The frame dates precisely from the end of the sixteenth century and includes a narrow edging, bearing the inscription *Jesus Nazarenus Rex Judaeorum*, which encroaches on the painting. The edging, which seems nonetheless always to have been part of

Holbein's painting, includes, between the words of the inscription, five angels bearing the instruments of the martyrdom: the shaft, the crown of thorns, the scourge, the flogging column, the cross. Integrated afterward in that symbolic framework, Holbein's painting recovers the evangelical meaning that it did not insistently contain in itself, and which probably legitimized it in the eyes of its purchasers.

Even if Holbein's painting had originally been conceived as a predella for an altarpiece, it remained alone; no other panel was added to it. Such isolation, as splendid as it is gloomy, avoided Christian symbolism as much as the surfeit of German Gothic style, which combined painting and sculpture but also added wings to altarpieces, aiming for syncretism and the imparting of motion to figures. In the face of that tradition, which directly preceded him, Holbein isolated, pruned, condensed and reduced.

Holbein's originality, then, lies in this vision of Christly death that is devoid of pathos and is intimate on account of its very banality. Humanization thus reached its highest point: the point at which glory is obliterated through the image. When the dismal brushes against the nondescript, the most disturbing sign is the most ordinary one. In contrast to Gothic enthusiasm, humanism and parsimony were the inverted products of melancholia.

And yet such originality is affiliated with the Christian iconographic tradition that came out of Byzantium.[7] Around 1500, there were depictions of the dead Christ spread throughout central Europe, under the influence of a Dominican mysticism, whose major representatives in Germany were Meister Eckhart (c. 1260-c. 1328), Johannes Tauler (c. 1300-61) and especially Heinrich von Berg, who called himself Heinrich Suso (c. 1295-1366).[8]

Grünewald and Mantegna

Holbein's vision should also be compared to that of Matthias Grünewald in his *Dead Christ* of the Isenheim Altarpiece (1512-15), which was removed to Colmar in 1794. The central panel representing the Crucifixion shows Christ bearing the paroxystic marks of martyrdom (the crown of thorns, the cross, the countless wounds), even including putrefaction of the flesh. Here Gothic expressionism reaches a peak in the exhibition of pain. Grünewald's Christ, however, is not reduced to isolation as is Holbein's. The human realm to which he belonged is represented by the Virgin,

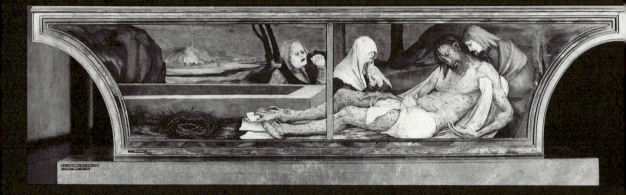

M. Grünewald, Dead Christ, 1512-1516
(Colmar, Unterlinden Museum).

Andrea Mantegna, *Cristo in Scurto*, 1480
(Milan, Brera Museum).

who falls into the arms of John the Evangelist, and by Mary Magdalene and John the Baptist, who bring compassion into the picture.[9]

The predella of the same Colmar altarpiece painted by Grünewald displays a Christ somewhat different from the one in the *Crucifixion*. It is an *Entombment* or *Lamentation*. Horizontal lines take the place of the *Crucifixion*'s verticality, and the corpse appears more elegiac than tragic – it is a heavy, soothed body, dismal in its calm. Holbein might simply have inverted the body of Grünewald's dying Christ by placing the feet toward the right and eliminating the three mourners (Magdalene, the Virgin and John). More sober than the *Crucifixion*, the *Lamentation* already suggests the possibility of a transition in Gothic art toward Holbein. However, Holbein certainly goes much farther than the temporary quieting down shown by the Colmar master. Doing something more poignant than Grünewald, with bare realism as his only means, Holbein is also more engaged in a struggle against the father–painter, since it seems that Grünewald was very much inspired by Holbein the Elder, who had settled in Isenheim, where he died in 1526.[10] Holbein thoroughly calms the Gothic upheaval, and while his art skims the contemporary burgeoning mannerism, it suggests a classicism that avoids infatuation with an unballasted empty form. He forces the weight of human grief onto the image.

Finally, Mantegna's famous *Cristo in scruto* (c. 1480, at the Brera Museum in Milan) may be considered the precursor of the quasi-anatomical vision of the dead Christ. With the soles of the feet turned toward the viewers and the foreshortened perspective, Mantegna's corpse imposes itself with a brutality that verges on the obscene. Nevertheless, the two women who appear in the upper left-hand corner of this painting introduce the grief and compassion that Holbein puts aside precisely by banishing them from sight or else creating them with no mediator other than the invisible appeal to our all-too-human identification with the dead Son. It is as if Holbein had integrated the Dominican-inspired Gothic grief, filtered through Suso's sentimentalism, just as Grünewald's expressionism displays it, and frees it of excess as well as of the divine presence that presses down with all its guilt-provoking, expiatory weight upon Grünewald's imagination. Also, it is as if Holbein had picked up the anatomical and pacifying lesson taught by Mantegna and Italian Catholicism, less sensitive to man's sin than to its forgiveness, and influenced more by the bucolic embellishing ecstasy of the Fransciscans than by Dominican dolorousness. And yet, always heedful of the Gothic spirit, Holbein maintains grief while humanizing it, without following the Italian path of negating pain and glorifying the arrogance of the flesh or the beauty of the beyond. Holbein is in another dimension: he makes commonplace the Passion of the crucified Christ in order to make it more accessible to us. Such a humanizing gesture, which is not without a modicum of *irony* toward transcendence, suggests a tremendous amount of mercy with respect to *our* death. According to legend, the corpse of a Jew recovered from the Rhine would have provided Holbein with a model....

The same half-ghoulish, half-ironic verve reached its climax in what must now be termed pure grotesque when, in 1524, while staying in the south of France, Holbein received a commission from the publishers Melchior and Gaspard Treschel in Lyons to execute a *Danse Macabre* in a series of woodcuts.[11] This dance of Death, drawn by Holbein and cut by Hans Lutzelburger, was published in Lyons in 1538. It was reproduced and circulated throughout Europe, presenting renascent mankind with a picture of itself that was both devastating and grotesque, adopting François Villon's tone through images. From the newborn and lower classes to popes, emperors, bishops, abbots, noblemen and young lovers — all of humanity is in the grip of death. Clasped in the arms of Death, no one escapes its grip, a fatal one to be sure, but here anguish conceals its own depressive force and displays defiance through sarcasm or the grimace of a mocking smile, without triumph, as if, knowing it is done for, laughter is the only answer.

Death Facing the Renaissance

We easily imagine Renaissance man as Rabelais depicted him: imposing, perhaps somewhat funny like Panurge, but boldly launched in the pursuit of happiness and the wisdom of the divine bottle. Holbein, on the other hand, proposes another vision — that of man subject to death, man embracing Death, absorbing it into his very being, integrating it not as a condition for glory nor a consequence of a sinful nature, but as the ultimate essence of his desacralized reality, which is the foundation of a new dignity. For that very reason, the picture of Christly and human death in Holbein is intimately connected to *In Praise of Folly* (1511) by Desiderius Erasmus, whose friend, illustrator and portrayer he became in 1523. It is by acknowledging his folly and looking death in the face — but perhaps by facing his mental

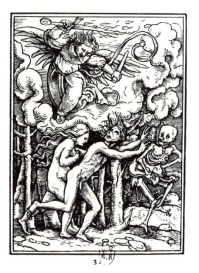
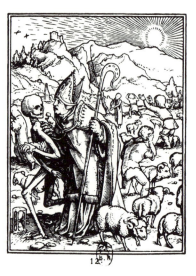
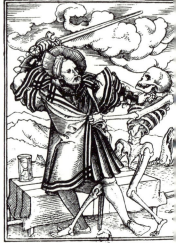

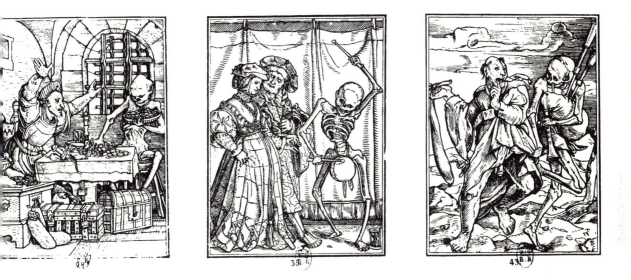

M. Mezian after Holbein, *Simolachri, Historie e Figure de la Morte*, 1549
(Paris, Bibliothèque nationale).
From left to right:
Adam and Eve are driven from paradise.
The bishop.
The gentleman.
The rich.
The noble woman.
The idiot.

risks, his risks of psychic death – that man achieves a new dimension: not necessarily that of atheism but definitely that of a disillusioned, serene and dignified stance. Like a picture by Holbein.

The Protestant Affliction

Did the Reformation influence such a concept of death, and more specifically, such an emphasis on Christ's death at the expense of any allusion to the Redemption and Resurrection? Catholicism is well-known for its tendency to stress the "beatific vision" in Christ's death without dwelling on the torments of the Passion, underscoring that Jesus had always had the knowledge of his own Resurrection. Calvin, on the other hand, insists on the *formidabilis abysis* into which Jesus had been thrust at the hour of His death, descending to the depths of sin and hell. Luther had already described himself personally as a melancholy being under the influence of Saturn and the devil: "I, Martin Luther, was born under the most unfavorable stars, probably under Saturn," he wrote in 1532. "Where there lives a melancholy person, the devil has drawn his bath.... I have learned from experience how one must behave during temptation. Whoever is besieged with sadness, despair or any other deep affliction, whoever harbors a serpent in his conscience must first hold to the consolation of the divine Word, and then when eating and drinking, he will seek the company and conversation of pious and Christian people. In this manner things will be better for him."[12]

As early as his ninety-five *Theses Against Indulgences*, Martin Luther formulated a mystical call to suffering as a means of access to Heaven. And if the idea of man's generation through grace is found next to this immersion in pain, the fact remains nevertheless that the intensity of one's faith is geared to one's ability for contrition. Thus: "As long as hatred of self abides [i.e., true inward penitence], the penalty of sin abides, viz., until we enter the Kingdom of Heaven" (thesis 4); "God never remits guilt to anyone without, at the same time, making him humbly submissive to the priest, His representative" (thesis 7); "A truly contrite sinner seeks out and loves to pay the penalties of his sins; whereas the very multitude of indulgences dulls men's consciences, and tends to make them hate the penalties" (thesis 40); "Christians should be exhorted to be zealous to follow Christ, their Head, through penalties, deaths and even hell" (thesis 94).

Lucas Cranach the Elder became the Protestants' official painter, while Dürer sent Luther a series of religious engravings. But a humanist such as Erasmus was wary at first about the Reformer. Afterward, he became more and more reticent about the radical changes proposed in *On the Babylonian Captivity of the Church of God*, particularly with respect to Luther's thesis according to which human will was a slave to God and the devil. Erasmus agreed with the Occamistic position that free will constituted a means of access to salvation.[13] In all likelihood, Holbein must have felt closer to his friend Erasmus than to Luther.

Iconoclasm and Minimalism

Theologians of the Reformation such as Andreas Karlstadt, Ludwig Haetzer, Gabriel Zwilling, Huldreich Zwingli and others, including Luther himself although in a more ambiguous fashion, began waging a real war against images and all representational forms or objects other than words or sounds.[14]

Basel, a commercial city but also a flourishing religious one, was overrun by the Protestant iconoclasm of 1521-23. Reacting against what they thought were the papacy's materialistic, paganistic excesses and abuses, the Wittenberg reformers sacked churches, pillaged and destroyed images and all material representations of faith. In 1525, the Peasants' War provided the occasion for a renewed destruction of artworks. A great "idolomachy" took place in Basel in 1529. Although not a devout Catholic, Holbein was distressed by it as an artist, especially as one who had painted wonderful Virgins: *The Adoration of the Shepherds* and *The Adoration of the Magi* (the two wings of the Oberried Altarpiece, Freiburg-im-Breisgau, Munster, 1520-21), the so-called "Solothurn Madonna" (1521), and later the *Meyer Madonna*, also known as the "Darmstadt Madonna," painted for burgomaster Meyer (1526-30). Basel's iconoclastic climate caused the painter to flee: he left for England (probably in 1526), carrying a letter from Erasmus that introduced him to Thomas More and contained the well-known statement: "Here the arts are cold: he goes to England in order to scrape together a few angelots."[15]

It should be noted, however, that in both camps — reformers and humanists — a tendency arose to intensify the confrontation between man and suffering death, giving evidence of the truth of, and a challenge to, the shallow mercantilism of the official Church.

Nevertheless, even more so than his illustrious friend Erasmus, and in contrast to the Catholic martyr that Thomas More became at the end of his life, Holbein probably experienced a true revolution in, even an erosion of, belief. While keeping up appearances, this curbing of faith within the strict dispassionateness of his profession seems to have led him to integrate, in his own particular way, various aspects of the religious and philosophical currents of his time — from skepticism to the rejection of idolatry — and remodel through art, for his own use, a new vision of mankind. The stamp of suffering (as in *Portrait of His Wife and His Two Elder Children*, 1528, Basel Museum, or the Amerbach diptych — *Christ as the Man of Sorrows*, and the *Virgin as the Mater Dolorosa*, 1519-20) and even more so the unimaginable and invisible landscape of death ("The Ambassadors," 1533, which includes the anamorphosis of a tremendous cranium in the lower part of the picture) compelled Holbein's attention as the main ordeal of the new man and undoubtedly of the artist himself. Nothing seems desirable anymore, values collapse, you are morose. Well, that state can be made beautiful, one can make the withdrawal of desire seem desirable, and as a consequence what might have looked like abdication or morbid dejection will henceforth be perceived as harmonious dignity.

From a painterly standpoint, we are facing a major test. The problem is to give form and color to the nonrepresentable — conceived not as erotic luxuriance (as it appears in Italian art, most particularly in the representation of Christ's Passion) but rather as the nonrepresentable conceived as the dissipation of the means of representation on the threshold of their extinction in death. Holbein's chromatic and compositional asceticism renders this competition between form and death, which is neither dodged nor embellished but set forth in its minimal visibility, into its extreme manifestations constituted by pain and melancholia.

In 1530, having returned from England to Basel in 1528, Holbein converted to the Protestant church after asking, as recorded in the Christian Recruitment registers, for "a better explanation of the Holy Communion before he would go." His conversion, founded on "reason and information," as Fritz Saxl noted,[16] exemplifies the ties he maintained with the Lutherans. Some of his drawings display a clear choice in favor of the spirit of reformation within the Church but without joining the fanaticism of the Reformer himself. Thus, in *Christ as the Light of the World*, in the diptych on Leo X, the cover of the first Lutheran Bible published in Basel, and the illustrations for Luther's Old Testament, Holbein was expressing a personal opinion rather than illustrating an encompassing dogma. In a woodcut depicting Luther, the Reformer appears as a *Hercules Germanicus* but the artist actually represents his fear, his horror and an *atrocitas* of fanaticism.[17] Erasmus's world appears to suit him more than Luther's. Holbein's famous portrait of Erasmus (1523) gave posterity the definitive image of the humanist; when we think of the author of *The Praise of Folly*, do we not always give him the features that Holbein the Younger imprinted on him? Even more to the point, the intimacy of both men with death should be kept in mind.

"Mors Ultima Linea Rerum"

Holbein's famous series, which I have already mentioned, the *Danse Macabre*, explored with exceptional variety the seemingly limited theme of an individual's encounter with death. But what diversity there is, what vastness of space within those scaled-down miniatures and this topic! Holbein took up the same theme again on a dagger's sheath, inserting the deathly dancers in a concave, bounded space. And again in the *Alphabet with the Dance of Death*, where each letter is accompanied by a human figure grappling with Death. It is difficult not to link such an obsessive and unburdened presence of Death in Holbein with the fact that his friend Erasmus's patron saint was the Roman god Terminus, and the motto on his medal bearing that god's likeness read, "*Terminus Concedo Nulli*" or "*Concedo Nulli Terminus*," meaning, "I yield to none," and also, in the medal's circumference, "Contemplate the End of a Long Life" (in Greek) and "Death is the Ultimate Boundary of Things" (in Latin). *Mors ultima linea rerum* might indeed be the motto of the *Dead Christ* of Basel — if it were not the motto of Horace and Erasmus.[18]

The coldness, the restraint and even the unsophisticated appearance of Holbein's art have often been emphasized.[19] It is true that in his time the change in the painter's status is responsible for this change in style that is characterized by the dissolution of the atelier system, the concern for one's own career, a kind of biographical effacement in favor of a nascent mannerism that was taken with affectation, plane surfaces and slopes, that he was nevertheless able to link to his feeling for space. Protestant iconoclasm also left its mark. Holbein disapproved of it, he even fled from it when he left Basel for England; but without, however, giving in to any form of exaltation. In fact, he absorbs the spirit of his time — a spirit of deprivation, of leveling, of subtle minimalism. It would be inaccurate to reduce the trend of the period to a personal tendency for melancholia, even if the latter can be seen in the demeanor of the figures from various countries or social circles which he was fond of painting. Nevertheless, such personality and period features converge: they end up locating representation on the ultimate threshold of representability, grasped with the utmost exactitude and the smallest degree of enthusiasm, on the verge of indifference.... In fact, neither in art nor in friendship is Holbein a committed person. The disgrace of his friend Thomas More doesn't bother him and he stays with Henry VIII. Erasmus himself is shocked by such cynicism, which is perhaps only an aesthetic and psychological aloofness: the coldness and emotional paralysis of the melancholiac. In the addendum to a letter to Bonifacius Amerbach, dated March 22, 1533, Erasmus complains about those, including Holbein, who impose upon his patronage, take advantage of their hosts, and disappoint those to whom he has recommended them.[20]

Cynical or Aloof

Was Holbein, the enemy of iconoclasts and one who had escaped the destruction of images during the Protestant fury in Basel, an iconoclast of ideals? Had the distant, aloof, accomplished ironist become a sort of amoralist out of loathing for any kind of pressure? Was he a devotee of disenchanted non-pressure (*dé-pression*), including the extinction of all artifice at the heart of a gloomily, scrupulously mannered artifice? Appreciated in the nineteenth century, disappointing in the eyes of twentieth-century artists, he may perhaps come closer to us in the part ironic, part gloomy, part desperate, part cynical light of his *Dead Christ*. Living with death and smiling about it, in order to represent it, was perhaps not the way to blaze the trail for a humanistic ethic of Goodness. Neither does it lead to martyrdom for the Protestant faith; rather it heralds more clearly the technician's amoralism without consideration for the beyond, one who seeks a form of beauty somewhere between deprivation and profit. Paradoxically, out of this arid spot, out of this desert from which all beauty should be missing, he compresses disturbance into a masterpiece of colors, forms, spaces....

Indeed, his minimalism maintains a powerful, expressive seriousness that one understands readily when one contrasts it with the stately but haughty sadness, incommunicable and somewhat artificial, of the Jansenist *Dead Christ* by Philippe de Champaigne (at the Louvre).[21]

In short, was he neither a Catholic, a Protestant, nor a Humanist? A friend of Erasmus and Thomas More, but subsequently very much at ease with Henry VIII, their fierce, bloodthirsty foe. Fleeing the Protestants of Basel but also accepting their praise when he returned from his first trip to England, and perhaps converting to Protestantism. Willing to stay in Basel but leaving again for England to become the official painter of a tyrannical king who had put to death a number of his former friends, whose portraits he had so carefully done. When one follows these events, about which Holbein has left no biographical commentary (in contrast to Dürer, for instance), and when one scrutinizes the stern faces of his models, gloomy and straightforward, treated without any complacence, one seems to detect the character and the aesthetic position of a disenchanted verist.

Can Disenchantment Be Beautiful?

At the heart of a Europe in upheaval, the quest for moral truth was accompanied by excesses on both sides, while the realistic taste of a class of merchants, artisans and navigators promoted the rule of strict discipline, but one already corruptible by gold. The artist refused to cast an embellishing gaze at such a world of simple and fragile truths. If he embellished the setting or the clothing, he banished the illusion of having grasped the personality. A new idea was born in Europe, a paradoxical painterly idea – the idea that truth is severe, sometimes sad, often melancholy. Can such a truth also constitute beauty? Holbein's wager, beyond melancholia, is to answer yes, it can.

Disenchantment transformed into beauty is particularly perceptible in feminine portraits. The somewhat despondent serenity of the "Solothurn Madonna," whose prototype was the painter's wife, was followed by the clearly distressed and downcast representation of the wife in the *Portrait of His Wife and His Two Elder Children* (Basel, 1528). The female portraits done in England do not depart from the assumption of deprivation to the point of desolation. Certainly, the kingdom's tragic history under Henry VIII lends itself to it, but while the people simultaneously feared and adored their king, Holbein retains a gloomy vision of his time. Such indeed is the series of wives in which the delicacy of the features and the strength of character vary, but all maintain an identical, somewhat frightened or doleful stiffness; see, for instance, the *Portrait of Queen Jane Seymour*, the *Portrait of Anne of Cleves*, the *Portrait of a Lady* (once thought to be Catherine Howard), as well as the *Portrait of Edward, Prince of Wales* (1539) whose lowered eyelids suffuse the swollen cheeks of a child's innocence with held-back sorrow. Only perhaps the slight mischievousness — or is there more irony than pleasure here? — of *Venus and Cupid* (Basel, 1526) and *Laïs of Corinth* (Basel, 1526), whose model may have been the painter's illegitimate wife, frees these two paintings from such sternness, without, however, leading Holbein's brush into the realm of jolly, carefree sensuality. Among the portraits of men, the gentleness of mind as in the *Portrait of Erasmus of Rotterdam*, the noteworthy elegance of aristocratic handsomeness, also a thoroughly intellectual one, in the *Portrait of Bonifacius Amerbach* (Basel, 1519), as well as the sensuality in the *Portrait of Benedict von Hertenstein* (1517, at the New York Metropolitan Museum of Art) interrupt the continuous vision of a mankind always already entombed. You don't detect death? Try harder, it can be found in the lines of the drawing, in the composition; it is transformed into the volume of objects, faces, bodies, as with the anamorphosis of a skull at the feet of "The Ambassadors" (*Double Portrait of Jean de Dinteville and Georges de Selve*, London, 1533).[22]

An Expenditure of Colors and Laid Out Forms

It is not my purpose to maintain that Holbein was afflicted with melancholia or that he painted melancholiacs. More profoundly, it would seem, on the basis of his oeuvre (including his themes and painterly technique), that a *melancholy moment* (an actual or imaginary loss of meaning, an actual or imaginary despair, an actual or imaginary razing of symbolic values including the value of life) summoned up his aesthetic activity, which overcame the melancholy latency while retaining its trace. Because Magdalena Offenburg was the model for his Basel *Venus* (done before 1526), because of his *Laïs of Corinth*, and because of the two illegitimate children he left in London, one may imagine that the young Holbein had a secret and intense erotic life. Charles Patin was the first to emphasize Holbein's dissipated life, in his edition of Erasmus's *In Praise of Folly* (Basel, 1676). Rudolf and Margot Wittkower endorsed that interpretation and made a spendthrift of him: he was to have squandered the considerable sums he was assumed to have received at the court of Henry VIII buying wild, opulent clothing, so much so that he left only a derisory legacy to his heirs....[23] There is no real evidence to prove or disprove such biographical assumptions, except for the legend of Magdalena Offenburg's own dissipated life. The Wittkowers, moreover, insist on ignoring the painter's work and consider it unimportant that his pictures do not in any way reflect the erotic and financial extravagance that they ascribe to him. From my point of view, that personality trait — assuming it is confirmed — in no way invalidates the depressive center his work reflects and overcomes. The economy of depression is supported by an omnipotent object, a monopolizing Thing rather than by the focus of metonymic desire, which "might account for" the tendency to protect oneself from it through, *among other means*, a splurge of sensations, satisfactions, passions, as elated as it is aggressive, as intoxicating as it is indifferent. It will be noted, nevertheless, that the common feature of these expenditures is *detachment* — getting rid of it, going elsewhere, abroad, toward others.... The possibility of unfolding primary processes, spontaneously but with artful control, appears, however, as the most effective way of overcoming the latent loss. In other words, the controlled and mastered "expenditure" of colors, sounds and words is imperative for the artist–subject, as an essential recourse, similar to "Bohemian life," "criminality" or "dissoluteness" alternating with "miserliness," which one observes in the behavior of such skylarking artists. Hence, very much like personal behavior, artistic *style* imposes itself as a means of countervailing the loss of the other and of meaning: a means more powerful than any other because it is more autonomous (no matter who his patron is, isn't the artist master of his work?) but, in fact and fundamentally, analogous with or complementary to behavior, for it fills the same psychic need to confront separation, emptiness, death. Is not the artist's life considered, by himself to start with, to be a work of art?

The Death of Christ

A depressive moment: everything is dying, God is dying, I am dying. But how is it possible for God to die? Let us briefly return to the evangelical meaning of Christ's death. Theological, hermetic and dogmatic accounts of the "mystery of redemption" are numerous, complex and contradictory. While the analyst cannot accept them by examining them, he or she might try to discover the meaning of the text as it unfolds within his or her hearing.

There are words of Christ that foretell His violent death without referring to salvation, while others, on the contrary, seem immediately to point to and hence serve the Resurrection.[24]

In Luke's context, "serving" refers to "serving at the table," then shifts to "giving his life," a life that is a "ransom" (*lutron*) in Mark's gospel.[25] This semantic shift clearly sheds light on the status of the Christly "sacrifice." He who provides food is the one who sacrifices himself and disappears so that others may live. His death is neither murder nor evacuation but a life-giving discontinuity, closer to nutrition than to the simple destruction of value or the abandonment of a fallen object. A change in the idea of sacrifice obviously takes place within those texts, one that claims to establish a link between men and God through the mediation of a donor. While it is true that giving implies deprivation on the part of the one who gives, who gives of *himself*, there is greater stress placed on the *bond*, on assimilation ("serving at the table") and on the reconciliatory benefits of that process.

Indeed, the only rite that Christ handed down to his disciples and to the faithful, based on the Last Supper, is the oral one of the Eucharist. Through it, sacrifice (and concomitantly death and melancholia) is *aufgehoben* — destroyed and overcome.[26] A number of commentators question René Girard's thesis, which postulates the abolition of sacrifice by Christ and in Christianity, thus also bringing to an end the very notion of the sacred.[27]

The significance one can extract from the word "expiate" is in keeping with such a supersession: *expiare* in Latin, *hilaskomai* in Greek, *kipper* in Hebrew, which imply more of a reconciliation (to be favorably disposed toward someone, to let God be reconciled with oneself) than the fact of "undergoing punishment." It is indeed possible to trace the meaning of "to reconcile" to the Greek *allassō* (to make different, to change with respect to someone). This leads one to see in the Christian expiatory "sacrifice" the offering of an acceptable and accepted gift rather than the violence of shed blood. The generous change of the "victim" into a saving, mediating "offering" under the sway of a loving God is without doubt, in its essence, specifically Christian. It represents something new for the Greek and Judaic worlds, something of which they were unaware, or else, in light of their own worship they viewed it as scandalous.

Nevertheless, one should not forget that a whole ascetic, martyrizing and sacrificial Christian tradition has magnified the victimized aspect of that offering by eroticizing physical and mental pain and suffering as much as possible. Is that tradition no more than a simple medieval deviation that betrayed the "true meaning" of the Gospels? That would be setting little store in the anguish expressed by Christ himself, according to the Evangelists. How can we understand it when it is so powerfully asserted, alongside the oblatory assurance of an oblatory gift made to a father who is also oblatory, equally present in the Gospels' text?

Hiatus and Identification

The break, brief as it might have been, in the bond linking Christ to His Father and to life, introduces into the mythical representation of the Subject a fundamental and psychically necessary discontinuity. Such a caesura, which some have called a "hiatus,"[28] simultaneously provides an image and a narrative for the many separations that build up the psychic life of individuals. It provides image and narrative for some psychic cataclysms that more or less frequently threaten the assumed balance of individuals. Thus, psychoanalysis identifies and relates as the indispensable condition for autonomy, a series of separations (Hegel spoke of the "work of the negative"): birth, weaning, separation, frustration, castration. Real, imaginary or symbolic, these processes necessarily structure our individuation. Their nonexecution or repudiation leads to psychotic confusion; their dramatization, on the contrary, is a source of exorbitant and destructive anguish. Because Christianity set that rupture at the very heart of the absolute Subject — Christ; because it represented it as a Passion, as an interdependent opposite of his Resurrection, his glory and his eternity, it brought to consciousness the essential dramas that are internal to the becoming of each and every subject. It thus endows itself with a tremendous cathartic power.

In addition to displaying a dramatic diachrony, the death of Christ offers imaginary support to the nonrepresentable catastrophic anguish that characterizes melancholiacs. It is well known that the so-called "depressive" stage is essential to the child's access to the realm of symbols and linguistic signs. Such a depression — parting sadness as a necessary condition for the representation of any absent thing — reverts to and accompanies our symbolic activities unless its opposite, exaltation, reappropriates them. A suspension of meaning, a night without hope and eclipse of perspectives including that of life, then the reawakening in the memory of the recollection of traumatic partings, thrusting us into a state of withdrawal. "My God, my God, why hast thou forsaken me?" Moreover, serious depression or paroxystic clinical melancholia represents a true hell for modern individuals, convinced as they are that they must and can realize all their desires for objects and values. The Christly dereliction presents that hell with an imaginary elaboration; it provides the subject with an echo of its unbearable moments when meaning was lost, when the meaning of life was lost.

The postulate according to which Christ died "for all of us" appears often in the texts.[29] *Huper, peri, anti*: the words mean not only "because of us" but "in favor of us," "in our stead."[30] They go back to the "Songs of the Servant of Yahweh" (in the "Book of the Consolation of Israel," Isaiah 40-55) and even earlier to the Hebraic notion of *ga'al*: "to free by purchasing back goods and people that have become alien property." Thus, *redemption* (repurchase, liberation) implies a substitution between the Savior and the faithful, which opened the way for many interpretations. One of these is a compelling one in the analyst's literal reading: the one that suggests an imaginary *identification*. Identification does not mean delegating sins or shifting their burden to the person of the Messiah. On the contrary, it calls for a total implication of the subjects in Christ's suffering, in the hiatus He experiences and, of course, in His hope of salvation. On the basis of that identification, one that is admittedly too anthropological and psychological from the point of view of a strict theology, man is nevertheless provided with a powerful symbolic device that allows him to experience death and resurrection even in his physical body, thanks to the strength of the imaginary identification — and of its actual effects — with the absolute Subject (Christ).

A true initiation is thus elaborated at the very heart of Christianity, which takes up again the deep intrapsychic meaning of initiatory rites that were anterior or alien to its domain, and gives them new meaning. Here, as elsewhere, *death* — that of the old body making room for the new, death to oneself for the sake of glory, death of the old man for the sake of the spiritual body — lies at the center of the experience. But, if there is a Christian initiation, it belongs primarily and entirely within the imaginary realm. While opening up the entire gamut of complete identifications (real and symbolic), it allows for no ritual ordeal other than the words and signs of the Eucharist. From that standpoint, the paroxystic and realistic manifestations of asceticism and "dolorism" are, indeed, extreme positions. Beyond and above that, the implicitness of love and, consequently, of reconciliation and forgiveness completely transforms the scope of Christian initiation, by giving it an aura of glory and unwavering hope for those who believe. Christian faith appears, then, as an antidote to hiatus and depression, but one which includes hiatus and depression and starts from them.

Could it be superegoistic voluntarism that maintains the image of an oblatory Father, or is it the commemoration of an archaic paternal figure risen from the paradise of primary identifications? The forgiveness inherent in redemption condenses *death and resurrection* and presents itself as one of the most interesting and innovative instances of trinitary logic. The key to the nexus seems to be primary identification: the oral and already symbolic oblatory gift exchanged between Father and Son.

For individual reasons, or else on account of the historical crushing of political or metaphysical authority, which is our social fatherhood, the dynamics of primary identification at the foundation of idealization can run into difficulty – it can appear as deprived of significance, illusory, false. The only thing then surviving is the meaning of the deeper workings represented by the Cross: that of caesura, discontinuity, depression.

Did Holbein become the painter of a Christianity stripped of its antidepressive quality that derives from the identification with a rewarding beyond? At any rate, he leads us to the ultimate edge of belief, to the threshold of nonmeaning. The *form* (of art) alone gives back serenity to the waning of forgiveness, while love and salvation take refuge in the execution of the work. Redemption would simply be the discipline of a rigorous technique.

Representing "Severance"

Hegel brought to the fore the dual action of death in Christianity: on the one hand, there is a natural death of the natural body; on the other, death is "infinite love," the "supreme renunciation of the self for the sake of the other." He sees in it a victory over the tomb, the *sheol*, a "death of death," and emphasizes the dialectic that is peculiar to such a logic. "*This negative movement, which belongs to Spirit only as Spirit*, is inner conversion and change...*the end being resolved in splendor, in the feast honoring the reception of the human being into the divine Idea.*"[31] Hegel stresses the consequences of this action for representation. Since death is represented as being natural, but realized only on the condition that it be identified with its otherness, that is, with a divine Idea, one witnesses "*a marvellous union of these absolute extremes,*" "*a supreme alienation of the divine Idea . . . 'God is dead, God himself is dead' is a marvellous, fearsome representation*, which offers to representation the deepest abyss of severance."[32]

Leading representation to the heart of that severance (natural death *and* divine love) is a wager that one could not make without slipping into one or the other of two tendencies: Gothic art, under Dominican influence, favored a pathetic representation of natural death; Italian art, under Fransciscan influence, exalted, through the sexual beauty of luminous bodies and harmonious composition, the glory of the beyond made visible through the glory of the sublime. Holbein's *Body of the Dead Christ in the Tomb* is a rare, if not unique, accomplishment, which situates itself at the exact point where this severance in representation, of which Hegel speaks, occurs. The Gothic eroticism of paroxystic pain is missing, just as the promise of the beyond or the renascent exaltation of nature are lacking. What remains is the tightrope — as the represented body — of an economical, sparing graphic rendition of pain held back within the solitary meditation of artist and viewer. To such a serene, disenchanted sadness, reaching the limits of the insignificant, corresponds a painterly art of utmost sobriety and austerity. It presents no chromatic or compositional exultation, but rather a mastery of harmony and measure.

Is it still possible to paint when the bonds which tie us to body and meaning are severed? Is it still possible to paint when *desire*, which is a bond, collapses? Is it still possible to paint when one identifies not with desire but with *severance*, which is the truth of human psychic life, a severance which is represented by death in the imagination and which melancholia conveys as symptom? Holbein's answer is affirmative. Between classicism and mannerism, his minimalism is the metaphor of severance: between life and death, meaning and nonmeaning, it is an intimate, slender response to our melancholia.

Before Hegel and Freud, Pascal confirmed the sepulcher's invisibility. For him, the tomb is Christ's hidden abode. Everyone looks at Him on the Cross, but in the tomb He hides from His enemies' eyes, and the saints alone see Him, in order to keep Him company in an agony that is peace.

Christ was dead, but seen on the Cross. He is dead and hidden in the sepulcher.

Christ has been shrouded only by saints.

Saints alone enter there.

That is where Christ assumes a new life, not on the Cross.

It is the final mystery of the Passion and the Redemption.

On earth Christ was able to rest nowhere but in the sepulcher.

His enemies ceased working on him only in the sepulcher.[33]

Seeing the death of Christ is thus a way to give it meaning, to bring him back to life. But in the tomb at Basel, Holbein's Christ is alone. Who sees him? There are no saints. There is, of course, the painter. And ourselves. To be swallowed up by death, or perhaps to see it in its minimal, dreadful beauty, as the limit inherent in life. "*Christ in grief... Christ being in agony and in the greatest sorrow, let us pray longer.*"[34]

Painting as a substitute for prayer? Contemplation of the painting might perhaps replace prayer at the critical place of its appearance — where nonmeaning becomes significant, while death seems visible and livable.

Like Pascal's invisible tomb, death cannot be represented in Freud's unconscious. It is imprinted there, however, as noted earlier, by spacings, blanks, discontinuities or the destruction of representation.[35] Consequently, death reveals itself as such to the imaginative ability of the self in the isolation of signs or their banalization up to the point of disappearing: such is Holbein's minimalism. But as it grapples with the erotic vitality of the self and the jubilatory abundance of exalted or morbid signs conveying Eros's presence, death calls for a distant realism or, better yet, a grating irony: this brings forth the "danse macabre" and disenchanted profligacy inborn in the painter's style. The self eroticizes and signifies the obsessive presence of death by stamping with isolation, emptiness or absurd laughter its own imaginative assurance that keeps it alive, that is, anchored in the play of forms. On the contrary, images and identities — the carbon copies of that triumphant self — are etched with inaccessible sadness.

Now that our eyes have been filled with this vision of the invisible, let us look once more at the people Holbein has created: heroes of modern times, they stand straitlaced, sober and upright. Secretive, too: as real as can be and yet indecipherable. Without a single impulse that betrays *jouissance*. No exalted loftiness toward the beyond. Nothing but the sober difficulty of standing here below. They simply remain upright in a void that makes them strangely alone. Self confident. And close.

NOTES

1. Fyodor Dostoyevsky, *The Idiot*, trans. David Magarshack (New York: Viking Penguin, 1955). (Author's emphasis.)

2. *Ibid.*, pp. 418-20. (Author's emphasis.)

3. "Incorporated within the present frame above the painting and running its full length is an inscription, with Angels with Instruments of the Passion, JESVS NAZARENVS REX IVDAEORUM, executed with brush on paper, almost certainly contemporaneously with the painting. An attribution to Holbein himself, while not certain, is not to be ruled out, even though the Angels recall the work of his recently deceased brother, Ambrosius." John Rowlands, *Holbein* (Boston: David R. Godine, 1985), p. 127.

4. The relation of height to width is 1:7, but if the plate affixed to the lower margin of the picture is included the relation becomes 1:9.

5. See Paul Gantz, *The Paintings of Hans Holbein* (New York: Phaidon, 1950), pp. 218-20.

6. See "Der Leichnam Christi im Grabe, 1522," in *Die Malerfamilie Holbein in Basel*, ed. Joseph Gautner, Ausstellung im Kunstmuseum Basel zur Fünfhundertjahr Feier der Universität Basel, 1960, pp. 188-90.

7. See ch. 7, "Nerval, *El desdichado*," of my *Soleil noir: Dépression et mélancolie* (Paris: Gallimard, 1987).

Before Holbein such a representation of the body fully stretched out can be seen, for instance, in Pietro Lorenzetti's *Deposition* in the lower church at Assisi. One finds the same position, but turned in the opposite direction, in the recumbent Christ in the murals (c. 1450) of the Blansingen church near Basel. About 1440 the master of the *Heures de Rohan* depicts a stiff, bloodied image of the dead Christ but accompanied by Mary's mercy. Villeneuve's *Pietà* with the Christ in profile should be compared with that series. See Walter Überwasser, "Holbeins Christus in der 'Grabnische,'" *Festschrift für Werner Noack* (1959), pp. 125ff.

One should also mention the sculpted *Christ in the Tomb* in the Freiburg cathedral and another sculpture in the Freising cathedral (1430), presenting a recumbent Christ quite similar in position and proportions to Holbein's painting, leaving aside, of course, the anatomical knowledge of the body characteristic of the Renaissance artist.

8. Concerning religious feelings in Germany at the end of the Middle Ages and their influence on painting, see Louis Réau, *Mathias Grünewald et le retable de Colmar* (Nancy: Berger-Levrault, 1920).

9. See Wilhelm Pinder, *Holbein le Jeune et la fin de l'art gothique allemand* (Cologne, 1920).

10. See Überwasser, "Holbeins Christus."

11. The Death theme recurs throughout the Middle Ages and finds a particularly receptive audience in northern European countries. In his prologue to the *Decameron*, on the other hand, Boccaccio banishes all interest in such gloominess and exalts the joy of living.

Thomas More, on the contrary, whom Holbein met through Erasmus, speaks of death as Holbein might have done on the basis of his *Dead Christ*: "We joke and believe death to be far removed. It is hidden in the deepest secrets of our organs. For since the moment you came into this world, life and death go forward at the same pace." See A. Lerfoy, *Holbein* (Paris: Albin Michel, 1943), p. 85. Shakespeare, as is well known, excels in the tragic and magical intertwining of death themes.

12. Martin Luther, *Tischreden in der Mathesischen Sammlung*, vol. 1.122, p. 51, as quoted by Jean Wirth, *Luther, étude d'histoire religieuse* (Geneva: Droz, 1981), p. 130. Translator's note: translation from the French, with the help of the German text in *Tischreden*, ed. Walther Rehm (Munich, 1934), p. 324. For the subsequent quotations I have used the translation by Bertram Lee Woolf of the ninety-five theses in *Reformation Writings of Martin Luther* (London: Lutterworth Press, 1952), vol. 1, pp. 32-43.

13. See Erasmus's *De libero arbitrio* and Luther's answer, *De servo arbitrio*. See John M. Todd, *Martin Luther, a Biographical Study* (Westminster, Md.: Newman Press, 1964) and R.H. Fife, *The Revolt of Martin Luther* (New York: Columbia University Press, 1957).

14. See Carl C. Christensen, *Art and the Reformation in Germany* (Columbus: Ohio University Press, 1979), Charles Garside, Jr., *Zwingli and the Arts* (New Haven: Yale University Press, 1966). One should note within the same tradition the extensive iconoclasm of H. C. Agrippa von Nettesheim's *De incertitudine et vanitate scientiarum et artium atque excellentia verbi Dei declamatio* (Antwerp, 1531; French translation, Leiden, 1726).

15. See Christensen, *Art and the Reformation*, p. 169.

16. See Fritz Saxl, "Holbein and the Reformation," in *Lectures* (London: Warburg Institute, University of London, 1957), vol. 1, p. 278.

17. *Ibid.*, p. 282.

18. See Erwin Panofsky, "Erasmus and the Visual Arts," *Journal of the Warburg and Courtauld Institutes* 32 (1969), pp. 214-19. Like Terminus, Erasmus yields to nothing; or still, according to another interpretation, it is Death itself, like Terminus, that does not yield.

19. See Pierre Vaisse, Introduction to *Holbein le Jeune* (Paris: Flammarion, 1972).

20. See Panofsky, "Erasmus," p. 220.

21. Philippe de Champaigne's dead Christ lying on a shroud resembles Holbein's painting with regard to the Savior's solitude. The painter eliminated the Virgin who was present in J. Bonasono's print after Raphael, which is Champaigne's source. Nevertheless, while also coming close to Holbein

through the coloring's rigor and restraint, Champaigne remains at the same time more faithful to the sacred texts (showing Christ's traditional wounds, the crown of thorns, etc.), and colder, distant, even hardened. The Jansenist spirit shows in that vision, as do the recommendations of late-sixteenth-century theologians (Borthini, Paleoti, Gilio) to avoid expressing pain. See Bernard Dorival, *Philippe de Champaigne (1602-1674)*, 2 vols. (Paris: Léonce-Laguet, 1978).

22. See Gantz, *The Paintings of Hans Holbein*.

23. See Rudolf and Margot Wittkower, *Born Under Saturn, The Character and Conduct of Artists: A Documented History from Antiquity to the French Revolution* (New York: W.W. Norton, 1969).

24. Thus, on the one hand: "And Jesus said to them, 'The cup that I drink you will drink; and with the baptism with which I am baptized, you will be baptized' " (Mark 10.39); "He said to them, 'You will drink my cup' " (Matt. 20.23); " 'I came to cast fire upon the earth; and would that it were already kindled. I have a baptism to be baptized with; and how I am constrained until it is accomplished!' " (Luke 12.49-50); and especially the famous quotation that signals the loss of hope, "Eli, Eli, lama sabachthani?" that is, "My God, my God, why hast thou forsaken me?" (Matthew 27.46; cf. Mark 15.34). All biblical references follow *The New Oxford Annotated Bible*, Revised Standard Version, 2d ed. (New York: Oxford University Press, 1971).

There is on the other hand the message of glad tidings: "For the Son of Man also came not to be served but to serve, and to give his life as a ransom for many" (Mark 10.45); "But I am among you as one who serves." (Luke 22.27).

25. See Xavier-Léon Dufour, "La mort rédemptrice du Christ selon le Nouveau Testament," in *Mort pour nos péchés* (Brussels: Publication des Facultés Universitaires Saint-Louis, 1979), pp. 11-45.

26. See A. Vergote, "La mort rédemptrice du Christ à la lumière de l'anthropologie," in *Mort pour nos péchés*, p. 68.

27. René Girard, *Des choses cachées depuis la fondation du monde* (Paris: Grasset, 1978).

28. See Urs von Balthasar, "La Nouvelle Alliance," in *La gloire et la croix* (Paris: Aubier, 1975), vol. 3, p. 2.

29. See Rom. 5.8, "But God shows His love for us in that while we were yet sinners Christ died for us"; and also, "He who did not spare His own Son, but gave him up for us all" (Rom. 8.32), and "And walk in love, as Christ loved us and gave himself up for us, *a fragrant offering and a sacrifice to God*" (Eph. 5.2); in similar fashion, see Mark 10.45, 14.24; Matt. 20.28, 26.28; Luke 22.19; and 1 Peter 2.21-25.

30. See Dufour, "La mort rédemptrice."

31. G.W.F. Hegel, *Lectures on the Philosophy of Religion*, trans. E.B. Speirs (New York: The Humani-

ties Press, 1962), vol. 3, p. 93. (Author's emphasis.)

    32. *Ibid*. (Translation emended, author's emphasis.)

    33. Blaise Pascal, "Le Sépulcre de Jésus-Christ," no. 362, in *Pensées de M. Pascal sur la religion*, ed. Zacharie Tourneur (Paris: Editions de Cluny, 1938), vol. 2, p. 101.

    34. See n.33; the text is from Pascal, "Le Mystère de Jésus," no. 297, *Pensées*, vol. 2, p. 12.

    35. See Julia Kristeva, "Un contre-dépresseur: la psychanalyse," *Soleil noir*.

From *Soleil noir: Dépression et mélancolie*, Paris, Gallimard, 1987.
English translation forthcoming from Columbia University Press.

Translated by Leon S. Roudiez.

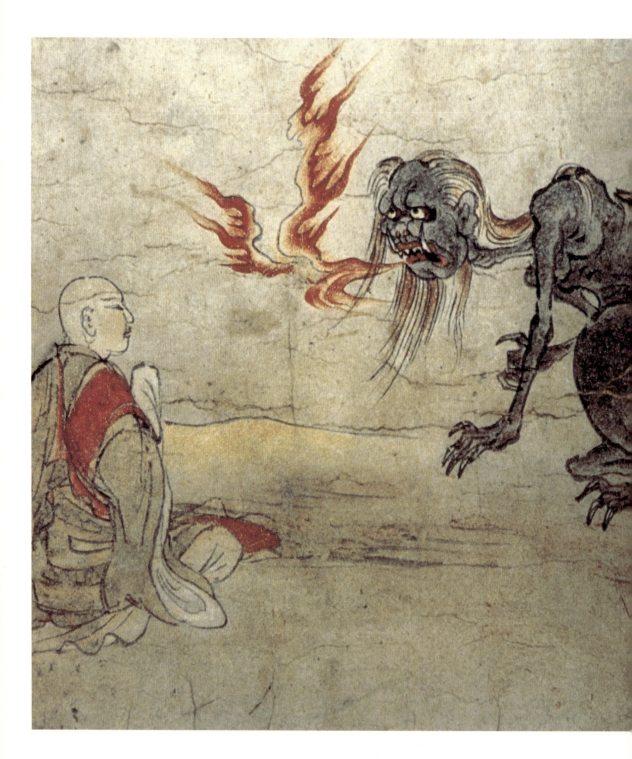

Monk and *gaki*.

Hungry Ghosts and Hungry People:
Somaticity and Rationality in Medieval Japan

William R. LaFleur

One dog barks at nothing
ten thousand others
pass it on
            — Japanese aphorism*

Excretion is not simply a middle term between two appropriations.
          — Georges Bataille, "The Use Value of D.A.F. de Sade"

The Somaticity of Specters

Invisible bodies, no doubt by definition, can be done away with much more easily than visible ones. Since angels, ghosts, demons, ancestors, ghouls and the like take up no physical space in our empirical world, the liquidation of them involves no bloodletting, leaves no corpses, and calls for no official inquiry. Whenever such invisible bodies are being deleted from the "chain of being" long believed in by a given people, that act of erasure is a sure sign that the aspiration to be recognized as "modern" has gotten strong among them. Aquinas lived when larger philosophical problems were still linked to positions adopted concerning the bodies of angels; soon therafter, angelic bodies and, in fact, all references to such beings, fell completely out of discussions considered properly philosophical. In this kind of move, modernity was finding — and founding — itself.

The loss was, of course, widely seen as a gain. The discarded was obscurantism, something for which the medieval mind, it was assumed, had had a penchant; the

---

*W.S. Merwin, *Asian Figures*, New York, Atheneum, 1975, p. 38.

winner was rationality, a precious commodity now free at last to come into its own and to claim the new, modern age for itself. The bond was tight between modernity and rationality; the invisible adhesive making it so was the assumption that it was necessary and natural, not contingent – and, most certainly – not itself a story.

Now even to suspect an *element of the fabricated* in modernity's account of itself – let alone read it in Lyotard's terms as "grand narrative" – is, of course, to feel oneself already somewhat loosened from that epoch and the spellbinding story it had been telling about itself. And to query that is also to become newly curious about what the life of the mind was like before the modernity narrative caught us in its spell and had us convinced that the modern's own relationship with rationality was privileged. Now the jump from the medieval to the modern looks less like a chasm and more like a gully – or, more accurately, a series of them. Medieval mentalities, we are increasingly apt to discover, were what they were, not because real rationality or a method peculiar to the sciences was not yet theirs, but merely because the store of information at their disposal was much smaller than it later became for moderns and for ourselves (whatever we are). With the incremental growth of specific knowledge came a gradual reduction in the distance between the known and the unknown; medieval thinkers simply had to make long, often very bold, jumps in places where later peoples got by – and continue to get by – with shorter and shorter ones.

This brings us, with recharged curiosity, back to the invisible bodies in medieval thought and to noticing that they frequently show up in overtly philosophical texts and in ways that seem natural to the discourse there. To explain their presence as "illogical" is circular; to attribute it solely to concessions to folk belief and/or the pressure of religious authorities – as if the medieval thinkers really knew otherwise all along! – is to charge bad faith without clear evidence of such. To the medievalist, then, the nexus between invisible bodies and rationality becomes problematized anew. Ghosts and ghouls may be odd in any age; historical inquiry is interested in why they are less odd in one era than in another. To delineate that difference is the reason for my attempt here to recover – without reclaiming – the intellectual whereabouts of a specific kind of invisible body that had a large role in the life of the mind in medieval Japan. The body on which I focus this inquiry is that of the *gaki*, an important component in the development of medieval Japanese Buddhist thought. Being Buddhist, it had its origin in India, where the concept of such beings (termed *preta* in Sanskrit) was first articulated. Along with the expansion of Buddhism, this figure too climbed out of India, spread not only southward but also eastward along the Silk Route. The evidence is clear that it gained for itself a secure niche in the minds of the peoples of southeast Asia but also among the Chinese, Koreans and Japanese.[1]

"Hungry ghost" is the usual but rough rendering of these terms into English. The concept, it is worth noting, has been something of an embarrassment to modern Buddhists, including persons of the West who like their Buddhism rational and empirical; although these ghosts pop up all over the tradition, such persons dismiss them as external to "real" Buddhism, things that the popular mind dragged in during weak moments when the Buddhist philosophers — with their usual vigilance for maintaining the rational — were dozing.

I doubt that this is the way to go. It assumes a notion of pure rationality, one easily separable from the folk mind and from the larger social correlates of any view or theory. My own account will not ignore the interestedness of the Buddhist ecclesiastical authorities; nor will it deny the folk their due. It will, on the contrary, suggest how hungry ghosts, as beings with bodies, were — at least for medieval Japan — an important reed that was woven into many places in a cognitive basket that was used to try to hold a lot of things together. To play a role in a synthesis intended to satisfy philosophers, ecclesiastics, a privileged aristocracy, a wary government and a vast "folk" — this was what the concept of the hungry ghost was expected to do. Appeals to some level of demonstrability were part of the argument for it all; it was what passed for "science" in its day.

And for a long time it worked. When it fell apart that happened not because the Japanese discovered rationality but because better and fuller information about the world gradually became more than the old basket could hold. At the same time, contradictions built into the old container's structure became undeniable and finally unmanageable. Improved information about things, combined with a growing awareness of the old paradigm's structural stresses, were both enough to drastically relativize its importance. This meant it had to be reassigned. Whereas in the medieval period, the concept of hungry ghosts had been part of the best science of the day, in the modern it slipped increasingly into a much more narrow domain, one for which the nineteenth-century Japanese invented a new word, *shūkyō* or "religion." The coinage made a small cage. In it were placed notions like that of the hungry ghost – now something no more than a vivid metaphor for strictly internal and private realities.[2]

Back home in medieval Japanese thought, however, it had been the somaticity of these creatures that was important. There, they had certainly not been merely symbols of events of psychic pain or hyperbolic representations of greed. Without a body – different from man's and ordinarily invisible to humans, to be sure – these creatures would have made no sense. It is, in fact, the *bodily interaction* between humans and ghosts which was crucial for the medieval people who concern me here.

The classic sources in the Buddhist scriptures are unambiguous about that somaticity; the *preta/gaki* are depicted as the real, discrete, and fully embodied occupants of a distinct rubric in the taxonomy of being. Their somaticity is so much a part of them that it is also the locus of their misery. For the hungry ghost is not just periodically hungry. Hunger is in its name because it is constituted by hunger, not merely conditioned by it. For other kinds of beings – mankind, animals and the like – hunger will come and go but for the *gaki* there is only an ongoing, unalleviated gnawing of the stomach and parching of the throat. When the Buddhist canon again and again depicts this creature as one "with a stomach as huge as a mountain but a throat as narrow as a needle," there may be hyberbole in the dimensions, but the antinomy of the structure is of central importance to the definition of this type. That body is this being's horrible dilemma: voracious appetites and absolutely minimal equipment cannot even begin to satisfy it. A painting from Sung China shows it well.

Within the classically defined Buddhist understanding of the "chain of being," this creature had a position only one rung above that of the creatures in hell. Because transmigration through multiple lives was simply assumed to be true, those beings born as hungry ghosts received that fate as retribution for gross moral faults in anterior lives. Their torture was punitive, much like that of the creatures of hell.

The nuance of difference between this fate and that of hell's inhabitants is, however, interesting. Whereas hells are prisons, the hungry ghost was in a place without walls. Because the locus of its punishment was coextensive with its own body and, in fact, constituted that body, the need for walls was gone. These damned were free to wander the world at will because they could never escape their own bodies. The need for hell's externally applied instruments of torture also fell away: the scimitars, corkscrews and hot irons of generic hells. Gone too was the need for a small

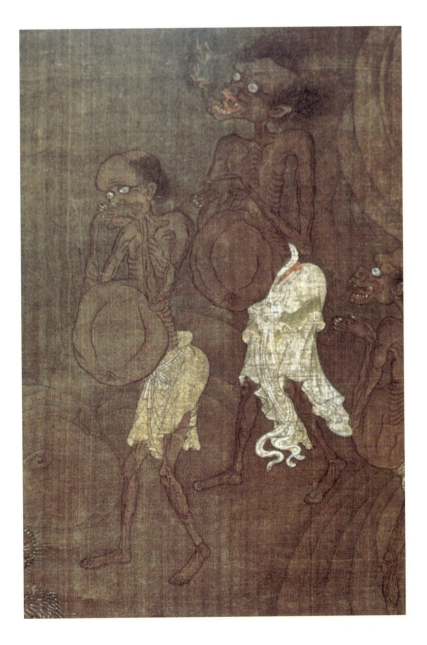

Hungry ghosts from a Sung painting.

z o n e

army of keepers and torture-dispensing thugs. In the case of the hungry ghost, it is not what is done to the body that causes pain but the received structure of the body itself that virtually hurt like hell.

Science and the Fate of Feces

The visual evidence on which I concentrate is drawn primarily, but not exclusively, from two extant scrolls of twelfth-century Japan, sequentially arranged pictures that depict hungry ghosts in a variety of activities. These scrolls, now housed in the Japanese National Museums of Tokyo and Kyoto, are known as *Gaki-zōshi*, inasmuch as "*gaki*" is the Japanese rendering of the Chinese characters for "hungry ghost" and "*zōshi*" pinpoints the documentary/evidential nature of pictures such as these.[3] The scenes in them, still vivid and captivating after seven hundred years, tell us more than any other resource about *gaki* bodies and how they were imagined by the medievals.

On many points, the ancient Indian Buddhist scriptures and the medieval Japanese totally agreed. For instance, each holds that the hungry ghost, while occupying a distinctly separate place in the taxonomy of being, is a form of existence into which a human being could be reborn with terrifying ease. With karmic transmigration assumed, a slip downward in the taxonomy was often the price to be paid for moral turpitude. This doubled the horror. Not only were humans encompassed by invisible *gaki* in their present life, but they faced the dire possibility of dying and being reborn as such in the next one. And that personalizing of the horror also proximized it; given the fact that such an eventuality might at any given time be no more than one die-and-rebirth event away, there was a "Gregor Samsa" factor here. The terror was real and total. Finding oneself transformed into a body so utterly alien was potentially as close as the other side of one heart failure, one fatally complicated childbirth, one entrapment in a burning building or any other of the many means of sudden death.

Terror was part of argument. Dull minds, it was assumed, needed powerful fillips to see reality. Some ascetics may have gotten clairvoyant through their disciplines and were in possession of "heaven's eye" (*tengen*); they could see how the whole system worked and could literally see the bodies of the *gaki*.

But lesser men and women needed stories and pictures to jog their minds.

Because terror was thought to be a facilitator rather than manipulator of such cognition, the *Gaki-zōshi*, for instance, were thought to be apertures into reality as it really is.

And medieval Japan gives ample instances of these pictures doing their intended work. In this, the hungry ghost scrolls were like the scrolls and screens depicting hell (*jigoku-zōshi*). The poet Saigyō (1118-90), who elsewhere depicted his reactions to hell-pictures, records his sense of horror in seeing portraits of *gaki* making and then eating their own children:[4]

Creatures who birth
babies every night, every day
and gulp them down as fast —
a prodigious realm showing
great feats of horror.

Dream-journey narratives, reports of people claiming to have returned from brief sojourns in other worlds and the picture-scrolls seem to have reinforced one another. A thirteenth-century text tells of a man who saw the realm of *gaki* and found them "looking just the way they are shown in pictures."[5]

The point seems clear. The horror shows, the real terror and the making of personal leaps into the Buddhist epistemic web were all connected. Medieval men, women and children learned about these aliens, at least in part, so that they might take the requisite steps in this world to avoid being reborn that way in the next. And undoubtedly the Buddhist temples collected both credence and revenues from this. There were very wealthy temples and elite monks who had personal and institutional reasons for wanting wide and deep public purchase of this view of reality.[6] Ideological closure was, to be sure, high on their list of desiderata.

However, to notice their patent, even blatant, interestedness does not remove the necessity of our trying to reconstruct how the medieval view of things "worked," how it felt as an episteme — and how and why it eventually fell apart. To see ideology at work here does not preclude the fact that the Buddhism of this epoch also proffered what was to be accepted as the best available *science* of the day. To detect the signs of manipulation does not negate the fact that these were also configurations of data and theory intended to present — even to the presenters themselves — the era's version of a cognitively satisfying schema of reality.

This calls for a scrutiny of the scrolls — and, I propose, at the nexus between *gaki* and feces in them. To look at the pictures is to look at the bodies of wraiths — but at wraiths most commonly in places where excrement and other bodily wastes will be found. *Gaki*, the pictures tell us, will invariably be present in latrines and cesspools. In an especially graphic scene from the scroll in the Tokyo Museum we are shown what is happening in a back alley of the capital. The exquisite realism of execution here reinforces the sense that it comprises an aperture into a reality ordinarily unseen — not just in the social sense (because the latrine was in a back alley) but, more importantly, in the ontological sense. The human defecators here are clearly blind to the presence of the *gaki* around them. The painting's viewer, a human like those portrayed, was meant to get the point: "So, too, you are blind to these things most of the time! And this is your rare chance to see what really exists. It is not to be missed!"

This might profitably be regarded as medieval art as ontological X ray. It purports to open the view to two things he or she ordinarily cannot see: first, that *gaki*, in fact, commingle invisibly with humans in their own world and, second, that men, women and children ordinarily live their lives oblivious to the gruesome beings hunched over next to them. The picture functions as aperture but then also reflexively as mirror. It provides a rare chance to really "see" *gaki* but also to get a glimpse of humans — the viewers themselves — living daily life in a condition of epistemic and visual occlusion.

But what the picture says about feces is as important as what it says about human myopia; the "science" is as much a part of it as are the psychology and religion. And that is because this offers the viewer a challenge to "verify" the entire schema's intelligibility. In a word, the viewer of the pictures was implicitly requested to conduct an experiment, one that involves heightened awareness of excrement: what can be observed about it, what is mystifying about it, and how the unknown can be turned into the known. The experiment is one that makes a lot of things "work" conceptually, by positing a cause-effect and strictly *physical* relationship between the voracious mouths of *gaki* and the empirically observable fact that excrement in latrines and in cesspools simply disappears at a fairly rapid rate.

The experiment was certainly circular. But the important thing is that what might be termed the "hungry ghost hypothesis" had a certain conceptual tidiness. Just by

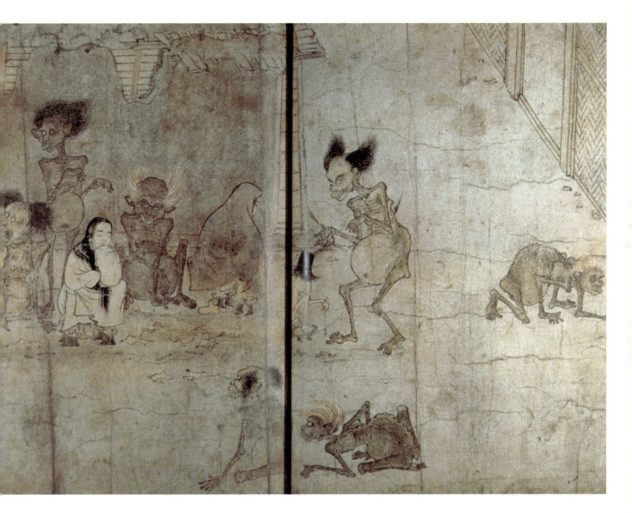

Street scene of defecators.

calling to mind a few basic things, the advocate of Buddhist explanations could show that what the sutras said made sense. Although the ghosts themselves were invisible by definition, humans could certainly observe the *effects* of their presence and actions in their own world: excrement had a limited street-life. It discolored, pulverized and then was gone. And it did so not instantly — but still more rapidly than many other discards in the streets. This rapid-but-not-too-rapid rate of disappearance was itself a source of curiosity but, fortunately, was explained by Buddhist science: the hungry ghost's needle-thin throat made impossible any instant consumption of excrement but, on the other hand, its intense craving guaranteed it would perform its scavenger role with all the energy it could muster. Even the rate of excremental decomposition seemed, in this quasi-empiricist fashion, to shore up the case for *gaki*'s existence. The scriptures explained what went on in the latrine and the latrine verified what the scriptures said. Even if circular it was the best science around just then. And the Buddhist institutions had much to gain from having the best books and explanations of the day.

Coprophagy is the key here. It receives highlighted treatment in the *Gaki zōshi* because of its centrality to the argument reconstructed here. A frame of the Tokyo scroll shows us what I would call a scene of "Coprophagite in Cesspool." This may well be our best peephole into the medieval mind at work here — but only if we repress or overcome our twentieth-century impulse to assume that the really interesting "mind" at work here is the unconscious one. It is, unaccustomed as we are to seeing it so, the *conscious* mind that needs excavation here.

There is irony in this. Precisely because of the cultural success of psychoanalytic theory and the widely held belief among us that to disclose the unconscious is to gain contact with what is fundamental, we in our time are now forced to exert considerable intellectual energy merely to reimagine what it would be like to have one's overwhelming curiosity directed to the mere physicality of shit — that is, its trajectory as material stuff into, through and out of our world. Ours is a case of having been blinded by insight — in this case, the most recent ones of our own sciences. The explanatory power of psychoanalytic discoveries and theories would ordinarily channel us into assuming that we know the meaning — a meaning in and for the human psyche — of the coprophagous ghosts in these pictures. It is, however, our own episteme that gives us cognitive problems here. Our total absorption of the

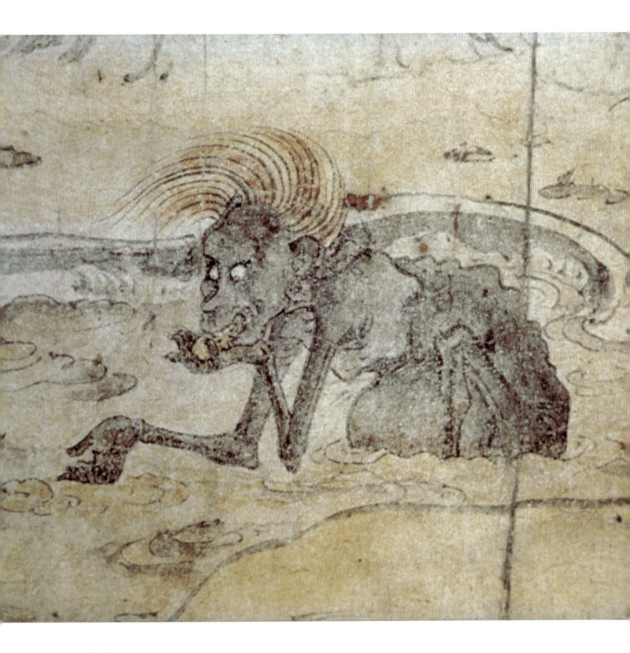

Gaki in cesspool.

modern discovery that it is really bacteria which effect the disappearance of feces turned our age's attention to the psychological meaning of such things, thus allowing for a twentieth-century slippage into a kind of cultural amnesia about the priority of questions having to do with the raw physicality of such things. The medievalist, however, must now recollect the intellectual shape of an era in which shit was still largely a substance whose physical properties and transformations were still matters of primary curiosity.

For us to squat for a moment – even if only mentally and through these X-ray apertures – on high-heeled wooden *geta* in a back alley of this street in the capital of medieval Japan may, perhaps, be what is needed to disclose something of the contingency (and maybe even the historical oddity) of intellectual life in the recent West. The painters of these pictures devoted, we must note, a good deal of scroll space to portraying excrement and its transmogrifications as some kind of stuff in our world. (This includes, to the joy of historians, pictorial evidence of the "shit-sticks" elsewhere found in East Asian texts.)[7] The overwhelming impression left by this is not that these people were unusually prurient or obsessed with scatological possibilities. Rather, it appears that their fascination was focused on *a question that needed explanation*. That is, they wanted simply to know what was happening to feces as feces – as they physically change and then disappear.

And where did this lead them? Given the state of information at their disposal, it brought them right to what I would call the "hungry ghost hypothesis." Here, the texts of Buddhism, already widely touted as giving authoritative information about everything and not limited to the narrow domain of "religion," had an explanation.[8] They spoke eloquently and in detail about a species of invisible beings, which hovered in and around humans and congregated in large quantities at latrines and other places of defecation. In a word, what we have identified as the work of bacteria was exactly what they saw as scavenging and clean-up duties performed by hungry ghosts.

And, of course, this explanatory scheme did not limit itself to shit. Thought to be physically rather than psychically related to us and our bodies, *gaki* performed a variety of distasteful but necessary tasks. Condemned by bad karma racked up in earlier lives, the hungry ghosts were forced to consume all the human body's excreta, effluvia and ejacula. Nasal mucus was certainly included. A portion of a *Rokudō-e* or "Painting of the Six [Buddhist] Courses," which derives from the thirteenth century and is in the possession of Shōju-raigō-ji Temple in Shiga, includes a very important section depicting hungry ghosts. Within this there is a temple scene, unfortunately worn with age. Just visible, however, is a monk who sits along the temple balustrade; the moment grasped is that in which he has turned from listening to the sermon indoors to face outward, holding his nose in a pincer of fingers and ejecting snot. Just below him is a shadowy hungry ghost with hands extended to catch the discharge.

Within this same portion of the painting is another section which has perplexed many. There is, I think, little that is puzzling here. The distinctly female ghost with outstretched "receptacle" hands, the manual action of the walking man, and the white globules that seem to fly into the air behind him all combine, I would suggest, to tell us this is a man engaged in ambulatory masturbation, and it is his semen that the kneeling, female hungry ghost is trying to catch in her hands.

In dying, of course, the entire body becomes a kind of ejecta. And exposed corpses, the medievals certainly observed, lose their form in much the same way feces do. The similarity of the decomposition pattern suggests that here too it is *gaki* that are at work — now not on a part but on the whole. The *Gaki zōshi* capture the point exactly in a scene set in a cemetery. The fate of feces was also, this suggests, structurally that of the fate of the body as a whole. The process is the same: wasted bodies are on large scale what body wastes are on a smaller scale.

The Ghosts in the System

The principal ancient source for what shows up in these scrolls is an Indian Buddhist sutra which had been translated into Chinese during the sixth century. Known in China as the *Cheng-fa nien-ch'u ching* (Japanese: *Shōbōnenjo-gyō*), it not only categorizes all beings in the universe but, within the rubric of the hungry ghost, further stipulates the existence of thirty-six subspecies. The hungry ghosts are typed as: ones with bodies like cauldrons, those with needle-thin throats, vomit-eaters, excrement-eaters, nothing-eaters, eaters of vapors in the air, eaters of the Buddhist dharma, water-drinkers, hopeful and ambitious ones, saliva-eaters, wig-eaters, blood-drinkers, meat-eaters, consumers of incense smoke, disease-dabblers, defecation-watchers, ones that live under the ground, possessors of miraculous powers, intensely burning ones, ones fascinated with colors, inhabitants of the beach, ones with

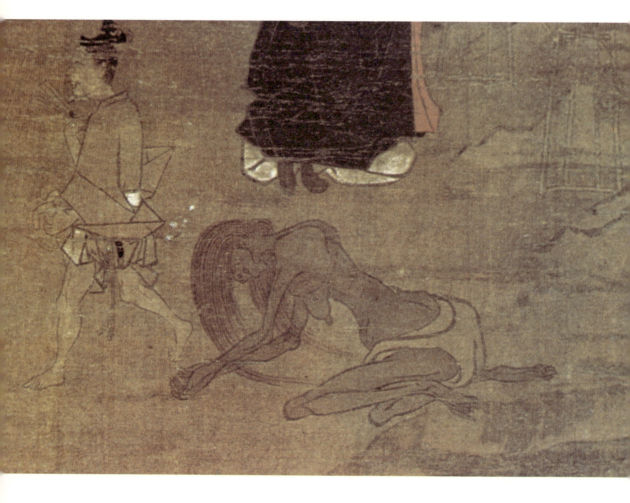

Semen catcher.

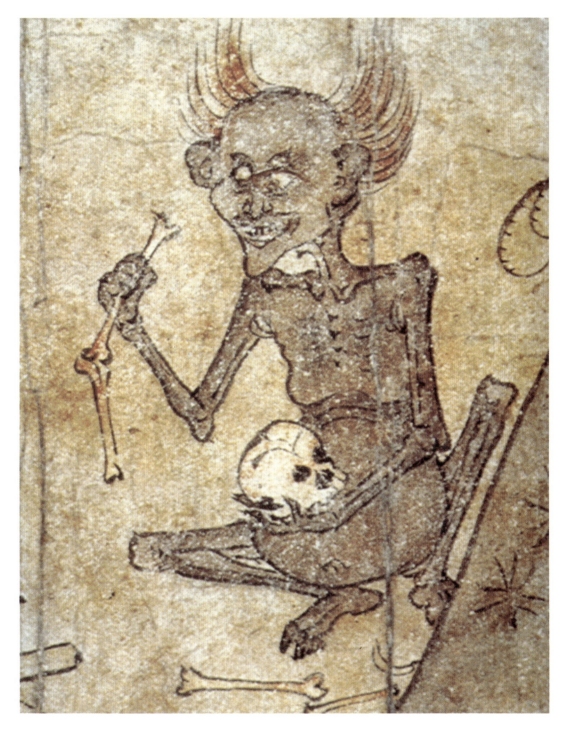

Gaki in cemetery.

zone

walking-canes, infant-eaters, semen-eaters, demonic ones, fire-eaters, those on filthy streets, wind-eaters, burning-coal consumers, poison-eaters, inhabitants of open fields, those living among tombs (and eating ashes), those that live in trees, ones that stay at crossroads, and those that kill themselves.[9]

On first reading, the list seems to be a chaos of categories — almost as if were vying to be that "Chinese Encyclopedia" which Foucault, in the opening pages of *The Order of Things*, said that he found, much to his own fascination, in Borges. Nevertheless, certain patterns exist in this seemingly motley array of types. Although there are exceptions, hungry ghosts in this list are largely classified by what they consume and where they choose to hunker down. And what they eat, aside from things like the Buddhist dharma and items such as "nothing," turn out to be things widely regarded as polluting and/or repulsive.

I am here, of course, less interested in what may or may not have been the principles informing the original Indian selection for this list than in the use to which the medieval Japanese put it. The treatment of *gaki* in the $\overline{Ojoyoshu}$, written in 985, stands in between the Indo-Chinese scripture and the twelfth-century scrolls.[10] There may be the making of a unified view in these earlier texts, but it is in the illustrated scrolls that the lineaments of a *system* are more clear than ever before. Far from being a picturing of types lifted at random from written sources, the selection of the artist seems to have been careful and calculated to have persuasive power. The presentation of the whole in a format that virtually begs the viewer to "verify" the hungry ghost hypothesis against things in his or her own experience seems designed to serve not just as a portrait but as an argument.

In the *Gaki zōshi*, we can see the hungry ghost hypothesis as it was stretched to provide "explanation" for other things beyond those that are body wastes and wasted bodies. For instance, the invisible ghosts were used to tell what is happening in cases where we would use language about oxidation. Here, in a most literal sense, we have the portrait of consumption, but it is a consumption of — rather than by — fire. The *gaki*, invisible but connected bodily to the visible world, is brought in to explain why flames and conflagrations die out — why, especially, airborne embers, meteors, and even lightning bolts seem suddenly to be "caught" in mid-course and then disappear from sight. The *gaki* is a consumer of fires. (Written texts say that in its blind, deluded passion to fulfill the hunger and thirst within, the *gaki* mistakes fire for food, thus incrementally aggravating its condition. This is why it both emits fire from its mouth and takes more of it into its body.)

And what works for fire works for water, too. Evaporation received its explanation this way: the hungry ghost, the texts were careful to point out, was not only voraciously hungry but unquenchably thirsty as well. One of the scenes of the scrolls is that of an ancestral pillar positioned at the gate of a Buddhist temple. Pious folk would pour water in a purification/memorial rite on the base of the upright stone that was topped with an icon of the Buddha (see below, *Unintentional Exposure*). The fascinating item here, of course, is the *gaki* lapping up the water almost as quickly as it is poured out on the stones. The rationale for this seems clear. What we would attribute to the evaporation of moisture was, for that time, an instance of patent, fully obvious involvement by hungry ghosts. What the theory was trying to explain, thus, was not limited to body wastes and things ordinarily thought of as "polluting," but was more ambitious, encompassing and inclusive.[11] The congeries of things given in the *Cheng-fa nien-ch'u ching* begin, in the *Gaki zōshi*, to look more like a unified, coherent pattern of mutually supporting instances – to that extent, at least, less like a list and more like a science. The making of these things into a pattern, and therefore "rational," was of prime importance here. That is what, I claim, the *Gaki zōshi* is all about.

To commence the argument with shit and other repulsive things was a smart move on the Buddhists' part. Explicating Bataille, Mark C. Taylor notes that "in the eyes of Reason, *das ganz Andere* is *grotesque*."[12] This means that those who profess mastery of Reason must, sooner or later, try to encompass all alterities. Since that is so, the Buddhist system-builders, precisely by *beginning* with all the bodily, nasty stuff – cadavers, specters, feces, etc. – were tackling the difficult things first rather than last. Their theory would, it seemed, take up and "place" the feces with alacrity. This also disguised what was happening. To have commenced with "mind" would have signaled to all that it was indeed "philosophy" as systematizer which was at work here.

The Buddhists' top-of-the-page treatment of the otherwise obdurate, heterologous things probably gained them extra points and a strategic advantage. What they were pushing as a system/philosophy was what, they obviously hoped, would demonstrate "consistent homogeneity...established throughout the external world by everywhere replacing a priori inconceivable objects with classified series of con-

zone

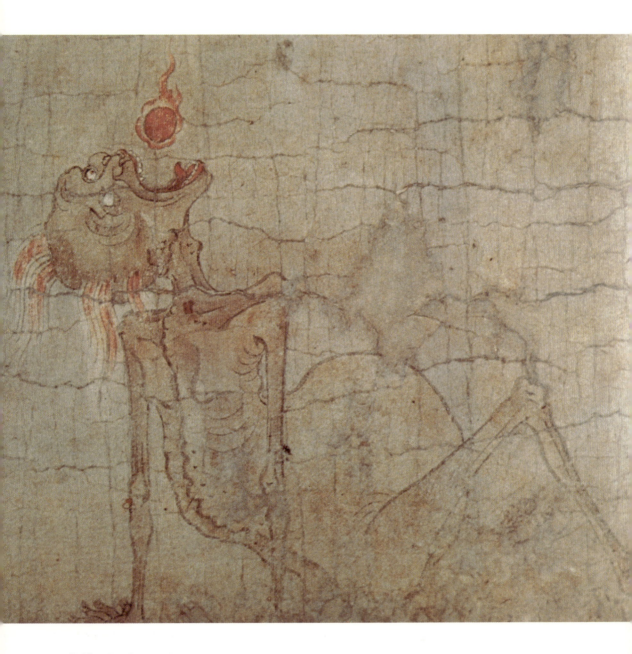

Gaki eating fire.

ceptions or ideas."[13] The lowest of the low was a good place to start; it made everything that followed — a hierarchy to be sure — look sensible. Within that hierarchy, all beings were arranged.

In Buddhism, as compared at least with medieval Christianity, discussions of comparative reality (ontology quantified) were less important than tight equations between moral performance and the weal or woe that followed from that performance. The principle of karmic reward or retribution serviced the system and the taxonomy of species-slots into which beings could be reborn, stretched from beings in hell, on the bottom, to those in heavenly realms, at the top. The nonfinality of death and the inevitability of transmigration were a priori assumptions of the whole scheme, but also things the apologists strove to "prove" again and again.[16]

The theory was that morally good lives could enable one to jump out of one species or rubric and into a better one; conversely, an immoral life could, after death, bring transpecifications downward. A lot depended, of course, on the assumption that the dead are reborn by a moral calculus. The central problem for this "science" was that the single most important operation, the transfer out of one life and into another, lay off the plane of the observable and in a place where it could not be seen. There seemed to be no way to demonstrate with any finality that a newborn was the rebirth of some person (or other sentient being) that had previously died. A quest to fill that embarrassing hole busied very good minds.

The hungry ghost performed, if not a perfect, at least an important role right there. Since the vulnerable point of the system lay in its dependence upon transactions in a domain just out of ordinary sight, the ghosts (also invisible) and their seeming interaction with a variety of substances (all visible) fit the need for at least "a weak proof." People's eyes told them that this stuff did, indeed, disappear; that much was empirical. The Buddhist doctors had, then, a theory sufficiently viable to let them press their detractors for something even slightly better. "Where," they might ask, "do you suppose the shit in the latrine eventually goes? Or the cadaver that lies exposed out in the public cemetery? Or the semen and menstrual blood that falls from the body to the ground? Or the water sprinkled on memorial stones or ground? Or even the flame that flies through the air and then suddenly disappears without a trace? How, in lieu of the *gaki* and its capacity for consuming such things, can these disappearances from sight be explained?" Skeptics would have been forced into coming up with better explanations and, since they knew nothing of oxidation, evaporation and the like, they obviously had none.

Thus, the hungry ghost hypothesis also became the hungry ghost "proof"; it had its own work to do in making the whole system seem sensible. The visible and the invisible were woven into one narrative: feces, karma, ghosts, feelings of terror, dreams of hellish tortures were all combined, interconnected and mutually supportive. No single item was foundational. As Wittgenstein held, "What stands fast does so, not because it is intrinsically obvious or convincing; it is rather held fast by what lies around it."[15] That there was a political/social impact in all of this is beyond doubt. Socially conservative forces in Japan's late Antiquity or early medieval period, for instance, had little trouble seeing the utility, to themselves and to their class, in a system holding that hierarchy was the invisible structure of the cosmos. An added boon for them lay in the teaching that every individual has the status deserved by him or her through good or bad deeds in earlier lives; upward mobility, moreover, ought to and must come through the death and rebirth of an individual — much preferable, to be sure, to any change, large or small, in the existing social system. The cosmology of six basic rubrics was a "ladder of being" that matched and reinforced an empirical social stratification, which ran the gamut from the emperor on down to people so low they were scarcely recognized as human. A graded system of court ranks was as finely stratified as the ranks in the cosmic ontology as taught by the Buddhist clergy. The one reinforced the other.

The social payoff for the well-off was clear. During the Heian period (794-1191), those around the emperor liked to be called the class "above-the-clouds," thus implicitly assimilating themselves to the "heavenly beings" rubric in the Buddhist cosmology; those on the bottom lived on dung heaps. And all were, according to doctrine, exactly where they were supposed to be. Those at the social apex lived elegant lives. Beautiful things were "naturally" theirs and, by contrast, were simply out of place in the lives of the lower classes. The tenth-century courtesan, Lady Sei Shōnagon, therefore, was merely expressing class candor when in *The Pillow Book*[16] she had a list of simply "unsuitable things" and among these was included: "Snow on the houses of common people. This is especially regrettable when the moonlight shines on it." Since the poor lacked the faculty to appreciate such beauty, the snow was wasting itself, she suggested, by indiscriminately falling on commoners' roofs.

Society's unequal — but karmically deserved — distribution of social status and wealth was, according to the system, "balanced" by a certain equalization in other areas. Illness and death, for instance, were no respecters of person and privilege. Even emperors die. Even members of the courtier class are prey to injury and disease — although apotropaic rituals by well-paid monks and religious functionaries might keep such things at bay.

Just as illness and death came to every class, so too did hungry ghosts. There may be great disproportion in the distribution of material wealth but, said the Buddhists, none in the way the invisible *gaki* were allocated to mankind. The aristocrats may wallow in wealth, but by virtue of being human, they had hungry ghosts all over them, even in the midst of their feasts. One frame of the Tokyo scroll showed how even the nobility had to suffer the presence of small, imperceptible *gaki* during their parties. What are the little beasties after? Crumbs of food left on the face? Saliva? Earwax?

We can only guess. What the painting's patrons were after, however, is much less difficult to discover. The intention of the painting was probably most focused on registering a point among viewers who were not themselves members of the upper-classes, persons surely curious about what went on in the houses of the fabulously rich. Here, they were given their window inside. But what they were meant to see is that, in spite of their wealth, the privileged suffer too — at least in *invisible* ways! Poorer or disadvantaged viewers of these pictures were meant to realize that, whatever imbalance existed in the distribution of visible wealth, there was a great egalitarianism in the sharing of the invisible presence of things like hungry ghosts. What, then, could possibly be the justice in any complaint against the way things were set up in the world? Philosophy and the status quo went hand-in-hand.

In this, everyone from emperors down to starvelings have, it was thought, precisely the lives they have karmically earned for themselves. What Max Weber had called India's "perfect theodicy" was alive and well in medieval Japan, providing, through this kind of mainline or cosmological Buddhism, a system to satisfy and support the privileged nobility and the clergy of the great urban temples. Everything fit. The system explained emperors and it explained shit. Philosophy as systematizer was doing what it does best — or worst. Even Hegel would have been impressed.

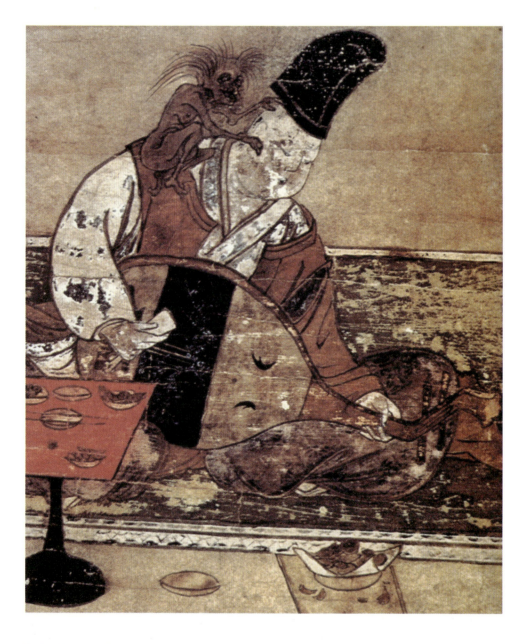

Party of aristocrats.

Unintended Exposure

The artist or artists who painted the *Gaki zōshi*, we must assume, were obliged to paint to fit the didactic purposes of the Buddhism of the mainline. Perhaps they were directly commissioned for this but, being temple painters, maybe they did so by habit or by habitus. Their role was not incidental. Hell, hungry ghosts, paradises and other nonempirical modalities were, through the medium of the artist's brush, to be brought forward for viewing by men and women who otherwise could not see such things. Those — especially the less privileged — who could "see" the *gaki* through these X-ray-like apertures, were also supposed to see and assent to the naturalness of the entire structure that lay both beyond the quotidian world and, reflexively, gave it its own hierarchical structure. To see the *gaki*, in part, was also to glimpse — and acknowledge — the whole.

Because the pictures had to be as convincing as possible, it followed that the more "real" such an artist could make it all seem, the more the state, the temples and the nobility would feel themselves well-served, well-protected and safer in their privileges. Art could make paradise and hell real for people who otherwise could not see such places; art could also make a miasma behind which the machinations of real power could hide. Culture and contingency would disappear offstage; nature and necessity would step out into the spotlight. This, then, put a premium upon *realism*. To represent the world of the *gaki* as continuous with the world of empirically observed humans and animals would, by the terms of the project, be expected to be the best way for this kind of art to achieve its goal.

And yet, it is precisely here that things began to come undone. Ironically, it was this grasping for the ultimate in realistic representation that seems to have turned this art into something very much other than what the establishment would have wished to have shown. Perhaps this is because a totally successful mix between ideology and reality is fundamentally impossible. In any case, in these paintings the quest for realism turned sour. What went "wrong," at least as the establishment would have seen things, is that the artists' eagerness for realism drew them away from the scriptures and away from Chinese prototypes and into the streets to find real-life models for their hungry ghosts. The result was that this art, intended to render visible what was ontologically out of sight, ended up showing all too vividly what was supposed to have remained socially invisible. It is, of course, possible that the artists connived with the poor to give them visibility, but a determination of that degree of intention cannot be read from the pictures. And in an important sense it hardly matters. The significant thing is that, even if inadvertent, what got lifted out of the hovels of invisibility and onto paintings that can still be seen today turn out to be some of the most poor, wretched and emaciated people of Japan's twelfth-century capital. And, placed frame by frame next to the lives of the privileged and well-fed nobility in these pictures, the gross social disparity is also rendered for all time and people to see.

For any artist seeking real models for the painting of hungry ghosts, twelfth-century Heiankyō, the old capital (where the city of Kyoto now is), provided starve-lings in abundance. The *Hōjōki*, an after-the-fact account reshaped into a classic literary text in the thirteenth century, details what a famine in the year 1181 had been like:

> The number of those who died of starvation outside the gates or along the roads may not be reckoned. There being no one even to dispose of the bodies, a stench filled the whole world, and there were many sights of decomposing bodies too horrible to behold. Along the banks of the Kamo River there was not even room for horses and cattle to pass.[17]

This literary text, one composed – significantly – after real political power had been successfully grabbed by members of the military class, is clear. During the time of the famine itself, however, we have no such vivid account in prose. The reasons for the contemporaneous silence are as clear as those for the next regime's willingness to see depictions of the stresses and malfeasance of the government it had undone.

And it is also for this reason that the scrolls, contemporaneous with the famine and the political woes of the old regime, become doubly interesting. Once we know about the famine, it becomes clear that the painters of the *Gaki zōshi* did not draw their materials from their imaginations; they worked from having seen hungry people and on the basis of having closely observed the bodily signs of advanced starvation. The gray pallor, the gaunt appearance, the wary look in the eyes of beggars subsist-ing on the edge of society and the edge of life: these things tell us that the painters of invisible *gaki* modeled their work on the bodies and behavior of visible people.

There was something almost clinical in the exactitude of bodily details. The hair, for instance, is quite remarkable in what it reveals. Although it shows up all over the *gaki* scrolls, the presence here of red and blond hair – in great quantities, in fact — is not fortuitous. The water-offering section of the Kyoto Museum scroll, discussed above, shows it vividly. In order to grasp what is so remarkable in this, it must be remembered that it was not until much later — during the sixteenth century, in fact — that the Japanese had their first glimpse of naturally red or blond hair. In the twelfth century, at the time of these pictures, no Dutchman or Englishman had yet come to Japan. Moreover, although it is possible that the painting of red-haired beings had been copied from Chinese sources, many of the representations of hungry ghosts in Chinese art give them the black hair ordinarily found on the heads of East Asian peoples (see Sung painting above). This may be because in such cases, the Chinese were doing stylized work, painting their hungry ghosts by combining their imaginations with the formulaic statements about such creatures in the Buddhist scriptures. The Japanese, by contrast, for some reason or another, seem to have taken to the streets to find models. Some art historians have assumed that the red hair on the *gaki* was a stylized motif to heighten their grotesqueness. I suggest that exactly the opposite was the case.

My point is that it is fairly easy to account for these otherwise anomalous hair colors in strictly medical terms. Although black hair is normal for East Asians, it is a fact that the hair of the severely hungry fails to retain its usual melanin, and thus often shows up as reddish or blond. Therefore, it would appear that the painters of these pictures had observed — and on these scrolls, were recording — the physical link between light-colored hair and acutely advanced human starvation. For a people who otherwise only saw hair that was black, the lack of pigment in that of starvelings would have been quite remarkable — as unusual and unnatural, for instance, as it is for black North Africans in the twentieth century. Starvation and severe malnutrition, however, alter what is "natural" in such cases. In fact, part of the pathology of such starvation — referred to as "kwashiorkor" by virtue of the adoption of a Ghanese word into Western medical vocabularies — is precisely such depigmentation of otherwise healthy, black hair. The drastic reduction in the protein throughout the body touches even the extremities; twelfth-century Japanese, like enfamined North Africans in our own time, would have discovered, no doubt to their horror, that the body starved for food changes it colors. Skin turns gray and normally black hair turns reddish or blond.

A recalcitrant reality, therefore, seems to have subverted official and socially

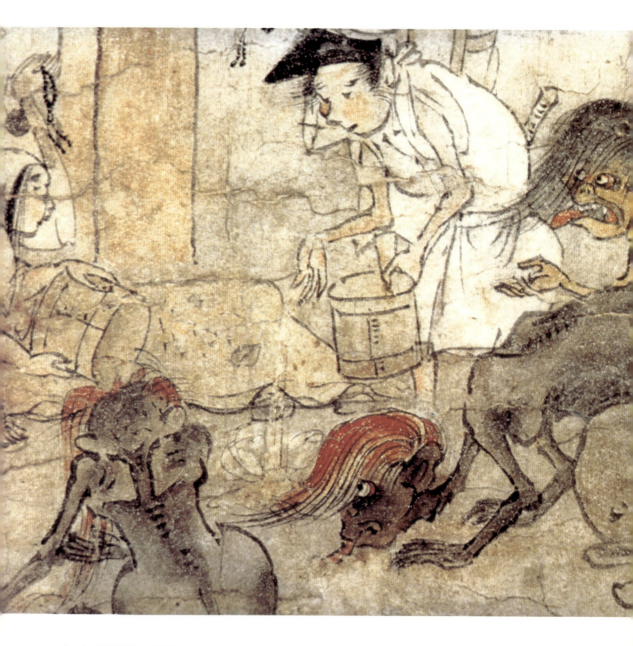

Gaki with bright red hair.

useful doctrine about the naturalness of sharp stratification in the universe and in society. What emerges clearly in these pictures is that there was an awesome disparity between the theory of things and the way they really were. The nub of this contradiction was the fact that what was happening on the streets was clearly very different from what the Buddhist-based "science" was saying should be the case.

The theory itself, of course, was bound to be implicitly placed in doubt by these things. According to it, the physiology of the hungry ghost was distinctive, unique. It comprised a discrete species, one actually epitomized in telltale fashion by the fact that its body was structured as a continuous defiance and reversal of a "law" that is built into the bodies of humans. The law in question was that the body demonstrates a quantitative proportionality between the intake of food and the size of the body's midsection. Normally, large amounts of food result in expansion of the body's girth; conversely, a reasonable reduction in intake produces a "reduced" body as well. What looks like a law of proportionality, one known to common observation, is at work in this.

The hungry ghost, by definition, has a body which not only defies that law but seems to embody its opposite. When the scriptures state repeatedly that the *gaki* possesses "a belly like a mountain but a neck like a needle," there is much more than Indian hyperbole and metaphor in this. The significant thing is that this *defines* the body of a certain kind of being; that being is known by the patent and *enstructured* disproportion or inverse relation between the stomach and the throat. The former bespeaks voluminous ingestion of food but the latter suggests the physical impossibility of that. The odd thing about the *gaki* is that, when compared with the human, it is a physiological oxymoron. It takes in an absolute minimum of food but shows the centrally defining characteristic — enormous girth — ordinarily associated with eating vast quantities.

This, however, is only anomalous from the human point of view. The sutras are saying in their metaphoric way that, in fact, the existence of the hungry ghost is structured by its own "law," one that in its content is the opposite of what governs the somatic life of mankind. Although humans did not ordinarily expect to see a hungry ghost, this was, at least in theory, the visual key to spotting one if seen. The reversal of the law operative for humans constitutes the law for creatures of another species altogether. This is the crux of differentiating them; the species were clearly distinct.

The streets of Heian-kyō, however, did not follow the logic of the texts and of Buddhist science – especially in conditions such as those which were to be found there during the famine of 1181. It was at such times that the bellies of starvelings swelled – not with food but, as we now know, with the gases that accumulate in the severely malnourished when the linings of the stomach walls decompose. This condition, edema, is probably the most sure sign of the kwashiorkor syndrome. Today we recognize it, understand it and when possible seek to prevent it.

In twelfth-century Japan, however, edema and the widespread presence of the kwashiorkor syndrome within urban society appear to have had in them the makings of a fundamental epistemological crisis. In a word, the categorical distinction between man and not-man was getting all confused. The supposedly patent truth of the fundamental taxonomy was being undermined. This was because very hungry *human beings* – humans with families, humans known to their fellows, humans even with names – were bit by bit showing in their bodies the telltale feature of hungry ghosts. At first, when there was little to eat, the bodies of these people simply thinned, thereby retaining the proportionality factor. But then, when the condition got really severe, their stomachs swelled and bloated even while the body frame remained little more than skeletal. But all of this was happening where it was not supposed to be happening – namely, within the bodies of humans known to be such.

Really acute starvation, therefore, revealed a patent and gross contradiction between the theory and observable reality. Visible realities were upsetting the theory. The starvelings of Heian-kyō were indubitably human but showed the bodily signs of the *gaki* species. To those who may have wondered on occasion about the viability of the whole theory, this probably fanned further, deeper skepticism. If the taxonomy was in trouble at this point, there would eventually be signs of trouble all the way down the line.

Fecal Matter/Fecal Mind

There is something hard, irreducible and unassimilable about these people in the pictures. They dirty the intentions of the paintings' privileged patrons. Here, these hungry human bodies stand and squat like surds in the very system they were meant to serve. Here is where the epistemic fracture between the ideology and the reality becomes salient. The X ray turns out differently than expected. Intended to render the metaempirical as real and, conversely, to conceal the power plays of muscle and mind that had stitched this world together, the pictures let the facts of fabrication out. Perhaps it is the chasm between reality and ideology that makes this happen. Or maybe it is an instance of what Bataille referred to as "the intellectual process [which] automatically limits itself by producing of its own accord its own waste products, thus liberating in a disordered way the heterogeneous excremental element."[18]

In the *Gaki zōshi*, there is much more expression of the problem than resolution of it. Some features of the painting leave only a tantalizing ambiguity. The scene that is the last one viewed as the Kyoto Museum scroll is unrolled is one that raises questions without giving answers. It portrays monks feeding *gaki*, who come running pell-mell from the woods to get the food offered. We can wonder whether people, especially the wealthy, saw an element of exemplary behavior in this — and whether they drew from it any applications in terms of feeding the starving in their own society.

The inscribed text that accompanies the picture gives little help in answering this. It tells only that the giving of food to hungry ghosts was a practice established by Ānanda, a direct disciple of the Sakyamuni, and the formula for continuing to do so. The suggestion, if any, is primarily that of ritual and, in fact, *segaki*, a service of giving food to *gaki*, still exists in Japan today. (Today in Japanese temples, the food ritually left out for hungry ghosts will be a few grains of cooked rice — most usually eaten by birds or small animals. The chants and their punctilious performance receive the emphasis.) Inasmuch as this scene in the scroll reflects a concurrent practice, it probably tells us that it was invisible *gaki* rather than visible people who were fed in *segaki* ritual contexts.

The theodicy of karma, as Max Weber noted, is a powerful one. Its social correlates are clear, strong and hard to contravene when supported by the powerful. Much of Buddhism — at least, that which was involved with articulating the structure of the cosmos and upholding the stratification of society — took over that portion of the Indian heritage almost without question. This is not, however, to say there was no other type. In fact, within Buddhism itself, there was another tradition which offered a *critique* of that view of karma. Early Buddhists were critical of caste, said

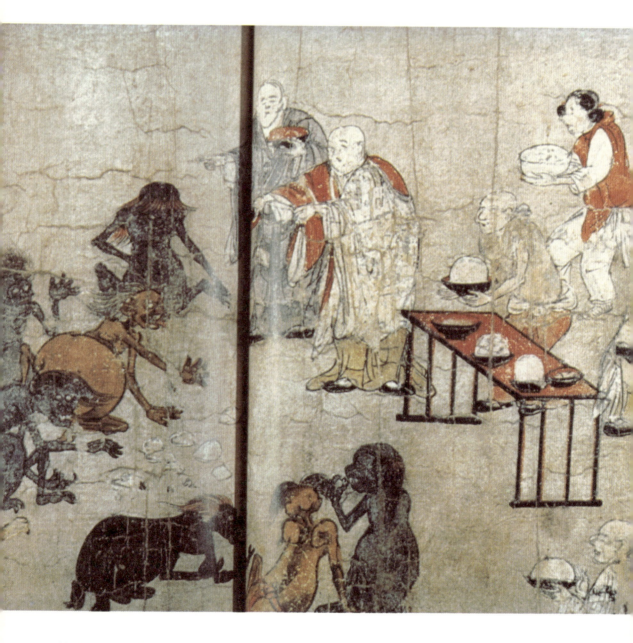

Monks and feasting *gaki*.

no aware person need be fated by karma, stressed egalitarian themes, and celebrated compassion as a central virtue.

Some philosophers, pushing the dialectical possibilities in classical Buddhist logic, clearly saw that the hierarchies, both ontological and social, were contingent and constructed. Since their view of reality included no place for a deity, the notion of anything as entirely self-dependent — and in that sense, foundational for a system — struck them as absurd.[19] The carryover of this, especially into Chinese Zen, rendered notions such as "holiness" and "purity" suspect; the critique of these concepts turned to iconoclasm and humor. The *Record of Lin-chi* refers to the sutras as good paper for use in the toilet. With reference to the great Buddhist systems under construction, this Buddhist work refers to them as nothing more than "fashioning models and creating patterns out of illusory transformations."[20] To the classic question "What is the Buddha?" one answer became "a shit-stick."

There was, then, this *doubleness* in the tradition of Buddhism by the time of the troubles of twelfth- and thirteenth-century Japan. Yet, the ethical and social correlates for the critical, antihierarchical philosophical position were hard to come by. They showed up only sporadically. Siagyō (1118-90), a monk-poet, thought the court life of the capital decadent and found something terribly artificial in the court poets' refusal to write about anything socially unpleasant. He broke the taboo by composing verse about the horrors of war and poems that showed sympathy for the grinding poverty of fisherfolk in rural areas — in spite of their karma. The strong-minded Buddhist Nichiren (1222-82) condemned the decadent and consumptive lives of the nobility. Both he and his contemporary Dogen (1200-53) questioned the long-standing view that karma consigns women to a status inferior to that of men. Shinran (1173-1262) and Ippen (1239-89) expressed compassion for the ordinary poor and celebrated personal nobility in the unlettered, impoverished and diseased.

Was it ordinary pusillanimity, then, that kept Japanese Buddhism from reaching out for a more systematic restructuring of society? Or was it due to a keen sensitivity, one often cultivated in Buddhism, to the proclivity for producing only ironic results — especially whenever there are systematized efforts to supplant a given system with another? It is difficult to say.

What seems clear, however, is that those medieval Japanese Buddhists — thinkers and poets — who were skeptical about the naturalness and necessity of the whole karmic/hierarchical structure focused more on what they had found as insight than as social blueprint. Among them, though, Ikkyū (1394-1481), a Zen cleric and poet, was probably the most penetrating. Coddled, celebrated and drastically "tamed" by the distorting memory of later generations — so that he became reduced to little more than a charmingly "eccentric" Zen figure from the past — Ikkyū had, in fact, consistently tried to tear off what struck him as an entire fabric of social lies. He rankled his fellow Buddhists, fulminating against the corrupt and power-craving practices of the great temples. Scatology, eroticism and a deliberate mixing of the pure and impure mark his poems. Whether declaring his deep hatred of temple incense or celebrating the sexual, body "nectars" of Mori, the blind woman he loved, Ikkyū assaulted both the conventions and the power-structure of his age. The whole hierarchical structure of deferred karmic rewards and punishments seemed contrived to him. And when, in 1461, he witnessed starvation — not unlike that of 1181 — in the countryside and city, he wrote a poem that, in effect, collapsed the categories and said what the visible hungry ghosts really were:[21]

Starvation in 1461

The pain and hunger penetrates my body,
The hungry ghosts I see are real people.
Through all its existence the body is a house aflame.
Misery mounts up to the highest heaven.

NOTES

1. Melford E. Spiro, *Burmese Supernaturalism* (Englewood Cliffs, NJ: Prentice-Hall, 1967), pp. 33-39.

2. Alasdair MacIntyre noted, correctly I think, that in moving from the medieval to the modern, "the specific character of religion becomes clearer at the cost of diminishing its content." See his "Is Understanding Religion Compatible with Believing?" in *Rationality*, ed. Brian R. Wilson (Oxford: Basil Blackwell, 1977), pp. 62-77.

3. The best reproduction of all these materials is in *Rokudo-E*, with photography by Keizō Kaneko and text in Japanese by Toru Shimbo (Tokyo: Mainichi Shimbunsha, 1977). See also Mieko Murase, *Emaki: Narrative Scrolls from Japan* (New York: The Asia Society, 1983).

4. Saigyo, *Sanka-shū* in *Nihon Koten Zensho*, vol. 78, ed. Yoshi Ito (Tokyo: Asahi Shimbunsha, 1971),

poem 980; p. 150. (Author's translation.)

5. Mujū Ichien, "Shaseki-shū," trans. Robert E. Morrell, in *Sand and Pebbles* (Albany: State University of New York Press, 1985), p. 115.

6. William R. LaFleur, *The Karma of Words: Buddhism and the Literary Arts in Medieval Japan* (Berkeley: University of California Press, 1983). My definition of "medieval," when applied to Japan, is also explained there.

7. Hideo Kuroda, *Sugata to Shigusa no Chūseishi* (Tokyo: Heibonsha, 1986), pp. 130-36.

8. On this, see my "Paradigm Lost, Paradigm Regained: Groping for the Mind of Medieval Japan," *The Eastern Buddhist* n.s. 18.2 (Autumn 1985), pp. 99-113.

9. *Taishō shinshū daizōkyō* (Tokyo: 1924-32), vol. 17, p. 92a-b.

10. "Genshin's Ojo Yoshu: Collected Essays on Birth into Paradise," trans. A.K. Reischauer, *Transactions of the Asiatic Society of Japan* 2d ser., 7 (1930), pp. 46-49.

11. This is a point of difference from Mary Douglas's important study, *Purity and Danger* (London: Routledge and Kegan Paul, 1966).

12. Mark C. Taylor, *Altarity* (Chicago: The University of Chicago Press, 1987), p. 125. Also, Georges Bataille, *Visions of Excess: Selected Writings 1927-1939*, ed. and trans. Allan Stoekl (Minneapolis: University of Minnesota Press, 1985), p. 99.

13. Bataille, *ibid.*, pp. 95-96.

14. See *The Karma of Words*; and W. LaFleur, *Buddhism: A Cultural Perspective* (Englewood Cliffs, NJ: Prentice-Hall, 1988).

15. Ludwig Wittgenstein, *On Certainty*, ed. G.E.M. Anscombe and G.H. von Wright, trans. Denis Paul and G.E.M. Anscombe (New York: Harper and Row, 1969), p. 21e.

16. Ivan Morris, ed. and trans., *The Pillow Book of Sei Shōnagon* (New York: Columbia University Press, 1967), vol. 1, p. 50.

17. Donald Keene, ed. and trans., *Anthology of Japanese Literature* (New York: Grove Press, 1955), p. 202.

18. Bataille, *Visions of Excess*, p. 97.

19. LaFleur, *The Karma of Words*, pp. 20-25, 80-100.

20. Ruth Fuller Sasaki, trans., *The Recorded Sayings of Ch'an Master Lin-chi Hui-chao of Chen Prefecture* (Kyoto: The Institute for Zen Studies, 1975), p. 22.

21. James H. Sanford, trans., "Zen-Man Ikkyū," *Harvard Studies in World Religions* 2 (Chico, CA: Scholars Press, 1982), p. 184.

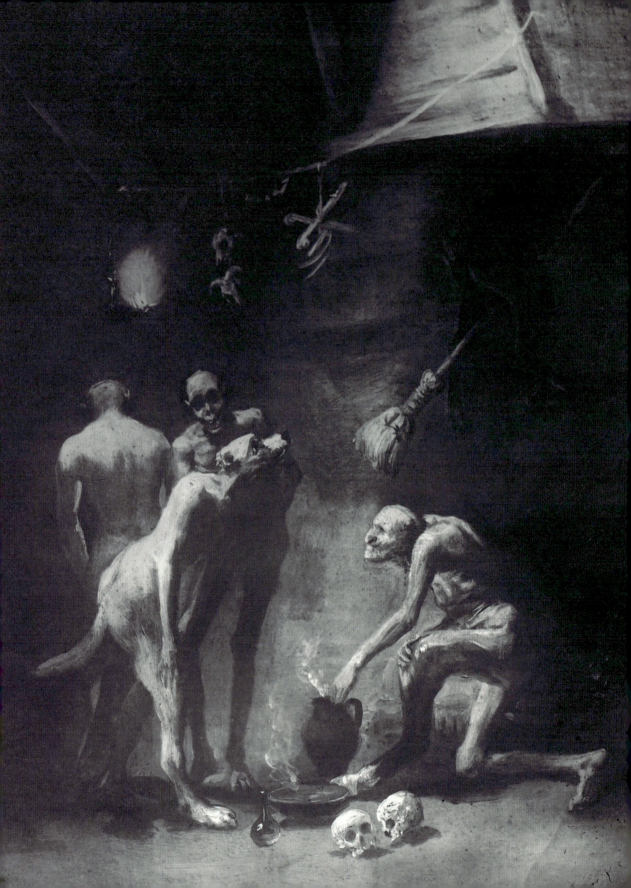

Metamorphosis and Lycanthropy
in Franche-Comté, 1521-1643

Caroline Oates

The free county of Burgundy, a French-speaking province of the Holy Roman Empire, lay between Switzerland and the kingdom of France, to which it was finally joined in 1674. Mountainous and densely wooded in many areas, Franche-Comté had a large wolf population until quite recently and, during the sixteenth and seventeenth centuries, an unusually large number of werewolves. Records of criminal proceedings and accusations against some nineteen people suspected as werewolves between 1521 and 1643 are summarized in the second part of this essay.[1] Some of these — Michel Verdun and Pierre Burgot (1521), Gilles Garnier (1574) and the werewolves tried by Henri Boguet in Saint-Claude (1598-99) — are already reasonably familiar to modern readers, thanks to descriptions of their cases in contemporary printed works. Other, less sensational cases were only brought to light more recently by the work of historians in the region's criminal archives.[2] These trials raise many questions: What events led to accusations and arrests of suspects? What did people believe about werewolves and their transformations? What happened to the human body? What explanations accounted for the reported and confessed metamorphoses? How did courts of law deal with suspected werewolves and what evidence justified convictions? In an attempt to answer some of these questions, and to set the trials in the rhetorical and historical context necessary to an understanding of the events which took place, this preliminary section will consider: 1) the information supplied by witnesses and suspects; 2) rationalizing theories of transformation; 3) how courts of law dealt with these cases.

Witnesses and Suspects

Trial records are usually fragmentary and provide only a very partial account of events. Some give details about the incidents that prompted an accusation but make no mention of the cause of the supposed transformation. Others specify how the transformation was effected, but do not indicate the circumstances of arrest. In some cases, little more than the name of the accused and the date of the trial is recorded. Nevertheless, when the statements of events and explanations given in these documents are considered collectively, sufficient similarities emerge to form a loose model of what was thought about werewolves and, to some extent, to fill the gaps in individual cases. Whether or not we accept the validity of the premises, there were logical grounds for accusations against werewolves, and most cases describe or presuppose the following stages:

1. An encounter with a wolf. Accusations generally arose from incidents known or thought to involve wolves; such events were often perceived as extraordinary and aroused speculation and suspicions.

2. Signs. People had reasons for suspecting particular individuals, and several cases mention signs interpreted by witnesses as indicating the werewolf's identity and confirming that transformation had occurred.

3. Explanations. Many reports show that both witnesses and accused not only believed transformations possible, but could also explain, in ways that they accepted as plausible, which people were able to transform themselves and how they did so.

Encounters with Wolves

It has been suggested that trials of werewolves during this period were inspired by the crimes of mass murderers.[3] Although human involvement in some of the deaths recorded in these trials cannot always be ruled out, and although some of the accused may well have been killers, the hypothesis is unconvincing. It was not without reason that common murderers were not accused; in most cases, there was evidence that wolves had been involved in the attacks that led to accusations. Often, witnesses had seen wolves during or shortly after an attack, and the bodies of victims also bore the marks of wolves' claws and teeth.[4] Nor were all attacks fatal, at least not immediately, and frightened or injured victims described their four-footed attackers (Perrenette Gandillon, 1599; Verjuz, 1599; Chastellan, 1643). But if human werewolves rather than real wolves were suspected, it was because people saw signs which seemed suspicious. Very often, witnesses perceived, or later remembered, something unusual or extraordinary in the animal's appearance or behavior: an especially large or ferocious wolf (Edict, 1573); a wolf with no tail; human toes or fingers seen on the wolf's body (Gaillard, 1598; Perrenette Gandillon, 1599); a wolf following a person (Verjuz, 1599). Observed abnormality indicates that the animal was understood to be something other than a normal wolf, and perhaps therefore a werewolf.[5]

In some instances, the wolf's very act of attacking a human being, or even simply entering a village, was seen as extraordinary and aroused suspicion of a werewolf (Edict, 1573; Peasant, 1573). In view of the fact that wolves normally avoid human contact, and human flesh does not usually feature in a wolf's diet, *any* encounter with a wolf near human habitation, especially if it attacked people, could seem *unusual* or *abnormal*, and worthy of explanation.[6] Uncharacteristic behavior in wolves could be explained in a number of ways. At the beginning of the sixteenth century Johann Geiler von Kaisersberg said that werewolves were wolves that ate people, and there were seven reasons for this: hunger, rabies, old age, experience (or perhaps "taste"), madness, the Devil or God.[7] That these were human beings transformed was just one of a range of possible explanations, and one that was especially favored in Franche-Comté.

Signs

Individuals were not accused of being werewolves without cause. An event, sign or circumstantial evidence usually led to suspicion of a particular person. In some cases, an incident involving a wolf occurred shortly before or after a meeting or dispute with a suspected witch, and (because witches were understood to be able to transform themselves into any shape they wished) the two events were seen as causally related (Gaillard, 1598). On other occasions, the arrest of a witch in the area may have been enough to arouse suspicion that the witch was also responsible for fatal wolf attacks (Saint-Claude werewolves, 1598). Equally, the unexplained absence of a person, especially a known witch, at the time of an attack could result in an accusation (Edict, 1632).

Wolves seen attacking people and livestock were often pursued, and hunting sessions were organized in areas where wolves frequently caused problems. A significant number of accused werewolves are known to have been apprehended during such hunts by bands of men who, having lost sight of the wolf, came upon individuals, often beggars or vagrants, whose presence in the forest seemed suspicious (Peasant, 1573; Stumpf, 1589 [see figure 2]; Valeur, 1605; Chastellan, 1643).

The arrest of a werewolf, or of a witch similarly accused, often aroused or confirmed suspicions of human participation in other wolf attacks in the area. Bereaved families came forward with information about their mauled, dead or disappeared children, and witnesses volunteered evidence of wolves' activities to prosecutors during their inquiries. It is not surprising, therefore, that accused werewolves were often charged with several crimes of this kind.[8]

Many cases include further signs which were understood as confirmation of the suspicion, proof that transformation had occurred and definite identification of the suspect. A suspect's disappearance or attempted escape could be sufficient (Perrenette Gandillon, 1599; Valeur, 1605). One suspect, caught during a wolf hunt, was found in possession of strange pots of ointment (Peasant, 1573), while another was said to have turned back into a man, before the eyes of a witness, after being struck with a special stick (Chastellan, 1643). And just as something unusual in the appearance or behavior of a wolf might arouse the thought that it was a werewolf, so too could the physiognomy, expressions and gestures of a human suspect betray readable signs of a dangerous alter ego (Pierre Gandillon, 1599; Verjuz, 1599; Chastellan, 1643).[9]

Explanations

Transformations do not just happen. They happen to specific people, for particular reasons, by means of a certain process and often in special circumstances. Many accounts, particularly confessions, provide some form of explanation of what causes a person to become a werewolf, why and how transformation occurs and what happens to the human body.

Who is transformed. According to numerous medieval sources, werewolves were people who were predisposed to assume the form of a wolf at certain times, and whose capacity for transformation was imposed on them by destiny, fate or other circumstances beyond their control (involuntary, monomorphic metamorphosis). Becoming a wolf is often represented as uncontrollable or inevitable, and despite the better nature of the person, who is to be pitied as well as feared.[10] In some parts of Europe werewolves were seen rather differently. In the mid-sixteenth century, Caspar Peucer recorded the Livonian belief that werewolves were the enemies of witches and were compelled to assemble in spirit in the form of wolves around Christmas. He relates an incident involving a man from Riga who was identified as a werewolf after falling on the floor in a trance during a banquet and, when he finally returned to his senses, telling of his battle with a witch in the form of a butterfly.[11] In 1692, a self-avowed good werewolf named Thiess resolutely insisted during his trial in Jürgensburg that he and his fellow werewolves fought the witches three times a year in order to ensure a good harvest for their community.[12] Comparison with the Friulian *benandanti* studied by Carlo Ginzburg and with related beliefs in central Europe and the Balkan peninsula suggests that the Livonian werewolves belonged to a similar shamanistic agrarian fertility cult. *Benandanti* and other soul-voyaging witch-fighters, visionary emissaries to the dead and purveyors of communal fertility were usually people born with a caul, teeth, extra toes or other signs of election, and were often initiated or summoned to take up their tasks by another member of the group or by a messenger. On certain days (especially Thursdays) they would assemble in spirit, often in the form of animals, to combat the witches, after which their spirits would return to their bodies, which had lain motionless all the while, and they would often be exhausted on waking.[13]

Besides their transformations, occasional details in some of the Franche-Comté trials are reminiscent of such shamanistic beliefs. Pierre Burgot (1521) and Georges Gandillon (1599) said they were summoned to the assembly or initiated by another member of the group. Groz Jacques (1598) spoke of attending the sabbath in spirit; Georges Gandillon was also said to have fallen into a trance one Maundy Thursday, which left him exhausted, just as Burgot and the Saint-Claude werewolves (1598) were all weary after their transformations. But the echoes are only very faint, and there is nothing to suggest that the werewolf was seen in any positive way by local people, whether as a victim of witchcraft or fate, as a being with two natures or as a special person with a community function. All of these suspects were understood to be witches, and as such, knew how to transform themselves into wolves or any other shape which suited their purposes (voluntary, polymorphic metamorphosis).[14] There is no evidence that any of the suspected werewolves in Franche-Comté, unlike Thiess and the *benandanti* of the Friuli, saw themselves as destined to be werewolves or obliged to fulfill a social function, nor that they were seen as such by other people. Most of the trials resulted from accusations and denunciations by other members of the community, hunts were organized in response to public pressure and there are indications that, by the beginning of the fifteenth century, people in this part of Europe had nothing good to say about werewolves and saw them as witches intent only on harm.[15]

Purpose. Unlike the medieval werewolves whose transformations resulted from a natural compulsion or destiny and were, therefore, devoid of any purpose, those who controlled their own transformations were often said to have specific motives: to frighten or harm someone in particular (Verjuz, 1599; Chastellan, 1643); hunger (Burgot, 1521; Garnier, 1573); revenge (Gaillard, 1598); to gain money (Burgot; Gaillard); or simply to kill and eat people.

How to transform. Transformation is activated by a special process or mechanism, which may be any one or more of the following:
- Disrobing (Burgot, 1521; inversion in Verdun's transformation while clothed).
- Anointing the body with a magic salve (Burgot & Verdun; Peasant, 1573; Groz Jacques, 1598; Georges Gandillon, 1599; etc.).
- Donning a wolfskin (figure 1; Burgot, 1521; Georges Gandillon, 1599).[16]
- Other magic garments or objects (Stumpf's magic girdle, figure 2).[17]

These and other gestures or devices to account for the process of transformation are nonspecific and interchangeable. Accused werewolves were undoubtedly asked how they achieved their transformations, and those who confessed seem to have answered such questions with any of a range of familiar or logical explanations. This interpretation is supported by the fact that in trials involving more than one werewolf, suspects sometimes accounted for their transformations in different ways (Burgot and Verdun, 1521; the Gandillons, 1599). Furthermore, no pots of ointment, wolfskins, magic belts, etc., ever seem to have been produced in court as material

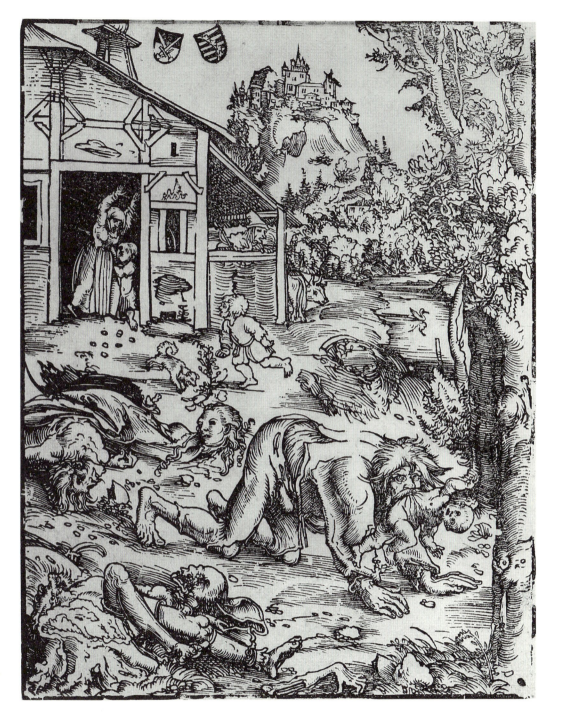

zone

Figure 1: Lucas Cranach the Elder, Cannibal or Werewolf, ca. 1510-15
(New York, Metropolitan Museum of Art).

evidence in support of such confessions. Some suspects, however, were accused *because* they were found in possession of strange ointments or other objects which witnesses took to be devices for effecting transformations (Peasant, 1573).[18]

Status of transformation. Reported transformations in Franche-Comté generally posit a total mutation of the human flesh into that of an animal; the animal form replaces the human form (Chastellan, 1643). This is explicit in those cases where transformation is said to be effected by putting on a special skin or garment (figures 1 and 2; the Gandillons, 1599).[19] Human attributes, such as toes or fingers, on the body of the animal also indicate that there is only one body, but two shapes (Gaillard, 1598; Perrenette Gandillon, 1599).

Transformation in spirit or "in ecstasy" presupposes two distinct bodies: a human body that lies motionless as if dead while the spirit journeys forth in another, animal form. Although there are occasional references to transvections or attending the sabbath in spirit while the human body lies at home in bed (Groz Jacques, 1598; Georges Gandillon, 1599), ecstatic transformations do not feature in any of these cases.[20] But the idea was neither new nor limited to any one area, and it was particularly important to demonological theories of transformation.[21]

Stories about Werewolves

In his *Discours des sorciers* (1602), Henri Boguet recorded the following incidents:

> In 1588, near Apchon in Auvergne, a hunter was attacked by a large wolf, and during the struggle, he cut off one of the wolf's paws which he put in his bag. Later, at the castle of a gentleman who had asked the hunter for a part of what he caught, he opened his bag and drew from it not a wolf's paw, but a human hand. There was a ring on one finger, which the gentleman recognized as belonging to his wife. She was found in the kitchen nursing her mutilated limb, and soon confessed that it was she who, in the form of a wolf, had attacked the hunter. She was later burned at Riom, and Boguet heard of the incident from "one who may be believed" who was in the area two weeks after it happened.
>
> A horseman riding near the castle of Joux saw several cats in a tree. He discharged his carbine at them, and out of the tree fell a large ring with several keys attached, which he took with him to the nearest village. At the inn, he asked for dinner, and when neither the landlady nor the cellar keys could be found, the horseman showed the keys he

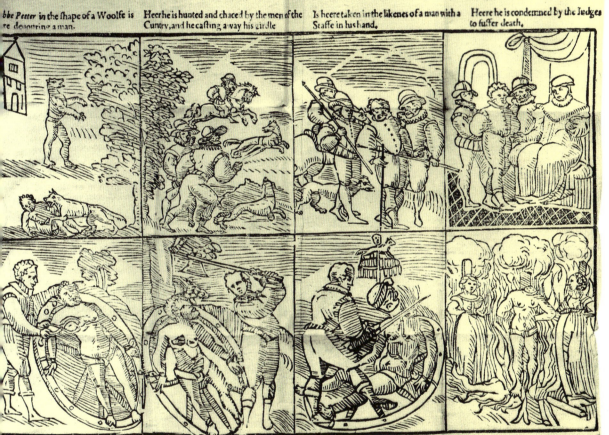

bbe Peeter in the shape of a Woolfe is
re deuouring a man.

Heere he is hunted and chaced by the men of the
Cuntry, and he casting away his girdle

Is heere taken in the likenes of a man with a
Staffe in his hand.

Heere he is condemned by the Iudges
to suffer death.

is heere laide on a Carte wheele
d his flesh pluckt from his bones
th hot pincers.

Heer he hath his legges and armes
broken vpon a Cart wheele with
a woodden Axe.

He hath heer his head strook from his body and stuck vpon
a hye pole with the picture of a Woolfe, and 16. peeces of
wood, resembling the 16. persons which he had slaine.

Heer is his body with his daughter and gossip
burned to ashes. Thus he liued and dyed in
the likenes of a woolf, and shape of a man.

Figure 2: A True Discourse Declaring the Damnable Life and Death of
One Stubbe Peeter, London, 1590.

313

had recently acquired to the landlord, who recognized them instantly. His wife soon reappeared, injured in one thigh, and duly confessed that she had been to the witches' sabbath and had lost the keys when she was shot.[22]

Such stories were by no means new to Boguet's time. More than a century earlier, Jacob Sprenger and Heinrich Institoris, authors of the *Malleus maleficarum*, had heard of a similar happening near Strasbourg. A man was attacked one day by three very large cats, and defended himself by striking them with his stick. Later that day he was arrested, accused of beating and causing severe injuries to three women of the town. When he reported the struggle with the three cats, he was released, but the three witches were not pursued.[23]

Not unlike our contemporary legends of vanishing hitchhikers and albino alligators in the sewers, these stories are related as true events; names, locations and guarantees of the informant's reliability are often supplied to ensure credibility, and plausibility is enhanced by explanatory details and proofs of the extraordinary phenomenon.[24] As in the tried cases, these stories all involve encounters with animals, often described as somehow unusual (particularly large or fierce, and so on). In each case, the explanation of the cause and process of transformation is encapsulated in the charge of witchcraft. More conclusive than in any tried case, however, is the evidence which confirms that transformation occurred and identifies the suspects. Injuries inflicted on the animal's body reverse the transformation and produce corresponding injuries or mutilations on the human body, thus revealing the identity of the attacker and providing visible and indisputable proof that the animal and the witch were one and the same. Predictably, this phenomenon, known as "repercussion," seldom features in trial documents; a rare instance from the records of a court in southwest France concerns a peasant who killed his wife in 1609. He claimed he had been attacked by a goat one night, and to defend himself, stabbed it several times in the belly with his dagger, only to find the dead body of his wife, a suspected witch, lying at his feet. Some of the neighbors confirmed that she was a witch, but others disagreed, and the court eventually banished the husband for murder.[25]

Although repercussion was not among the evidence in any of the documented trials discussed here, it certainly found its way into orally transmitted reports of some of the same cases, as the original stories were transformed in the retelling and acquired the more definite proofs typical of popular narratives. Boguet included it in his version of the trial of Burgot and Verdun (1521), although it does not appear in Johann Wier's more extensive and probably more reliable summary. The same trial was probably the original source of a story that Léonard Du Vair heard from Cardinal de Granvelle, one of Franche-Comté's most illustrious sons. A hunter from the region of Poligny saw a wolf one day and shot it with an arrow. Following the trail of blood, he traced the wolf to a house, where he discovered a woman tending an injured man, who was wounded in precisely the same part of the body as the wolf had been. The hunter informed the magistrate in Poligny, who had the man arrested and tortured until the truth was known. The suspect confessed that, using a certain ointment made by demonic arts, he had assumed the form of a wolf. "To this day," wrote Du Vair, "there is a record of this case written on a parchment attached to the door of the Dominican friars' church of that town."[26]

A striking illustration of this transformation of reports can be seen in two different woodcuts depicting the arrest and execution of Peter Stumpf of Bedburg, near Cologne in 1589. An illustration in an English pamphlet of 1590 (figure 2) shows a werewolf attacking a child and being chased by hunters, who then capture Stumpf in human form and bring him before the magistrate. The accompanying text, probably quite closely related to a record of the trial, states that as soon as the wolf disappeared from view, the hunters encountered Stumpf pretending to be out for a stroll in the woods. The encounter was seen as suspicious, and he was accordingly arrested and imprisoned. Shown the rack, he confessed that he was the werewolf who had killed sixteen people, and that he, his daughter and mistress were all witches.[27] The same story is depicted in a single-leaf woodcut by Johann Negele, published in Augsburg in 1589, only a short time after the trial (figure 3). Here, the werewolf is shown attacking a man who retaliates by lopping off one of the wolf's paws. The hunters' encounter with Stumpf in suspicious circumstances has been omitted, rendered unnecessary by the visible evidence of the werewolf's identity, namely, the repercussion of the same mutilation on the man's body. The images of his execution thus show that his left hand has been severed, and the accompanying verse describes how he was discovered at home in bed, nursing his telltale injury.

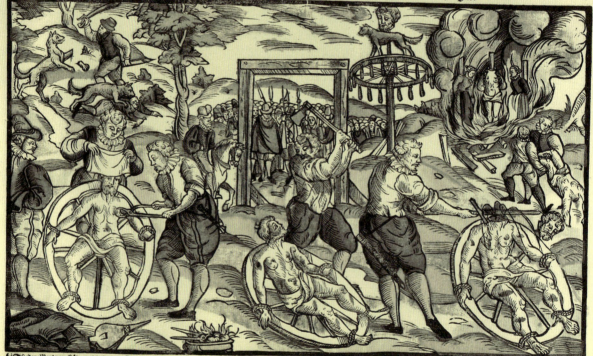

Figure 3: Execution of Peter Stumpf. From Johann Negele, *Warhafftige und wunderbarliche Newe Zeitung*...(Augsburg, 1589).

Theories of Transformation

Not everyone shared the belief that human bodies or spirits could assume animal forms. Such beliefs had been roundly condemned by medieval churchmen armed with the certainty that the human being, created by God in His own image, was immutable unless God Himself decided otherwise. The most well-known statement on this subject was the concluding phrase of a late ninth-century text, known as the Canon Episcopi:

> Whoever therefore believes that anything can be made, or that any creature can be changed to better or worse or be transformed into another species or likeness, except by God himself who made everything and through whom all things were made, is beyond doubt an infidel.[28]

Other learned authors, however, convinced though they were that the human body could not really be transformed, nevertheless refused to state categorically that reports of transformations were totally unfounded. Having heard accounts from "persons worthy of belief," Saint Augustine elaborated an explanation that, by defining the supposed transformation as an illusion, allowed for the real occurrence of an incident of this kind without compromising Christian doctrine. The so-called transformation, he said, affects neither the body nor the soul, but a third part of the human being, which he called the *phantasticum* – a spectral double that could go forth while the person lay asleep, dreaming the things encountered by the phantom. The illusory transformation, "if it happens at all," is the work of demons who give the *phantasticum* some visible appearance so that onlookers would see an animal.[29]

In the thirteenth century, William of Auvergne, Bishop of Paris, gave a similar explanation for the experience of a man who thought he was a werewolf. A holy man exposed the demonic illusion by summoning the wolf and locating the man, hidden away and in a profound sleep, to show that there was no transformation and that man and animal were two separate beings. William asserted that a demon caused the man to fall asleep and dream he was a wolf, while the same demon possessed a real wolf and made it attack people. This theory, like Saint Augustine's, accounts for "ecstatic" transformations involving two separate bodies and a comatose victim.[30]

Saint Thomas Aquinas suggested that if such things ever happened, it was by demonic illusion, which could be caused in two ways: 1) The Devil could interfere with the faculties of perception and the imagination so that things might be perceived as other than they really were. 2) He was also capable of fashioning an apparent body by molding air into some particular shape; he could use this to give himself a visible form (for the Devil had no physical body), or by surrounding a real body with it, he could make something appear to be another thing. Saint Thomas's theory admitted the possibility of a single body appearing to be transformed without being physically altered but did not suggest human collusion with the demon.[31]

Malleus maleficarum

Similar explanations were to be offered by fifteenth-century demonologists attempting to account for the alleged and confessed transformations of witches. Now seen as enemies of the faith and servants of the Devil, witches were held to be capable of causing real harmful effects by occult means with the assistance of demons.[32] Once this intimate link between the witch and the Devil had been established, even the most fantastic feats attributed to witches — transformations and transvections — came to be considered as potentially true events, caused by the Devil in return for the witch's service. The doctrinal position on this subject, however, was still that of the Canon Episcopi, which denied that there was any reality in such events. The authors of the *Malleus maleficarum* found a solution to the contradiction.[33] The Canon Episcopi, they said, had long been misunderstood; it referred only to the impossibility of *substantial* transformations, that is, alterations of the substance or essence that defines a living creature as human. It did not mention *accidental* transformations, changes occurring in those parts which are not essential to the definition of a human being. Illness, for example, or the process of aging, can radically alter the appearance of a person without bringing about any essential change. Judgment, perception and sense impressions can equally be prone to change in certain circumstances — by intoxication, for instance. Nor did the Canon exclude illusory or apparent transformations; the authors proposed that demons were capable of causing these by interfering with the humors and faculties of perception. They could move images stored in the memory and present these to the faculties of sight (as in a dream) so that a person would see something other than it really was. Alternatively, they could disturb and cloud people's judgment so that they understood things to be other than what they were. Because of their pact, demons could make witches think they were transformed and appear to be so in the eyes of others. Equally, they could cause witches to imagine such things while their bodies were lying hidden, and the demons themselves would assume the form of animals. Their theory thus accounted for apparent transformations "in ecstasy" (with the witch asleep and hidden) as well as those of the whole body (with the witch actually present where the illusory animal was seen).

Repercussion was not easy to explain. Sprenger and Institoris suggest that when the illusory transformation occurred "in ecstasy," the demons (who were invulnerable) would receive the injuries inflicted on their animal forms and swiftly transfer the same injuries onto the bodies of the sleeping witches. But when the transformation was an illusion of the eyes and the imagination, which the Inquisitors thought more probable, then the witches were present in person, and since their animal shape was only an illusion, nothing protected their real bodies from the blows. This theory provided a logical explanation which allowed for the witch's presence where the animal was seen, rather than presupposing an absent dreamer who, it could be argued, was innocent of any actual crime.

What they had to say about werewolves was rather different. Sprenger and Institoris briefly discussed the wolves that steal and eat babies, and cannot be captured by any means. These beasts, they said, were either real wolves possessed by demons, or illusions caused by witches (with demonic assistance) who made their victims imagine they were wolves. Thus, according to one of the most frequently quoted demonological works of the time, the werewolf was seen as a *victim* of witchcraft, suffering an imaginary, "ecstatic" transformation, and not as a witch and active servant of the Devil.[34]

Jean Bodin

Bodin was quite exceptional in arguing that the human body could be physically transformed into that of an animal. Although this perception of metamorphosis was similar to that of many witnesses involved in trials, few people publicly agreed with him, and many authors refuted him quite categorically.[35] Bodin dismissed the Canon Episcopi with an alternative definition of the substance or essence of human beings.[36] The real essence of a human being, he said, was not physical form, but the rational faculty. All animals have bodies and senses, but only humans have reason, and it is this which defines them as human and distinguishes them from other animals. If the body is altered but reason remains unimpaired, there is, therefore, no transformation of the "true form." He drew evidence for this from one of the typical proofs of many metamorphosis narratives, which insist that the persons transformed preserve their human reason, although their bodies are those of animals.[37] Bodin did admit that the phenomenon might be illusory, but the fact that spectators saw animals, that the animals bit ferociously and ran very fast and that human bodies carried the marks of blows inflicted on the bodies of the animals all led him to conclude that transformations were often more than illusions. Furthermore, he continued, if men have the ability to create hybrid plants and to transform iron into steel, why should we find it strange that Satan changes one body into the appearance of another, given the great power he has in the natural world?

Hallucinations

Even during the period when witches and werewolves were regularly admitting to fantastic transvections and transformations, there were those, like Reginald Scot and Pierre de l'Estoile, who thought it was all nonsense.[38] Other authors were less willing to dismiss out of hand the confessions made by convicted witches and suggested more naturalistic explanations. Some thought that the fantastic experiences confessed by witches might be hallucinations caused by drugs, and speculated about the contents and properties of the ointments so often mentioned in both stories and confessions.[39] Girolamo Cardano listed, among other substances, aconite (wolfsbane) and the fat from exhumed bodies of babies as ingredients for witches' ointments. He maintained that fantastic experiences were nothing more than hallucinations caused by the natural properties of these substances.[40] Della Porta listed the components of two types of ointment, one for transvections and the other for transformations: 1) sweet flag, cinquefoil, bat's blood and belladonna (deadly nightshade), mixed in oil; 2) aconite, celery, poplar leaves and soot, mixed in fat rendered down from a boiled baby. Vigorous rubbing of the skin, he continued, created heat and opened the pores which would facilitate the absorption of the ointment and increase the effect of the active ingredients (nightshade and aconite). Thus, he said, natural substances were responsible for the visions, flights and metamorphoses that witches claimed to have experienced.[41]

Jean de Nynauld

If hallucinations and drugged sleep might account for the confessions of suspected werewolves, they did little to explain the fact that people were being eaten by real wolves which, in many cases, had been seen by witnesses. In an effort to solve this problem, the physician Jean de Nynauld suggested both drugs *and* demonic assistance. Following Della Porta, he described in detail the properties of particular plants that might produce similar sensations. He also said there were two kinds of ointment: one type contained narcotics which induced sleep and hallucinations and simply caused witches to dream everything the Devil had promised; the other kind, without narcotics, merely disturbed the senses and put the witches more at the Devil's disposal, making them ready to undertake things they would not normally dare to do. While they were in this state, the Devil himself would transport them through the air to places far away. Nynauld himself had heard, and believed, a first-hand report of a fantastic transvection which suggested that the experience was more than hallucination. A surgeon who had treated him in Germany told how he had followed his aunt (a witch) to the sabbath on a broomstick, after anointing himself with a certain salve, and how on their return he had the misfortune to be dropped in the Rhine four leagues from home. According to Nynauld, the ointments themselves had no specific properties other than that of inducing a suitably receptive state for the Devil to work his illusions more easily. The Devil effected the illusory transformations by shrouding the witch in an airy body and by deceiving the witch's imagination and the eyes of spectators.[42]

These texts on witchcraft ointments should be read with caution: there may well have been people who experienced strange sensations or hallucinations caused by aconite and belladonna; shepherds could indeed have used wolfsbane in preparations to protect their sheep, and many suspects certainly confessed to using ointments. But, with the exception of the peasant arrested in 1573 precisely *because* he possessed suspicious pots of salve, there is no conclusive evidence that any of those tried as werewolves had actually employed such substances. Although suspects' homes would have been searched for material evidence, none of the trial records suggest that ointments were found in these cases. In most cases, the existence of any ointment at all is doubtful.

We should also be wary of accepting at face value the claim that witchcraft ointments contained the fat of babies. Again, there is no evidence to substantiate confessed use of this substance which, like eating babies, seems to be simply another typical but unfounded attribute of witches.[43] Witches from Antiquity onward were accused of eating babies or sucking their blood, and alleged employment of infant corpses in the manufacture of witchcraft salves is an extension of this accusation of cannibalism, in that human substance is understood to be absorbed not by mouth but through the skin. Without adequate evidence to confirm such accusations, the supposed cannibalism of witches should not be taken literally, but should be seen as the most serious charge that can possibly be levied against the perceived enemies of society.[44]

Lycanthropia

Another naturalistic interpretation, particularly favored by physicians, proposed that werewolves were persons suffering from a type of melancholy known as lycanthropy who simply imagined they were wolves and behaved accordingly. The diagnostic of *lycanthropia*, or *morbus lupinus*, was outlined by Marcellus of Sidon in the second century A.D. and was later repeated in a large number of sixteenth-century works. Those afflicted with this condition were said to be recognizable by certain visible symptoms:

> They are pale and sickly to look at, they have dry eyes and cannot cry. Their eyes are hollow and their tongue is dry; they do not salivate and are very thirsty; they have incurable sores on their legs due to dog bites and frequent falls.

It was said that such people tended to go out at night, frequenting cemeteries and imitating dogs and wolves in every respect, especially during February. The condition was held to be curable by good food, rest and baths, and sufferers were neither considered criminal nor ever seen in animal form by anyone else.[45]

Although *lycanthropia* was often proposed as a natural, nondemonic cause of supposed transformations, some authors stated that this and other types of melancholy could be caused by demons. It was also accepted that the Devil preyed on melancholics, and many witches were found to be suffering from melancholy. Thus, even if it were accepted that transformations were purely imaginary, and that sufferers of lycanthropy would not be mistaken for animals, there was still disagreement about the cause and moral implications of the delusion. If demonically caused, it could result from the sufferer's active complicity with the Devil.[46]

In the cases under consideration here, there is no suggestion that any of the accused manifested symptoms of this condition (or any other recognizable illness), whether naturally or demonically induced. Like Della Porta's conjectures, the medical explanation failed to account for the fact that witnesses saw wolves. Although the transformation is said to be purely imaginary, diagnosis depends more on visible physiognomical symptoms than on assessment of the patient's behavior and mental condition. In a sense, therefore, even imaginary transformations were understood to involve changes in physical appearance.

Henry Boguet

In Boguet's opinion, molded by previous demonology, popular stories and, above all, the confessions of the accused and evidence of witnesses, transformations were demonic illusions affecting the imagination of the witch and the eyes of the spectator, and did not involve any substantial alteration of the body or the soul. He rejected the notion of the spirit taking an animal form while the body lay immobile, on the grounds that the spirit could not be separated from the body without death occurring.[47] In cases where transformation was said to have happened "in ecstasy," he first considered that the witch actually would be lying hidden away, senseless and sleeping deeply after using some ointment. The Devil, meanwhile, would give himself the appearance of a wolf and attack people and animals, but would disturb the imagination of the witch, who merely dreamed of the transformation. The Devil himself would inflict any injuries on the witch's body.[48] Other authors, including Pierre de Lancre, questioned whether this experience necessarily implied guilt, since the Devil could feasibly cause such an illusion in the mind of an innocent person during sleep.[49] But Boguet held that such things did not happen to the innocent, and the events in question occurred only because of the witch's collusion with the Devil. Thus, even if it was not the witch but the Devil who actually carried out a killing, the witch participated mentally in the crime and was guilty of "damnable intention."[50]

But having heard the confessions of the accused and the testimony of witnesses, Boguet believed that in most cases it was the witch in person who appeared to be transformed and attacked people. The Devil gave his servants their ointments and wolfskins to wear and made them think they were really transformed. Like Nynauld, he believed that the ointments witches used had no specific properties other than to dull the senses so that the Devil could more easily work his illusions. He also deluded the senses of witnesses, so that they thought they saw wolves, rather than witches wearing wolfskins. Repercussion was easily explained if the witches committed the crimes in person, for their wolfskins and illusory forms would not protect them from injuries.[51] The Devil further endowed his servants with the abilities and appetites of wolves, making them swift, agile and ferocious; Clauda Jeanprost, who was old and crippled, was asked how she ran with the other wolves and said that the Devil carried her (1598). Boguet had several reasons for concluding that the witches themselves attacked people and that the transformation was totally illusory. Victims and witnesses sometimes saw through the illusion and identified human toes or hands on the wolf's body (Gaillard, 1598; Perrenette Gandillon, 1599). All of those whom he had examined confessed to being very tired after their transformations, which, he said, would not have been the case if they had been lying asleep all the while. Equally, the clothes of the children they killed were said to have been found completely whole and untorn, indicating that they had been removed not by wolves' paws and teeth, but by prehensile and therefore human hands.[52] The accused, moreover, were incapable of repeating their transformations in prison when Boguet asked them to demonstrate. Lastly, scratches on suspects' legs, faces and hands showed that they had been running through the woods like wolves. All of these things indicated to Boguet that human hands had been at work, that there was no real metamorphosis and that the werewolves committed the attacks themselves.

With this theory, it was possible to accept reported transformations as true events without compromising Christian doctrine, and to reconcile the contradiction between the testimony of witnesses who saw or suspected killers in wolf form and the confessions of the human beings accused of the same crimes. Without this theory, there could have been no werewolf trials, no matter how strongly the public felt, because the statements of witnesses and the confessions of the accused could not have been simultaneously true. Unless the supposed transformation could be plausibly explained, and unless it was accepted that it had been caused by demons with the collusion of the suspect, the accusation made no sense and there was no logical or demonstrable connection between the accused and the crime.

Werewolves and the Law

The ravages of wolves thought to be werewolves aroused considerable public concern and could occasionally provoke a lynching (Perrenette Gandillon, 1599). But no matter how strongly the public felt, an accusation against a werewolf could not have resulted in a conviction in a court of law without acceptable evidence of recognizable crimes. Only rarely were suspected werewolves tried simply as murderers, and since the supposed transformation could only be explained by demonic intervention, the prosecution of accused werewolves tended to involve not only the charge of murder in the form of a wolf, but also complicity with the Devil and witchcraft — and witchcraft was a capital crime. Article 109 of the *Constitutio Criminalis Carolina*, promulgated in 1532 by Emperor Charles V and applicable throughout the Empire, decreed that persons who caused harm by witchcraft should be punished with death by fire, and that judges should seek learned counsel where necessary. As H.C. Erik Midelfort has observed, the requirement that judges should take expert advice had profound consequences in that it brought the demonological ideas of jurists and theologians of the universities into the arena of secular justice (Pierre Gandillon, 1599; Chastellan, 1643).[53] The *Carolina* was later reinforced by further edicts promulgated in Brussels in 1604 which prescribed the death penalty for any person over the age of discretion who voluntarily attended the witches' sabbath or who caused illness by witchcraft.[54]

As an isolated province, far removed from the head of state in Brussels, Franche-Comté enjoyed considerable autonomy under the administration of the Parlement of Dole. This body functioned as a supreme court of appeals and exercised its authority over the administration of justice in the whole territory. The three grand bailliwicks of the province were in turn divided into smaller districts (*bailliages* or *prévôtés*), each with its own tribunal presided over by a lieutenant. As of 1586, the lieutenants were required to have a degree or doctorate in civil law at least, and had to be wise, skilled, sufficiently experienced for their duties and free from notoriety or criminal reputation. In each district, a *procureur fiscal* and an *avocat fiscal* were responsible for defending the sovereign's rights and authority and for prosecuting criminal offenses.[55] These courts had the authority to try and judge all criminal cases and to pronounce judgment in capital cases tried in the first instance in lower courts without powers of high justice. Sentences delivered by the *bailliages* could be either executed immediately or appealed to a higher court, whose decisions could in turn be appealed to the Parlement. The Parlement's judgment was usually final.[56]

The majority of suspected werewolves were tried in the secular courts, and the Inquisition's role seems to have been quite limited (1521; 1551; Verjuz, 1599). This may be attributed in part to the efforts of the Parlement of Dole to maintain control over all criminal proceedings in the territory. A decree of 1539 stipulated that Inquisitors were not to arrest or proceed against the sovereign's subjects without fully informing the secular officers.[57] The Inquisitor General of Besançon and his *procureur* were reprimanded by the Parlement in 1551 for their failure to do so in the case of Pierre Tornier (1551).

Criminal justice in the abbatial territory of Saint-Claude, in the south of Franche-Comté, had long been administered by religious officers under the abbot's control. Since the fourteenth century, cases warranting the death penalty had been handed over for judgment to a secular bench of *échevins*, or aldermen, who were periodically elected among the bourgeois of Saint-Claude. These men would formally receive the accused, examine the documents of the case, seek learned advice or order further procedure where necessary and deliver the appropriate judgment. The 1530s saw the creation of a lay *grand juge*, who had extensive powers throughout the territory of Saint-Claude; Henri Boguet held this office from 1596 to 1611. The *grand juge's* functions varied according to different districts, and in the town of Saint-Claude itself he heard all criminal cases, ordered arrests and supervised interrogations. The *grand juge* was nevertheless required to refer any case that warranted the death penalty to the *échevins*, who retained their rights as criminal judges of Saint-Claude, although the simple fact of handing over the case was a clear indication of the *grand juge's* opinion regarding sentence. Their decisions could also be appealed to the Parlement of Dole.[58]

Almost all of the accused were of the lowest social status — vagrants, beggars, shepherds and peasants, some of whom were not natives of Franche-Comté; and as of 1598, many were women. Several had no previous reputation as witches but were apprehended in suspicious circumstances during the chase of a wolf and brought directly before a magistrate; they only confessed to witchcraft during interrogation, when asked to explain their transformations (Peasant, 1573; Stumpf, figure 2; Valeur,

1605; Chastellan, 1643). Others, denounced as witches by members of their communities, were suspected as werewolves *because* they were known to be witches, and in these cases the suspect's activity as a werewolf was often just one of many other charges of witchcraft (Saint-Claude witches, 1598; Verjuz, 1599).

Officers who learned of crimes were expected to report them to the judge who would instruct the *procureur* to gather information in secret. The *avocat fiscal* would analyze the *procureur's* information and recommend whether to proceed with the case, and if so, whether the suspect should be summoned to appear before the court or seized immediately. Alternatively, the suspect might be arrested without prior consultation with the judge, if there were strong fears of evasion.[59] Boguet gave a detailed account of how a judge should proceed. He recommended that questioning should begin immediately after imprisonment, so that the Devil had no opportunity to assist suspected witches. Court officials, he said, should be hidden behind a curtain so that the accused would talk more easily. He advised judges to be firm but gentle, asking questions in quick succession, often repeating the same ones at intervals, since any variations in responses could indicate that the suspect was lying. Suspects were to be brought repeatedly for questioning and confronted at the earliest opportunity with any accomplices who might have accused them.[60]

Evidence fell into three classes, according to its weight in establishing guilt: full proofs, half proofs or proximate presumptions, and adminicules or minor indications of guilt. In witchcraft cases, these minor indications included: descendence from known or convicted witches; failure to react appropriately to a public accusation of witchcraft; possession of a damaged or defective rosary; requesting to be rebaptized; blaspheming and cursing; suspicious marks on the body; habitually downcast eyes; and the inability to shed tears. Such indications were enough to justify provisional detention. Of greater weight were half proofs among which were: attempts to escape; confessions made out of court; frequent association with a known witch; threats followed by actual effects; lying and variations in replies during interrogation; the accusation of accomplices; possession of suspicious powders or ointments; a longstanding reputation for witchcraft; the testimony of only one witness. Evidence of this kind, supported by minor indications, could be grounds for proceeding to torture, and could even justify a sentence of banishment, but not the death penalty, for which full proof was necessary.[61]

In normal procedure, the only acceptable proofs were: 1) the concordant testimony of at least two unimpeachable witnesses (the testimony of minors, convicted felons or mortal enemies was not admissible, members of one family counted as only one witness and women as half witnesses); 2) full voluntary confession of the accused, made without the application or threat of torture and not subsequently retracted. But because an act of witchcraft was usually committed in secret, and discovering the truth was particularly difficult, it was often treated as an extraordinary crime which warranted the use of extraordinary methods and the waiving of some of the normal rules of procedure. In such cases, torture might be used and the statements of persons who would not normally be acceptable as witnesses could be heard as evidence (Secrétain and Gaillard, 1598; Chastellan, 1643). The most important evidence in these trials was the confession of the accused, whether to specific acts of harmful witchcraft or dealings with the Devil and attending the sabbath.[62]

Just as physiognomical signs played their role in the diagnosis of a lycanthrope, the body of a suspected witch could also bear minor indications of guilt, and Boguet advised the examining magistrates to pay close attention to the gestures and expressions as well as the statements of suspects. Reluctance to look upward, for example, was one telltale sign. Others were more physiological — the inability to shed tears, for instance, or suspicious marks on the body. It was believed that the Devil sometimes left marks on the bodies of witches as a token of their allegiance. As a preliminary to an examination for such marks, the accused witch might be stripped and shaved. This humiliating process was enough in itself to persuade some suspects to talk (Secrétain, 1598); it also facilitated the search for powders, ointments or other material evidence which could be concealed in clothing or about the person. Examinations for these diabolic marks were to be carried out only by an expert surgeon, in the presence of a judge and other officers. The surgeon would test any unusual marks by pricking them with a needle, and if the suspect (usually blindfolded) felt no pain when pricked, or if no blood issued from the spot when the needle was withdrawn, the mark might be considered demonic.[63]

If no confession was forthcoming, Boguet suggested putting suspects in solitary confinement in a dark cell, and if this hardship still produced nothing, he recommended lodging them near others accused of the same crime, although this last tactic involved the risk that those who had already confessed might retract their confessions. As a last resort, torture might be applied. In Franche-Comté this generally took the form of the *strappado*, during which the accused would be hoisted in the air by a rope attached to a limb, then allowed to fall until brought to a halt with a jerk before the body touched the ground. Strict rules governed the use of torture. It was not to be applied unless there were strong presumptions of guilt (one or more half proofs supported by minor indications); suspects were not to be tortured more than three times, in measured bouts, and under the supervision of the judge. Confessions made under torture had to be confirmed later, outside the place of torture and once the suspect had been given time to recover. If the confession was retracted, it did not constitute full proof, but could justify further torture. If after three bouts of torture the suspects did not confess, or retracted their confession, they had to be released. Torture was only to be used in moderation, and it seems to have been used very sparingly, if at all, in most of the trials described below.[64]

On completion of this first stage of proceedings, the *procureur* would order a copy to be made of all the accumulated information, including his first report, the suspect's responses during questioning, records of formal confrontations with witnesses, surgeon's report, and so on, and the whole case would be reviewed, based on this enlarged file. This procedure, known as *recours et amplification*, was intended as a second inquiry, but in practice, since it referred back to the same evidence and the same witnesses' statements, it tended to confirm the findings of the first inquiry, rather than to add new information. The file was then passed to the *avocat fiscal*, who ordered the drafting of the indictment or *intendit*, summarizing all the accusations and grievances. The accused was given a copy of this document and had the opportunity to present the judge with any written evidence against the charges. There are no indications that any writings of the kind were offered in the cases described here; suspects are occasionally recorded as having simply held up their copy of the indictment (Jeanprost, 1598).[65]

If there were strong presumptions of guilt, but no full proof, the accused might be sentenced to banishment (Verjuz, 1599). If the evidence was insufficient, especially after a long detention, suspects could be released, although accused witches were rarely discharged absolutely and were often released "until recalled" at a later date if further information warranted it. If there was proof, in the form of a voluntary and confirmed confession and/or the testimony of the appropriate number of witnesses, plus supporting indications, sentence could be pronounced and, unless an appeal was made, executed immediately. For witches, the statutory penalty was death by burning, although this was usually preceded by strangling. Convicted were-wolves were often sentenced to exemplary punishments and tended to be burned alive: Garnier was dragged on a hurdle through Dole (1574) and Stumpf was given the pincers, broken on the wheel and beheaded before burning (figures 2 and 3), many others were burned alive, and always before large crowds of people.[66]

Suspected werewolves did not always confess: some were released or banished, and one woman was condemned on the evidence of witnesses (Couffin, 1574; Verjuz, 1599; Gaillard, 1598). Another confessed to certain charges of witchcraft but did not admit to being a werewolf (Secrétain, 1598). There is no easy explanation for the fact that many suspects did confess to crimes as werewolves. Actual or threat-ened torture may have prompted some confessions, but there is no evidence to con-firm the use or abuse of physical force in these trials. Gilles Garnier, on the other hand, confessed quite spontaneously in 1574. Some suspects may have eventually become convinced that they really had committed the crimes in question, others seem to have given up and resigned themselves to their fate. Sometimes the ordeals of imprisonment and interrogation were themselves sufficient to prompt a confes-sion (Secrétain, 1598).

The years 1598-99 mark the peak of werewolf activity in Franche-Comté, with nine trials and one lynching during these years. Eight trials were examined by Boguet, and he and his *procureur* André Vion, neither of whom was moderate where witches were concerned, must share some responsiblity for the high rate of confessions and condemnations: seven confessed to acts of witchcraft and six admitted to being werewolves as well; seven were burned alive and another died in prison.[67] Boguet was firmly convinced that a reputation for witchcraft was rarely undeserved, and his success in obtaining proof of this without torture in so many cases says much for the effectiveness of the techniques he recommended in his *Instruction*: fre-quent, rapid and repetitious questioning, solitary confinement, enlisting the aid of accomplices or even people pretending to be suspects to persuade others to con-fess, and so on.[68]

Nevertheless, Boguet's own contribution to this peak must be measured along-side other factors. The Parlement's 1598 edict on the hunting of wild animals, the deaths of children attacked by wolves in 1597-98, which are recorded in Boguet's cases, and the lynching of Perrenette Gandillon all indicate that wolves were caus- ing serious problems, that there was a panic about werewolves and that these trials were partly a response to public pressure. Furthermore, the trials at Saint-Claude also coincided with the beginning of Franche-Comté's most intense period of witch-hunting, between 1599 and 1610.[69] Nor was this wave of interest in werewolves limited to Franche-Comté; they were very much in the news elsewhere around the turn of the century, with trials occurring in France, Switzerland and Germany, and several discussions of lycanthropy appearing in print.[70]

But not all werewolf trials had the same results. Between August and November 1598, while Boguet was examining and handing over self-confessed werewolves to be condemned to death by the *échevins* of Saint-Claude, accused werewolf Jacques Roulet of Angers was brought on appeal to the Parlement of Paris, where he was judged mad and sent to hospital for two years.[71] During the same period, Jacques Verjuz was tried in Baume and Dole on charges similar to those brought against Clauda Gaillard in Saint-Claude; neither confessed but Gaillard was executed any- way, while the Parlement of Dole only confirmed Verjuz's sentence of banishment, despite the adverse testimony of many witnesses (1599). The difference between the judgments in Saint-Claude and Dole does not indicate that the high court judges were more lenient than Boguet was toward accused witches; it suggests rather that they were more scrupulous about the means of obtaining proof and more rig- orous in their interpretation of the evidence. It was the magistrates' increasing caution with regard to evidence in such cases rather than their disbelief in the real- ity of werewolves which brought about the decline and eventual cessation of trials and condemnations of werewolves. The edicts of 1632-34 and the decision in Chastellan's case in 1643 show quite clearly that public concern about werewolves was shared by high court judges and legal experts. But the trials of werewolves would never again reach the same frequency as in 1598-99, and only isolated cases occurred after this time. The "group" activities of the Saint-Claude werewolves did not recur, and the werewolf reverted to its former status as a more or less solitary criminal.

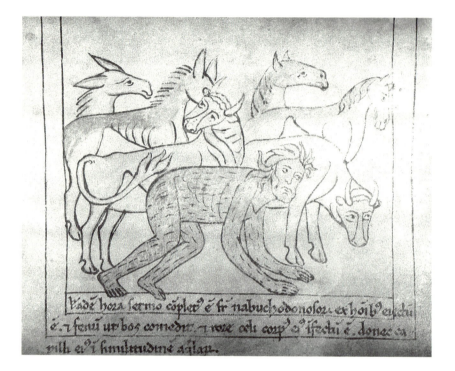

Nebuchadnezzar cast out among the beasts. From the illuminated
manuscript of the Bible of King Sancho of Fuerte, Spain, 1194-97
(Amiens, Bibliothèque communale).

one

Trials of Werewolves and Edicts
on Wolf Hunting, 1521-1643

1521   Pierre Burgot (called Groz Pierre), and
Michel Verdun of Plasne; Philbert Montot

Pierre Burgot and Michel Verdun, executed at Poligny in December 1521 for crimes
of heresy, witchcraft and murder in the form of wolves, were already famous by
the time Johann Wier published a summary of their confessions in 1563.[72] In the
presence of the Inquisitor General of Besançon, Jean Boin (or Bon), Burgot confessed
as follows:

On the day of the Poligny fair some nineteen years earlier, a terrific storm scat-
tered his sheep, and during his desperate search for them, he met three horsemen in
black, servants of the Devil. One of them tried to console Burgot with the promise
that his flock would be found if he swore allegiance to a master who would teach
him how to safeguard his sheep from wolves and other dangers. He even promised
money, although Burgot said he never received any. Burgot accepted the offer and,
renouncing God, promised to serve the Devil and to avoid Mass and holy water thereafter. Two years later, no longer employed as a shepherd, he forgot this promise and
went to church again as before. This continued for eight or nine years until Verdun
urged him to accompany him in paying homage to their master, which Burgot agreed
to do, so long as he would be given money.

Together, they went to an assembly at Chastel Charlon, where many people
danced, holding green candles which burned with a blue flame. Verdun made Burgot
take off his clothes and anointed him all over with a salve which transformed him
into a wolf – and Burgot was seized with horror at the sight of his fur, and his hands
and feet as paws. Verdun did likewise, and they both ran as fast as the wind. After
an hour or two, Verdun anointed their bodies again, and they turned back into men.
Burgot said he experienced such weariness after this experience that he could hardly
get up. Where he had said he was naked when he was transformed, and did not know
what happened to his fur when he returned to human form, Verdun claimed to have
turned into a wolf while he was clothed.

On one occasion, while in wolf form, Burgot attempted to kill a seven-year-old
boy, but when the child screamed loudly, he fled back to where he had left his

clothes and rubbed himself down with some herbs, as Verdun had taught him, to return to human form. Together, they had killed a woman who was picking peas, soon after which they were met by Monsieur de la Chusnée (who may have testified in this trial), with whom they spoke, but they were incapable of harming him.

Wier observed that Burgot and Verdun sometimes gave different answers to questions about the same incidents, but they both confessed the following:

As wolves, they killed and ate all but one arm of a four-year-old girl. Verdun said he liked the taste of human flesh, but Burgot claimed that it disagreed with his stomach. They strangled and sucked the blood of a third victim, and killed and ate a fourth, because Burgot was hungry. Their fifth victim was a girl of eight or nine whom they killed in a garden; Burgot said he broke her neck with his teeth because she had refused to give him alms. Finally, they killed a goat near the farm of Maître Pierre Bongré (who may also have testified – perhaps it was his goat), by biting it and cutting its throat with a knife. They further confessed that when they were wolves, they took great pleasure in coupling with wolverines, that their transformation never lasted as long as they hoped, and that they both possessed an ash-colored powder which they would rub on their left arms and hands and which killed any animal they touched.

In 1574, Daniel d'Auge reported having seen on the door of the church at Poligny a "fine description placed there as a perpetual reminder of two men of this town who, in 1521, renounced chrism and baptism to make themselves slaves of Satan, who made fine promises to make them great so that they willingly acquiesced to his offers and made themselves wolves whenever they felt fit, murdered and ate many little children, and then by using ointments turned themselves back into their original human appearance."[73]

Boguet added the name of Philbert Montot to the list of Poligny werewolves. It is not clear whether Montot was executed at the same time, although Boguet said he was, nor is it certain whether d'Auge's "fine description" was accompanied by a painting. But by Boguet's time a picture of not two but three werewolves had long hung at the church door, and "he who painted the three werewolves of Poligny represented them as each carrying a knife in its right paw." Boguet also adds that Michel Verdun was injured as a wolf by a hunter, who later found him in a hut where a woman was tending his wounds. Wier, whose account seems to be based on an official report, does not mention this incident, which Boguet may have heard or read elsewhere.[74]

Wier did not believe these men were guilty of murder. In his opinion, their supposed transformations were nothing more than hallucinations caused by drugs in their ointments, and full inquiries might even have revealed that the persons they said they had killed were still alive. While Wier may have been correct in assuming their innocence of murder, his hypothesis seems unlikely. Inquiries would definitely have been made, information gathered from people in the area and statements heard from witnesses. We know from other cases that when wolves had attacked children, and a suspected werewolf was apprehended, witnesses were only too willing to give information about wolf attacks, and bereaved parents came forward to testify.[75] It is extremely likely that the victims were dead, and that real wolves had been involved in some if not all of the killings.

Burgot was a shepherd, and perhaps Verdun was too, and as such they may well have made use of various "trade secrets," such as charms or more or less magical preparations intended to ward off evil and protect the animals in their care. The ointment that they said they rubbed on their hands and arms and used to kill any animals they touched may be just an inversion of the function and properties of the protection salve as described, for example, by the peasant arrested in 1573.[76]

1550   A Complaint about Wolves[77]

Officers of the *bailliage* of Amont complained to the Parlement of Dole in a letter of November 12, 1550, that wolves had eaten four children near Filain, and the ban on hunting meant that people could do nothing to catch the culprits. If all the game in the region were to be destroyed by allowing common people to hunt wolves, they continued, this was little compared with the harm the wolves were causing, "and the Court might well consider the perpetual sorrow now afflicting the fathers and families of those children."

1551   Pierre Tornier of Savigny-les-Montmorot[78]

Pierre Tornier obeyed a summons to appear before Fr. Melchior Molevy, Inquisitor General of Besançon, at the request of Simon Digny, *procureur* for the Inquisition, to answer charges of "several crimes, offenses and acts of witchcraft." Tornier was imprisoned and interrogated, and the Inquisitor ordered the arrest of the man's accomplices: his wife Marie Barnagoz, his sister Perrenette and Jeanne Guyenot. The accusations against them, now amplified by Pierre Tornier's statements, were that Marie Barnagoz and her husband, "transfigured into a savage wolf," had murdered two little children, and that with Perrenette and Jeanne they had committed some fourteen or fifteen murders and a multitude of other offenses and acts of witchcraft. The confessions of all four were heard and confirmed in the presence of the acting lieutenant and other officers of the *bailliage* of Montmorot. Before the sentence could be pronounced, however, the Inquisitor had to see the trial documents, which the officers refused to hand over in the absence of the lieutenant-general. Following the Inquisitor's complaint to the Parlement, the officers of Montmorot were ordered to conclude the trial as they ought to have done in the first place, and to administer justice in the proper manner in future. The Parlement also issued a sharp reprimand to the Inquisitor for his failure to observe the ordinance of 1539 by ordering the women's arrest without informing the secular officials.

The outcome of the trial is not known. Tornier's transformation into a wolf is simply stated, without further elaboration, but the accompanying charge of witchcraft provides an implicit explanation. The document does not specify whether more than two of the total of sixteen or seventeen murders were committed by the werewolf.

1573   September 3, Edict Concerning a Werewolf[79]
The Parlement of Dole had been notified that "a werewolf, as it is called," had been seen frequently in the region of Dole, and that it had caught and carried away a number of children. It had even tried to attack horsemen who had struggled with it at considerable risk to their own safety. In the interests of avoiding further damage, the court issued an edict granting special permission to inhabitants of the areas concerned to arm themselves with whatever they could and to pursue and kill "the said werewolf."

Extraordinary characteristics – the wolf's noteworthy daring and ferocity, its incursions into populated areas and its appetite for human flesh – aroused the suspicion that this was no ordinary wolf, but a werewolf.

1573 Arrest of a Peasant[80]

The diary of Lucas Geizkofler, a German student of law at the University of Dole, records the arrest and imprisonment of five peasants during the latter part of 1573. A wolf that had assaulted sheep in a nearby village was pursued by armed men, who followed it as it disappeared into the bushes. Instead of finding a wolf, however, they encountered a peasant carrying a bag. Asked if he had seen the wolf, the man replied that he had seen several, and if the hunters kept on running, they were bound to catch one. He declined their invitation to join the chase, because his bag was too heavy, and naturally, the men wanted to know what he was carrying. They soon found that the bag contained a quantity of little pots of ointment, and the peasant explained that when he rubbed this on his body and on the bodies of his sheep, there was nothing to worry about anymore. Taken immediately to the nearest judge, the peasant revealed that his friends also used the ointment, and all of them were arrested and brought to Dole.

The incident admirably illustrates how the chase of a wolf could easily lead to the capture of a human suspect. The hunters may have suspected that the man was a werewolf, and that the ointment was transformational salve, but this is by no means certain. Possession of pots of unidentified substances, especially if they were said to have occult, albeit beneficial properties, would probably have aroused suspicion anyway.

Geizkofler's diary also shows that wolves were causing serious problems in the area around Dole, that the wolves were understood to be extraordinary in character and behavior and that local people were convinced that these were werewolves in league with the Devil. A rumor was going around, he said, that nearby villages were infested with wolves as big as donkeys which ate people, especially women. Men shot at them in vain, and the vulgar people saw them as desperate sinners who had sold themselves to the Devil, who taught them how to turn into wolves to cause harm to people and livestock.

1574 January 7, Pierre Couffin of Saligney[81]

Pierre Couffin had been arrested and imprisoned on charges of "homicide committed on the persons of several children, eating and devouring of these in the form of a werewolf, and other crimes and offenses." Having heard the report of his interrogation, the court decided that Couffin should be released on bail, ordering him to hand over all his possessions as surety and to present himself at the court whenever he might be summoned, on pain of being convicted of the charges against him if he failed to appear.

Clearly, there was insufficient evidence to warrant further detention, and, unlike Gilles Garnier, also detained in the *conciergerie* of Dole during this month, on exactly the same charges, Couffin did not confess to being a werewolf.

1574   January 18, Gilles Garnier of Lyon[82]

The publication in three different places in 1574 of a pamphlet containing the Parlement's decree against Garnier made this one of the most famous trials of a werewolf. Garnier was a beggar who lived in a refuge with his wife Apolline and friends Jean Joly and Richard Estrabonne. All four were arrested around the beginning of December 1573 on the same charges of "homicide committed on the persons of several children, eating and devouring of these in the form of a werewolf, and other crimes and offenses." Apolline and the friends were presumably released, for no more is heard of them.[83] Without torture, Garnier confessed as follows:

Shortly after Saint Michael's Day 1573, in the form of a wolf, he attacked and killed "both with his hands like paws and his teeth," a ten- or eleven-year-old girl near the forest of La Serre. He removed her clothes, ate part of her thighs and arms, and, not content with this, also took a portion home for his wife. Around mid-day, eight days after All Saints, also in the form of a wolf, he strangled and fatally wounded "with his hands and teeth" another girl near the forest of La Ruppe; he had intended to eat her, but three people came to the rescue. About two weeks after All Saints, again in the form of a wolf, he killed a ten-year-old boy in a vine-yard near Gredisans, ate part of the thighs, legs and stomach, and dismembered one leg. On the Friday before Saint Bartholomew's Day, he attacked a boy of about twelve or thirteen near the village of Perrouze and dragged him into the woods nearby, where he killed him in the same way as the others; again he had intended to eat his victim, even though it was a Friday, but he was prevented by the arrival of would-be rescuers. On this occasion he was in the form of a man and not that of a wolf.

Garnier repeated his voluntary confession several times and was duly sentenced by the Parlement to be dragged through Dole on a hurdle and burned alive on January 18, 1574.

There is little doubt that real wolves were responsible for some if not all of the children's deaths. It is not certain whether there were witnesses who saw wolves or evidence of these animals' teeth and claws on the victims' bodies, and a human attacker on another occasion, or whether the details about the killer's shape were volunteered by Garnier himself. But there is ample evidence, in the edict of September 3, the other arrests and Geizkofler's diary, that real wolves were perpetrating attacks in the area, that many children had been killed or had totally disappeared and that the region was in the throes of a werewolf panic.

The order in which the crimes are listed in the decree might lead the reader to suppose that Garnier was caught in human form, in the act of killing the boy at Perrouze. In fact, this attack occurred on August 20, 1573, while the others, listed in their correct chronological order, took place around September 30, November 8 and November 15-16, respectively. The killing listed last, therefore, occurred well before the others, before the edict on hunting and more than three months before Garnier's arrest. This means that, contrary to the impression given by the decree, Garnier was not apprehended, in human form, while attacking the boy, and the circumstances of his arrest remain a mystery. But it is quite feasible that he may have been discovered in the woods in the same way as the peasant arrested in 1573, by beaters chasing killer wolves.[84]

The decree concerning Garnier makes no mention of witchcraft and offers no explanation for the supposed transformation. In an essay that accompanied the Sens edition of the decree, Daniel d'Auge supplied this explanation, saying that Garnier had confessed that he had made a pact with the Devil who, in return, had given him an ointment with which to transform himself into any shape he chose. But since the only source of this comment was a manuscript copy of the decree which had been glossed by various hands before it reached d'Auge, his information may not be reliable. We have already seen how Peter Stumpf's story was transformed in the retelling, and how Boguet's account of the Poligny werewolves adds proof in the form of repercussion although it was absent from Wier's more accurate description. Given that the decree *does* include Garnier's other crimes of intending to eat human flesh on a Friday, and feeding it to his wife, it is strange that the heinous crimes of witchcraft and demon worship should have been omitted, or anonymously included under the title of "other crimes and offenses." It seems more reasonable to suppose that they were not listed in the decree because Garnier did not mention them in his confession, and that the court chose to ignore the implications of witchcraft and concentrated on the murder charges, for which a full voluntary confession had been obtained. Such a reading suggests that the order in which the crimes are listed in the decree, and the implication that Garnier was caught *in flagrante delicto* in human form, may not have been accidental.

Reforms within the Parlement in the last months of 1573, instigated by the Duke of Alba, may have had some bearing on this trial. The main charge levied against the high court was that it conducted its business too slowly, and efforts were made to rectify this failing.[85] And while the Parlement was under pressure from above to perform its duties more efficiently, public concern and fears about wolves or werewolves attacking and killing children created pressure from below. Furthermore, the fact that Garnier was a beggar and too poor to pay the costs of the trial would also have been an incentive to conclude the trial as swiftly as possible.[86] It is small wonder, therefore, that Garnier's trial, lasting no more than seven weeks from arrest to execution, was dispatched with considerable speed, severity and publicity.

1598   January 25, Measures to Deal with Ferocious Animals[87]

The Parlement had been notified that in various parts of the region, wolves, bears and lynxes had recently taken to attacking domestic animals and even people, and that the communities were doing nothing to prevent these attacks because previous legislation prohibited the carrying of arms and imposed fines for unauthorized hunting. Officers suggested that the court should provide salaries for people to be appointed to hunt and kill these animals. The Parlement decided that the communities involved should appoint huntsmen and pay them ten francs to organize hunts for a certain time. Anyone taking part in the hunts would be allowed to carry arms and exempted from the prescribed penalties for hunting, so long as he did not abuse the privilege. The communities themselves would not only be responsible for the hunt organizers' premiums, but would also be held responsible for any "homicides" and other problems, as well as the cost of eventual damage if they did not take measures to capture these animals and prevent them from harming people.

The threat of penalties for communities failing to take appropriate precautions draws attention to the problem of enforcing observance of the prescribed measures. Many people concerned were reluctant to lose time earning a living or taking care of their regular business by taking part in the organized hunts, which brought risks of personal injury but little personal benefit to ordinary people, who stood to gain neither the premium nor anything to take home for dinner.[88]

Similar measures were also taken in France at this time to combat the depredations of wolves, and it has been suggested that this legislation and contemporary references to wolf attacks signal a marked increase in the wolf population around the turn of the century.[89] If this was the case, and wolf attacks on people were more frequent, it might explain the rise in the number of accusations and trials of suspected werewolves and the increased interest in lycanthropy during this period. Edicts encouraging armed bands to beat their way through the forests in pursuit of wolves and other wild animals certainly favored the capture of odd individuals who might be suspected as werewolves. But since the frequency of werewolf accusations and trials rose roughly in proportion to Franche-Comté's three main crises of witch-hunting, it is equally possible that more witch trials, rather than more wolf attacks, contributed much to the werewolf panic of 1598-1600; in which case, the panic itself may have helped to prompt the legislation by generating more discussion and focusing greater attention on regular, but not necessarily more frequent, animal attacks.[90]

1598 Jacques Bocquet (called Groz Jacques) of Savoy, Clauda Jeanprost (called Grand' Clauda Boisson), Clauda Jeanguillaume and Thievenne Paget (called la Micholette) of Orcières, Françoise Secrétain of Coyrières, Clauda Gaillard (called la Friboulette) of Ebouchoux[91]

All six were tried at Saint-Claude and examined by Boguet himself, on charges of witchcraft, transformation into wolves and murder. The chain of events that ultimately led to this group of witches and werewolves being brought to justice began on June 4, 1598, when Françoise Secrétain, aged about fifty-eight, requested lodging in the house of the Maillat family. Though at first reluctant to grant this request in the absence of her husband, Maillat's wife finally agreed. It is said that during the same evening, Secrétain gave a "crust of bread resembling dung" to eight-year-old Louise Maillat, and made her eat it, "strictly forbidding her to speak of it or she would kill and eat her." On Saturday, June 5, Louise became possessed and claimed that Secrétain had caused her illness. Secrétain, perhaps believing herself responsible, later paid a visit to Groz Jacques Bocquet to find out how to cure the child's possession [1].[92] Groz Jacques, who appears to have been a practicing witch, and whom Boguet described as "one of the great witches of his time," told her that if she took some bread from the Maillat home, kept it for three days and then fed it to the child, her possession would be cured [35]. Whether or not Secrétain carried this out, Louise Maillat did not recover, and on July 19, 1598, her parents took her to church to be exorcized. The following day, after the parents had spent the whole night praying, Louise delivered up her five demons and began to recover.[93]

But Secrétain had been publicly accused and was seized and imprisoned without delay, before she had a chance to escape. For three days she confessed nothing and claimed it was a crime to detain her. She was placed in solitary confinement in a dark, narrow cell, "and certain threats were used," but she still declined to confess [1-4]. It was noted that she shed no tears, always looked downward and had a defective rosary [39, 41]. The next day, she was stripped, shaved and examined by a surgeon, but no demonic marks were found on her body [43-44]. As soon as her hair was cut, however, she began her confession and added to it daily thereafter. She had caused Louise Maillat to be possessed by five devils [5]. She had given herself long before to the Devil in the form of a black man; she had copulated with him, when he was in the form of a dog, a cat or a hen (!), and his member had "burned her stomach" [7, 11-12]. She went to the sabbath astride a white stick, and there she danced and beat water to make hail, which sometimes fell in the wrong place [14-15, 21-22]. With Groz Jacques she had caused the death of a man by giving him a piece of bread sprinkled with a powder which the Devil had given them. She had also caused several cows to die by touching them with a wand and speaking certain words [23, 26, 29]. Secrétain was later accused as a werewolf by Groz Jacques, but she herself never confessed to this [4].[94]

Groz Jacques was arrested soon after Secrétain, and the same method of procedure was used with him [47]. When no marks were found on his body, he said that some witches did not have marks, which led Boguet to conclude that the Devil only marked those whose allegiance was doubtful [44]. Groz Jacques confessed that he had attended the sabbath in various places, and made hail, and he told Boguet that it was quite possible to go to the sabbath in spirit only [17]. He concurred with Secrétain's admission that they put a powder on bread to kill a man, and he also claimed to have caused animals to die by burying powders under a doorstep [23]. The Devil had asked him to give him one of his daughters, but Groz Jacques had refused [48].[95]

Shortly after the detention of Secrétain and Groz Jacques, a fourteen-year-old orphan named Christofle, of the village of Arinthod, publicly announced that they had taken her to the sabbath two years earlier, and she too was arrested [52]. More accomplices were named and arrested, witnesses added their testimony of grief and harm previously suffered, old grudges resurfaced and there were scores to be settled. Rolande du Vernoy claimed that because she had once refused Groz Jacques an egg, he had caused her chickens to die in a strange way, and then he had given her an apple which caused her to be possessed by two demons [33]. Groz Jacques in turn accused du Vernoy of being a witch, and both he and Secrétain said they had seen her at the sabbath [53]. Du Vernoy was also arrested and continued to be possessed in prison, obstinately refusing to confess for almost two years [53, 59]. Vengeance and spite may have inspired Groz Jacques's plea, shortly before his execution, that justice should be done to du Vernoy, for she would spoil everything if she escaped punishment [59].[96]

Between 1597 and 1598, wolves had attacked and eaten children of Claude Gindre, Claude Godard, Thievent Bondieu of Orcières and Anathoile Cochet of Longchaumois. Two children of Claude Bault of Longchaumois had also been attacked while picking strawberries; the girl was killed, but her brother escaped to tell the tale. The parents of all these children gave information, and the times and places of the attacks were verified. Groz Jacques, Clauda Jeanprost, Clauda Jeanguillaume and Thievenne Paget all confessed that, together, they had killed and eaten these children. When they went around as wolves, they said, the Devil also took the form of a wolf to lead them, and Groz Jacques confessed that he transformed himself by anointing himself with an ointment which the Devil had given him [47].[97]

It was Groz Jacques who persuaded Thievenne Paget to break her three-month silence. He had promised to do what he could to induce her to confess, and to this end was put in the room next to hers in prison.

And he fulfilled his promise; for after Thievenne had been but one night next to him she confessed, and stood so well to her confession that, by order of the Judge, a man was sent in to her the next day, and told her that he had been to the Sabbat with her, and told her particulars of it which he took from the confession of Groz Jacques and that of the other witches who had accused her.[48][98]

She said that the Devil had first come to her in the form of a man when she was distressed at losing one of her cows [8]. She had copulated with a demon in the form of a black man, and his member was cold and thin, and she claimed that this had happened three times while she was in prison [11-12, 46]. Sometimes on foot, and sometimes transported by the demon, she went to the sabbath where she made hail, and she had killed someone with a certain powder administered in cheese. She, too, admitted that she was one of the pack of wolves which had killed children at Orcières and Longchaumois.[99]

Clauda Jeanguillaume confessed that she had attended the sabbath, where she ate meat from a cauldron and made hail [21-22]. In addition to her participation in killing the children from Orcières and Longchaumois, she admitted that, in the form of a wolf, she had almost killed two other children, but had been prevented from inflicting any serious harm by the intervention of a dog – which she killed instead. Clauda Jeanprost was both old and lame. Boguet once asked her how she managed to run up and down hillsides with the other werewolves as she had confessed. She replied that Satan carried her [47]. She too had attended the sabbath, where cripples danced and everyone made hail [21]. Like the other werewolves, she said that they never ate the heads of their victims, because of the baptismal chrism, nor the right hand, as this was used to make the sign of the cross [9].[100]

On August 22, 1598, Françoise Secrétain was handed over to be judged by the *échevins* of Saint-Claude. Her indictment was read aloud by the *procureur*, and she confirmed that it was true, adding nothing except that during the previous two nights in prison, someone had burnt her head and hurt her. When asked, she could not say who had done this as she had neither seen nor spoken to the person. Boguet later remarked that the Devil was probably responsible [46]. The *échevins* appointed a day for her to reappear before them a week later, before which she was to be questioned again in prison. But they were not to pronounce sentence on that day; at least two further adjournments, September 3 and 12, 1598, were decided on, and the judges' final decision was ultimately preempted by Secrétain's death in prison, the precise date of which is unknown [45].[101]

The accused were given the opportunity to present written evidence against the charges, but most had nothing to offer, and both Françoise Secrétain and Clauda Jeanprost are recorded as having simply exhibited their copies of their indictments. The échevins received Clauda Jeanprost on August 28, 1598, and adjourned until September 12, but did not pronounce sentence until much later.[102] There are no precise records of the date of her execution, nor do we know exactly when Groz Jacques and the others were burned, but there are indications that they remained in prison for a considerable amount of time, perhaps as long as two years. Boguet remarked that it would have been fitting to burn all the werewolves together, but the Gandillon family were "hurried too quick to their execution," in April 1599 [47]. Rolande du Vernoy, who had appealed to the Parlement against an order for torture, was finally burned, after a long imprisonment, on September 7, 1600. Boguet stated that Groz Jacques "had been burned alive a few days before," and died contrite and repentant [59]. Thievenne Paget was burned along with Groz Jacques, Clauda Gaillard and Clauda Jeanguillaume, who had to be knocked unconscious by the executioner because she kept jumping from the flames [45]. Clauda Jeanprost had been executed some time earlier [48].[103]

Clauda Gaillard was accused by Christofle of Arinthod, who claimed to have seen her at the sabbath, but there was also information against her from the Perrin family [51]. It was said that Clauda Perrin had died, and Marie Perrin had fallen ill because Gaillard had breathed on them when they refused to give alms to her. Marie Perrin only recovered when her nephew Pierre challenged the witch to cure the harm [25, 35]. Jeanne Perrin testified that Gaillard had caused, and later cured, a sickness in one of her mares, and had also turned into a wolf in order to frighten her [51]. They had been walking together near the woods when Gaillard grumbled that Perrin had received more alms than herself, and went off into the bushes. As soon as the woman had disappeared, a wolf, with no tail and what seemed to be human toes on its hind paws, appeared from the same spot. It approached Perrin and frightened her so much that she dropped her money and fled, making the sign of the cross as she ran. When Gaillard later told her that the wolf would not have harmed her, Perrin suspected that the wolf had been none other than Clauda Gaillard herself [47].[104]

Gaillard never confessed but was nevertheless condemned to death on the basis of other evidence against her, namely: popular report that she was a witch; she shed no tears, although she tried; she blasphemed and uttered curses; there were discrepancies in her answers; she convicted herself by denying particular facts before she was accused; Christofle swore she had seen her at the sabbath; she was charged with particular acts of witchcraft by several people [48, 51]. There is a note of self-justification in Boguet's account of this decision, and not without cause. Only a single accomplice, who was also a minor, had accused her of attending the sabbath, and the witnesses who accused her of causing harm were mostly women from the same family who, although they agreed on the general charge of witchcraft, all testified to different, separate offenses [51].[105] If we compare the Parlement of Dole's decision in 1599 to banish Jacques Verjuz, whom a large number of witnesses had accused of causing illness or death in sixteen people, the sentence against Clauda Gaillard seems all the more severe.

In all of these cases, the process of transformation is attributed to the use of ointments and wolfskins supplied by the Devil. Although Groz Jacques had said it was possible to go to the sabbath in spirit only, there is no suggestion that any of the accused claimed to have been transformed "in ecstasy." Boguet understood from their confessions and the testimony of witnesses that the apparent transformation was an illusion caused by the Devil and that the witches themselves were running around attacking people. Their confessed tiredness after transformation, their scratched faces and the human toes or fingers glimpsed by witnesses on the wolves' bodies all proved this. Boguet further verified the illusory nature of the supposed transformation, asking some of the accused to demonstrate their ability to transform themselves. They were able to show him how they went about on all fours, but said that they could not turn into wolves because they had no ointment and no longer had their power in prison.[106] For Boguet, this simply confirmed that transformations were all illusory and that the werewolves had committed their crimes in person. Moreover, since God "will not permit the wicked, such as are witches, to have power over the persons of Judges," it was probably no surprise that they could not appear to be transformed in prison before the eyes of officers of the law [37].[107]

1599 Perrenette Gandillon, Pierre Gandillon (called Pètre) and Georges Gandillon of Nezen[108]
In 1597 or 1598, about three years before Boguet wrote his *Discours*, an adolescent

named Benoist Bidel was picking fruit in a tree when his younger sister was attacked beneath the tree by a wolf "which had no tail." He climbed down to help her, and the wolf turned to attack him instead; during the struggle, the boy was injured in the neck with his own knife. People came to his rescue and took him home to his father's house, where a few days later he died of his injuries. While ill in bed, however, he said that the wolf's paws had looked like human hands on the underside, but covered with hair on the backs. It was discovered later that the wolf was Perrenette Gandillon, who had made herself scarce immediately after the attack. She was found and killed by the peasants [47].[109]

Although the precise date of the lynching is unknown, it may have been this which led to the arrest — and execution, in April 1599 — of Perrenette's brother Pierre and his two children, Georges and Anthoina. They were all charged with "witchcraft, poisoning, murder, crimes and offenses," and were examined at Saint-Claude by Boguet. Pierre Gandillon's indictment, summarizing his admissions during questioning and the statements of witnesses and other accused witches, contained the following:[110]

He had renounced God and given himself to the Devil some fifteen years earlier. According to Boguet, this had occurred on an occasion when Gandillon was upset and angry that his scythe did not cut as well as his companions' scythes. The Devil had immediately appeared in the form of a goat and had won him over [8]. He had attended the witches' sabbath in several places, where he danced and ate meat with others. He also said that they coupled with demons — some in male form and others as women; the sabbath was always around midnight and he went there on foot [11, 16]. He had worshiped the Devil in the form of a large black ram, offering him candles and kissing his anus.[111]

He confessed that he had beaten water with a stick and had thrown in the air a powder given to him by the Devil, in order to make hail, which had severely damaged crops in the area of Nezen five or six times in 1598. He was commonly reputed to be a witch by those who knew him. He said he had received a wolfskin from the Devil which he had used to turn himself into a wolf about a dozen times over five or six years. He also told Boguet that he used an ointment when he transformed himself into a wolf. As a wolf, he had stolen and eaten several goats and other animals. Two years earlier, with an accomplice who was also transformed, he had attacked and injured the twelve-year-old daughter of Pierre Girard of Montadroit and a boy of the house of Bourgognon of Vescles. Two years before that, he and his accomplice, both as wolves, had attacked the child of Claude Butavant, but this man had forced them to abandon the attack. Pierre Gandillon also confessed that he sometimes turned into a hare. Boguet recorded that Gandillon had so many scratches on his face, hands and legs and was "so disfigured that he hardly appeared human, and horrified all who looked at him" [47].[112]

Georges and Anthoina (who was not accused as a werewolf) were tried during the same period as their father. Georges confessed that he had also renounced God and given himself to the Devil in the shape of a horned ram some fourteen years earlier. Boguet recorded that Georges succumbed to the Devil at a time when he was having difficulty driving some oxen [8]. Like his father, Georges had attended the sabbath where, with accomplices, he had beaten water with a stick of walnut wood to make hail. He, too, was reported to be a witch by all who knew him, and he showed Boguet the place on his shoulder where the Devil had touched him, although the mark had already disappeared [44]. He said that he had once transformed himself into a wolf at the instigation of his aunt Perrenette Gandillon, who had given him a wolfskin and rubbed his stomach with a certain ointment. His aunt had also transformed herself into a wolf. Georges told Boguet that he had never attacked any children, and that he had only killed goats with his aunt, including a goat belonging to his father, which they killed by mistake [47].[113]

Georges further informed Boguet that on the night of Maundy Thursday one year, he had lain in bed as if dead, and after three hours, he returned to himself with a start. It was said that strenuous efforts had been made to wake him during this time, and that he had made excuses for his deep sleep, attributing it to the previous day's hard work — but it was thought that he was really at the sabbath during this time. Attending the sabbath in spirit only, however, was irreconcilable with Christian doctrine, and for Boguet, Georges Gandillon was tired because he had been to the sabbath in person, while the Devil left an illusory shape in the likeness of Gandillon sleeping soundly. The fact that this sleeper could not be woken by any means was a sign that the Devil was at work [17].[114]

The Gandillons were handed over to the *échevins* on April 3, 1599, in the market square of Saint-Claude, where many people were present. Pierre Gandillon was asked if the indictment read out by the *procureur* conformed with what he had told the judge during interrogations. He begged for God's mercy, asked for justice to be done and stated that what he had told the judge was true – although he could not remember what he had answered. The *échevins* adjourned for three weeks, during which they examined all the documents and took counsel, as was required, from "wise persons and experts in law." On April 24, 1599, the three members of the Gandillon family and four others were sentenced to be burned alive and their bodies reduced to ashes on that very day.

1599   Jacques Verjuz of Baume-les-Nonnes[115]

After his trial by the Inquisition of Besançon on various charges of witchcraft, Jacques Verjuz was sentenced to perpetual banishment from Besançon and Franche-Comté on February 25, 1599, and he appealed to the Parlement of Dole. He had long been known as a witch by many people in Baume, and although he had been accused publicly, he had never tried to disprove the allegation. It was also said that he regularly slept with his mother. The illnesses of many animals and at least sixteen people, including his first wife and his brother-in-law, were understood to have been caused by his witchcraft. Sickness often ensued directly after a quarrel with Verjuz. Many of these people died, and the recovery of those who survived was usually attributed to counter-magic involving Verjuz: some recovered after eating soup made with nine different sorts of herbs picked from his garden, and one woman was cured after hitting him on the head. It is not clear whether Verjuz deliberately participated in administering these cures, but he does seem to have played upon his reputation and made threats which were construed as intent to cause harm by witchcraft.

Annette Trouvel de Court said that Verjuz had turned himself into a wolf one evening, and in this form he had accompanied her all the way to her village, with the intention of harming her. Nicole Gilbert also testified that one morning during the harvests in 1596, Verjuz had appeared before her, "with a hideous face," his eyes wide and sparkling like a cat's eyes, and his mouth wide open like the mouth of a wolf, and she thought he was trying to bewitch her.

On May 30, 1599, the Parlement of Dole acquitted him of four of the charges of causing illness by witchcraft and sentenced him to perpetual banishment for all of the other charges – including that of turning into a wolf.

The transformation into a wolf is presented here as just one of the many wicked attributes of a witch, rather than a career in itself. The incident shows how an encounter with a wolf did not have to be fatal to arouse the suspicion that it was a werewolf. It was enough that the encounter seemed abnormal.

1605   Jacques Valeur of Moissey[116]

In March 1605, two soldiers passing through the region saw a large wolf which they attempted to capture, near the village of Moissey. When the wolf disappeared from view, they continued on their way. Soon afterward, they met an odd-looking character carrying a bag, a pole and a bell, who took to his heels and ran as soon as he saw them. Finding this suspicious, the soldiers gave chase and soon caught up with him. He claimed to be a poor recluse by the name of Jacques Valeur. The soldiers decided to accompany him but he ran away again, and the next time they caught him, they took him to the nearest officers of the law.

Valeur was about fifty, was married, and had previously worked as a turner of skittle balls, but had recently taken to living alone as a hermit and a beggar because he suffered from severe headaches. His wife came to take care of his hut and garden, and to say her prayers, almost every day. Questioned about his attempts to escape from the soldiers, he explained that he had not tried to run away, but was simply running because it was a good remedy for his migraines. Rather than exculpating him, his description of his ailments seems to have further incriminated him, for he said that he suffered periodic blackouts lasting up to three hours and had no idea what he did during these bouts. Although at first he denied any criminal activity, he went on to disclaim responsibility for anything he might have done while he lost consciousness, and eventually he admitted that he frequently turned into a wolf and killed and ate children. He was condemned and burned at Dole.

Encountered and suspected as a werewolf in the same way as the peasant arrested in 1573, Valeur, with his unfortunate bouts of unconsciousness, was a perfect suspect. As he could not remember anything that happened during these periods, he himself could not be certain whether or not he had turned into a wolf and had eaten children.

1632-34   Edicts Concerning Wolves and Werewolves[117]

Reports had been received from various villages near Poligny, Salins and Arbois that wolves not only were attacking domestic animals but had even begun to assault people in the fields, killing some and seriously injuring others, "which raises the suspicion that these wolves are werewolves." In order to avoid further problems and damage, the court decreed on September 1, 1632, that for three months the communities concerned should pay for huntsmen to mount a continuous guard in the fields and to do their utmost to catch these wolves "dead or alive." The communities would also have to pay a premium of twenty francs for each wolf caught by the hunters, and it was to be understood by all involved that no one carrying arms against the wolves was allowed to abuse the privilege by infringing the regulations on hunting.

The court further ordered the inhabitants of these villages to raise the alarm by ringing the church bell as soon as a wolf was sighted, and to assemble the whole community in pursuit of the animal. They were also required to find out the cause of absence of anyone who did not appear at the sound of the tocsin, especially if any absentee was suspected of witchcraft or was otherwise notorious. Communities failing to satisfy these orders would be held responsible for any deaths and difficulties, as well as costs and damages arising from attacks. If they "caught or arrested any werewolves," the hunters were to take them straightaway to the sovereign's prisons in the area where the arrest took place, and lest anyone plead ignorance of the terms of this edict, the court ordered that it was to be published in every village at the exit from Mass, and a copy attached to each church door.

There are few texts that express so explicitly the fact that the Parlement of Dole shared the public suspicion that the fierce wolves were really werewolves. It is clear that these fierce wolves were understood to be humans using witchcraft to appear as animals, and that those humans were local witches whose absence from the general assembly might reveal their identity. The instruction to imprison the captured werewolves further emphasizes the supposition that a human being might be the culprit, rather than a real wolf. But there are also signs that the Parlement had doubts. Revisions and cancellations in drafting the phrase "which raises the suspicion that these wolves are werewolves" indicate that the court was not entirely happy with this suggestion — although the suspected nature of the beast is unmistakable in the rest of the edict.

The same text was published in an edict of August 25, 1633, regarding the ravages of wolves in the regions of Dole, Salins, Poligny and Arbois, but this time the phrase about the suspicion of werewolves was deleted. Nor was the phrase repeated in a subsequent edict of August 15, 1634, issued following complaints from villagers in the Doubs Valley that wolves were continuing to attack people, despite measures taken to prevent this in April of the same year.

1643   Claude Chastellan of St. Gervais, Savoy[118]

On October 27, 1643, Claude Chastellan was referred to the *échevins* of Saint-Claude who were to judge him for the crime of witchcraft, and he was formally received by them on October 31. They did not pronounce sentence until November 24. In the meantime, they transmitted the case "for neutral advice," into the hands of "advocates and persons expert in law." If the *grand juge*'s referral was a manifest sign of the death sentence he deemed appropriate, the *échevins*' recourse to "neutral counsel" was an equally clear indication that they had doubts about the case.

Chastellan was accused of transforming himself into a wolf and intending to attack and hurt a boy named Claude Tissot. Tissot testified that he had seen him in the form of a wolf, and that in this form, Chastellan had been chased. He was only brought to a halt when he was struck with a stick of ash wood. The blow caused him to change shape immediately, before Tissot's eyes, and to reappear as an ordinary man, crouching on his heels. Tissot was the only witness to this event, but four other witnesses gave concordant evidence concerning the manner in which Chastellan had been arrested. They all testified to his speed and his "extraordinary disposition for running away,...his glittering eyes, his hideous and terrifying face,... and other extraordinary postures and grimaces." It was also said that although he had been struck hard with an iron-shod pole and other sticks, he had neither been hurt by them nor brought to a standstill until struck with the stick of ash wood.

Without torture, Chastellan had confessed both in and out of court that he was a witch and had "committed the most abominable acts that such wayward and desperate persons are accustomed to commit." He had admitted that he had made a pact with the Devil, that he had been to the sabbath, where he danced, drank and ate and offered candles to the Devil, and that as a wolf he had killed and eaten children.

The advisors' report, which is entirely devoted to an assessment of the validity of the evidence, gives a clue to the cause of the *échevins*' uncertainty. The principal witness, Tissot, was under the age of fourteen, and in normal procedure minors were not acceptable as witnesses. The four adults had seen Chastellan's remarkable physiognomy and behavior (neither of which is surprising since he was being chased and beaten), but they had seen him neither transform himself nor harm anyone. The only indication that he might be a witch was his strange resistance to blows from anything but a stick of ash wood. Furthermore, although Chastellan had confessed that he was a witch and werewolf, there is no mention of any evidence of dead bodies, previous reputation for witchcraft or accomplices.

The expert advisors recommended that the testimony of a minor should be accepted here, because in "these atrocious crimes of divine and human lese majesty," where proof was "absolutely difficult," all kinds of witnesses were admissible, be they members of the same family, children or even disreputable persons. The statements of Tissot and the four adults, as well as Chastellan's extra-judicial confession, were, in the lawyers' opinion, sufficient indications of guilt to warrant torture, or even a condemnation. But when these were added to the confession he made in court, there was no doubt that "the truth of these crimes was sufficiently manifest" for the condemnation to proceed, because "in such abominable and occult crimes, the confession made in court passes for the whole truth, especially when supported by so many minor indications and presumptions of guilt." The *échevins* of Saint-Claude followed this advice, and Chastellan was strangled and burned on November 24.

All five witnesses were probably relating different moments of a single episode, during which they all chased the wolf that had frightened Tissot, striking at it in vain with their sticks and poles. Since Tissot alone claimed to have witnessed Chastellan's extraordinary reversion to human form after a blow from a stick of ash wood, this stick was presumably in the boy's hand at the time. Whatever he thought he had seen, Tissot certainly did not see the wolf turn into a man. Perhaps, during the pursuit of the wolf, Tissot simply came across Chastellan squatting in the undergrowth, supposed he was a werewolf, and beat him with his stick to prevent him from escaping until the others arrived to complete the capture.

The cause of transformation is implicitly explained by the charge of witchcraft. Third-party intervention in the mechanism needed to reverse the metamorphosis is exceedingly common, and effective gestures encountered elsewhere include: forcing the werewolf to look at light; touching it with a key; drawing three drops of blood; stabbing a paw with a cobbler's awl; cutting off a paw; shooting the were-wolf with a silver coin or bullet; the sign of the cross; exorcism. The details and specific actions may vary, but the function remains the same.[119] The werewolf here was not transformed in spirit or in ecstasy; his whole body was understood to be changed into that of a wolf. Chastellan was identified as a werewolf by an extraordinary sign – not by repercussion as in many stories, but by a remarkable invulnerability to harmful objects followed by an equally remarkable vulnerability to something less severe. His identity was also revealed by his behavior and features, his speed and agility and his fearsome expression, all of which were interpreted as signs of his animal alter ego and evil character.

NOTES

1. Other trials in Franche-Comté, France and Switzerland will be included in a more detailed examination of sixteenth- and seventeenth-century discussions of metamorphosis and lycanthropy in my forthcoming Ph.D. thesis, University of London, Warburg Institute. Unpublished sources in Franche-Comté were consulted thanks to an award from the University of London, Central Research Fund.

2. Of particular relevance to this study were: E.W. Monter, *Witchcraft in France and Switzerland: The Borderlands During the Reformation* (Ithaca, N.Y., 1976), pp. 143-51; Louis Duparchy, "La justice criminelle dans la terre de Saint-Oyend-de-Joux, aujourd'hui Saint-Claude (Jura), aux XVIème et XVIIème siècles," in *Mémoires de la société d'émulation du Jura* (1891), pp. 231-462; unpublished notes of Francis Bavoux, in the Archives départementales du Doubs (henceforth ADD), Série F "Fonds Bavoux"; and two articles by Bavoux: "Les loups-garous en Franche-Comté," in *Heures comtoises* 4 (1952), pp. 3-8, and "Loups-garous de Franche-Comté: Identification du refuge et observations sur le cas de Gilles Garnier," *Nouvelle revue Franc-comtoise* 1 (1954), pp. 43-50.

3. W.M.S. and C. Russell, "The Social Biology of Werewolves," in *Animals in Folklore*, ed. J.R. Porter and W.M.S. Russell (Cambridge, 1978), pp. 143-82, at p. 164.

4. Significantly, these are the only parts of a wolf's anatomy mentioned in the charges against Gilles Garnier, 1573.

5. Compare the signs of human intelligence that indicate the extraordinary nature of the wolves in: Marie de France, "Lai de Bisclavret" (c. 1160-70), in *Lais*, ed. A. Ewert (Oxford, 1944), pp. 48-57, "Lai de Melion," in *Lais anonymes des XIIème et XIIIème siècles*, ed. P.M. O'Hara Tobin (Geneva, 1976), and *Arthur and Gorlagon* (thirteenth cent.), ed. G.L. Kittredge, *Harvard Studies and Notes in Philology*

and Literature 8 (1903), pp. 149-274, esp. pp. 153-60.

6. See L.D. Mech, *The Wolf: Ecology and Behavior of an Endangered Species* (Minneapolis, 1970), pp. 289-94; E. Pulliainen, "Wolf Ecology in Northern Europe," in *The Wild Canids: Their Systematics, Behavioral Ecology and Evolution*, ed. M.W. Fox (New York, 1975), pp. 292-99; Jean Bodin was explicit: real wolves attack animals and werewolves attack people, *De la démonomanie des sorciers* (Paris, 1580), vol. 2.6, fol. 98.

7. Johann Geiler von Kaisersberg, *Die Emeis* (Strasbourg, 1516), fol. xli.

8. In 1598, near Angers, a vagabond named Jacques Roulet was accused of being a werewolf by a band of men who were chasing a wolf which they had found devouring the corpse of a boy. The wolf disappeared from view and the pursuers came upon Roulet, who admitted that he had killed the boy as a werewolf. Three other children who had recently been injured by wolves were brought to the court by their fathers and Roulet confessed to these attacks too: *L'incrédulité et mescréance du sortileige plainement convaincue* (Paris, 1622), pp. 785-90. Similarly, while the *procureur* of La Roche Chalais (near Bordeaux) was gathering information about wolf attacks, following Jean Grenier's arrest as a werewolf in 1603, several attacks were reported to him by parents and witnesses, and, when asked, Grenier duly claimed responsibility: de Lancre, *Tableau de l'inconstance des mauvais anges et démons*, ed. Nicole Jacques-Chaquin (Paris, 1982), vol. 4.2-4, pp. 211-34, at p. 215; see also C. Oates, "The Trial of a Teenage Werewolf, Bordeaux, 1603," *Criminal Justice History* 9 (1988). Unlike Jean Grenier, who was arrested *because* he had boasted, at a time when wolf attacks were occurring, that he could turn into a wolf whenever he liked, there is no evidence to suggest that any of the suspects in Franche-Comté was accused because he had claimed to be a werewolf, or imitated animal behavior, prior to being accused and arrested.

9. Compare the tradition that a werewolf's eyebrows meet in the middle: Montague Summers, *The Werewolf* (1933), pp. 118, 131. When suspects' features or gestures are described, the signs tend to be: wild eyes, awful grimaces, extreme ugliness, frantic movements and particularly unkempt, dishevelled and dirty appearance. Many of the signs mentioned are what we might reasonably expect to find in vagrants and other odd characters surprised in the woods. Physical or mental abnormality is sometimes implicit, but there is no evidence to support claims that suspects may have been suffering from congenital diseases causing psychosis, skin lesions, aversion to sunlight or excessive hirsutism; see L. Illis, "On Porphyria and the Aetiology of Werewolves," in *A Lycanthropy Reader: Werewolves in Western Culture*, ed. Charlotte F. Otten (Syracuse, N.Y., 1986), pp. 195-99.

10. Werewolves by destiny in: Marie de France, "Lai de Bisclavret"; *Arthur and Gorlagon*; Gervase of Tilbury, *Otia imperialia* (c. 1212), 3a, ch. 120, ed. F. Liebrecht (Hanover, 1856), pp. 51-52; *Evangiles*

des quenouilles (fifteenth cent.), ed. M. Jeay (Montreal, 1985), ch. 40, pp. 142-43. Werewolves caused by the fates: Burchard of Worms, *Decretorum libri XX* (c. 1008-12), vol. 19, ch. 5; "De poenitentia," in J.P. Migne, *Patrologia latina*, 140, col. 971. In Ireland, a curse causes a couple to become werewolves: Gerald of Wales, *Topographia hibernica* (1187-88), vol. 2, ch. 19, in *Giraldi Cambrensis opera*, 5 vols; ed. J.F. Dimock (London, 1861-91), vol. 5, pp. 101-07.

11. Caspar Peucer, *Les devins, ou commentaires des principales sortes de devinations*, trans. S. Goulart (Paris, 1584), vol. 4.9, pp. 192-205.

12. Carlo Ginzburg, *I benandanti* (Turin, 1966), pp. 37-40.

13. *Ibid.*, pp. 3-40; G. Klaniczay, "Shamanistic Elements in Central European Witchcraft," in *Shamanism in Eurasia*, ed. Mihály Hoppál, 2 vols. (Göttingen, 1984), vol. 2, pp. 404-22. Romanian werewolves are born with a caul or teeth or on Christmas Day, etc.: see Harry A. Senn, *Were-wolf and Vampire in Roumania* (Boulder, Col., 1982), pp. 25, 51-56. E. Le Roy Ladurie has also suggested that transformation beliefs surviving until the eighteenth century in parts of southwest France were the remnants of similar agrarian fertility cults: *La sorcière de Jasmin* (Paris, 1983), pp. 11-69.

14. Witches in many parts of Europe had long been considered capable of such diversity in transforming themselves or others: Circe transforms Ulysses' companions into swine in Homer, *Odyssey*, trans. A.T. Murray (Cambridge, Mass.: Loeb Classical Library, 1919), 10.229-43; Meroë's and Pamphile's are transformed in Apuleius, *The Golden Ass*, trans. W. Adlington (1566) (Cambridge, Mass.: Loeb Classical Library, 1915; repr. 1977), vol. 1.9, and 3.21; *striges*, or witches, appear as nocturnal birds of prey in Petronius Arbiter, *Satyricon*, trans. M. Heseltine (Cambridge, Mass.: Loeb Classical Library, 1913), 63; women or witches appear as snakes, dragons and cats in Gervase of Tilbury, *Otia imperialia* 1a, 15, 3a, 85, 113; witches transform themselves into cats and hares in Britain, and a Danish witch turns into a bull (see Summers, *The Werewolf*, pp. 193-203, 244-45); Rumanian witches turn into dogs, wolves, horses, millstones and cartwheels: see Senn, *Were-wolf and Vampire*, pp. 6-7.

15. Joseph Hansen, *Zauberwahn, Inquisition und Hexenprozess im Mittelalter und die Entstehung der grossen Hexenverfolgung* (Leipzig, 1900), p. 382, notes references to werewolves in a trial in Basel in 1407; in 1448, one Jacques de Panissière was tried in the Vaud region as a witch and werewolf: see Monter, *Witchcraft*, p. 149n.

16. Rather than acting as a simple disguise, the animal skin is usually understood as having the magical property of turning the person into what witnesses saw as a real animal. The fact that Cranach's werewolf (figure 1, c. 1510-15) is shown as a man wearing a wolfskin is probably attributable to the difficulty of representing a convincing metamorphosis without simply depicting an animal.

17. Peter Stumpf confessed that he transformed himself by means of a magic girdle, which the

wolf is wearing in the first two captions of figure 2. In the "Lai de Melion," the hero turns into a wolf when touched on the head with a magic ring.

18. Special times and places set apart are often necessary to transformations in tales and folklore: in the cemetery, at full moon (Petronius, *Satyricon*, 62); beyond a lake, for nine years (Arcadians) (Pliny the Elder, *Natural History*, 8.22); in the forest, for seven years (Gerald of Wales, *Topographia hibernica*, pp. 101-02); at Candlemas (*Evangiles des quenouilles*, pp. 142-43); around Christmas (Livonians) (Goulart, *Histoires admirables et mémorables de nostre temps*, Rouen, 1606, p. 249); Thursdays during the *quattro tempi* (Ginzburg, *I benandanti*, p. 4).

19. See also Job Fincel's story of a self-confessed werewolf of Pavia in 1541 who claimed that his fur grew on the inside of his skin (*versipellis* = "turn-skin") and who was so badly cut by curious people intent on verifying this claim that he died on the surgeon's table; reported by Johann Wier, *Histoires, disputes et discours*, ed. Bourneville and Axenfeld, 2 vols. (Paris, 1885), vol. 1.4, ch. 23, pp. 595-96.

20. Henri Boguet, *Discours des sorciers* (2nd ed., Lyon, 1606) (*An Examen of Witches*, trans. E.A. Ashwin, London, 1929, ch. 17, p. 47), gave the example of a man from Unau near Orgelet who denounced his wife as a witch because she had lain in bed as if dead one Thursday night. She could not be woken by any means, and when her husband tried to get out of bed to call the neighbors, he found he was unable to move his legs. This continued until cock crow, when his wife suddenly awoke. She said that she had slept extremely soundly because she had worked hard the previous day.

21. St. Augustine, *City of God*, trans. E. Matthews Sanford and W. McAllen Green, 7 vols. (London, 1965), 5.18.18, reported this story, told to him by "persons worthy of belief": the father of a man named Praestantius had fallen into a deep sleep after eating cheese, and could not be woken by any means. When he eventually awoke, he recounted his dream that he had been transformed into a horse and had carried rations to the soldiers' camp; these facts were later confirmed. Le Roy Ladurie, *La sorcière de Jasmin*, pp. 254-55n., found similar stories of soul voyages in animal form in a fourteenth-century Occitan source concerning Cathars, and the same concept survived in Gascon folklore until the nineteenth century.

22. Boguet, *Examen of Witches*, ch. 47, pp. 140-42.

23. Jacob Sprenger and Heinrich Institoris, *Malleus maleficarum* (1486-87) (Francofurti ad Moenum, 1580), 2.1, 9.

24. See Jan Harold Brunvand, *The Vanishing Hitchhiker* (London, 1983).

25. Cited by Le Roy Ladurie, *La sorcière de Jasmin*, p. 57.

26. Léonard Du Vair, *De fascino* (Paris, 1583), pp. 168-69.

27. Summers, *The Werewolf*, pp. 253-60.

28. See Joseph Hansen, *Quellen und Untersuchungen zur Geschichte des Hexenwahns und der Hexen-verfolgung im Mittelalter* (Bonn, 1901), pp. 38-39; and Edward Peters, *The Magician, the Witch and the Law* (Hassocks, Sussex, 1978), pp. 73-74.

29. St. Augustine, *City of God*, 18.18. See also Laurence Harf-Lancner, "La métamorphose illusoire: Des théories chrétiennes de la métamorphose aux images médiévales du loup-garou," in *Annales, E.S.C.* 1 (1985), pp. 208-26, and C. Oates, "Démonologues et lycanthropes: Les théories de la métamorphose au XVIème siècle," in *Métamorphose et bestiaire fantastique au Moyen Age*. Etudes rassemblées par L. Harf-Lancner (Paris, 1985), pp. 71-105.

30. Guilielmus Alvernus, Bishop of Paris, *De universo*, 2.3, ch. 13, in *Opera omnia* (Paris, 1674), p. 1043, col. 2.

31. *Summa theologica*, ed. P. Caramello et al., 4 vols. (Turin, 1948-50), vol. 1, 1a.114.4.

32. See Norman Cohn, *Europe's Inner Demons* (Brighton, 1975), and "The Myth of Satan and His Human Servants," in *Witchcraft: Confessions and Accusations*, ed. M. Douglas (London, 1970), pp. 3-16.

33. Sprenger and Institoris, *Malleus maleficarum*, 1.10 and 2.1, 8-9.

34. *Ibid.*, 1.10.

35. Among others, Claude Prieur, *Dialogue de la lycanthropie ou transformation d'hommes en loups...* (Louvain, 1596); Jean de Nynauld, *De la lycanthropie, transformation et extase des sorciers* (Paris, 1615).

36. Jean Bodin, *Démonomanie*, 2.6, fols. 94v-104.

37. For example Lucius's transformation in Apuleius, *The Golden Ass*, 3.26: "I that was now a perfect ass...did yet retain the sense and understanding of a man."

38. Reginald Scot, *The Discoverie of Witchcraft*, vol. 5.6, ed. B. Nicholson (London, 1886; repr. Wakefield, 1976), pp. 71-81, and Pierre de l'Estoile, *Mémoires-journaux*, ed. G. Brunet et al., 7 vols. (Paris, 1875-96), vol. 7, p. 151, concerning Jacques Roulet of Angers.

39. See Burgot and Verdun, 1521, for Wier's hypothesis.

40. Girolamo Cardano, *De Subtilitate* (Basel, 1557), p. 500.

41. G.B. Della Porta, *Magiae naturalis, sive de miraculis rerum naturalium libri IV* (Cologne, 1562), 2.27. He claimed to have put this theory to the test by observing a witch who volunteered to take part in the experiment. Della Porta and his companions left the room at the woman's request and watched through the keyhole as she undressed and rubbed her body with "a certain ointment" which caused her to fall into a deep sleep from which she could not be woken by any means. When she awoke, she recounted her travels across seas and mountains, and refused to believe their assertion that she had not moved from the spot, even when they showed her the bruises she had received while they tried to wake her.

42. Nynauld, *De la lycanthropie*, pp. 27-36.

43. See Otten, *A Lycanthropy Reader*, p. 27, for a discussion of the relative merits of babies' fat as a base for the active ingredients of witchcraft ointments.

44. See Cohn, *Europe's Inner Demons*, p. 54, and W. Arens, *The Man-Eating Myth: Anthropology and Anthropophagy* (New York, 1979), but also Anthony Pagden, "Cannibalismo e contagio: Sull'importanza dell'antropofagia nell'Europa preindustriale," in *Quaderni storici* 17.2 (1982), pp. 538-50.

45. Pseudo-Galen, in Claudius Galenus, *Opera omnia*, ed. C.G. Kühn, 20 vols. (Leipzig, 1821-33, repr. Hildesheim, 1965), vol. 19, pp. 719-20. On the same text in a fragment of Marcellus of Sidon, and its transmission by Aetius and Paulus Aegineta, see Wilhelm H. Roscher, "Das von der 'Kynanthropie' handelnde Fragment des Marcellus von Side," *Abhandlungen der königl. sächsischen Gesellschaft der Wissenschaften. Philol.-histor. Classe* 17.3 (1897), pp. 1-92. Early modern versions of the same diagnostic include: Wier, *Histoires, disputes et discours*, vol. 1, pp. 595-98; Martin Del Rio, *Disquisitionum magicarum libri sex* (Cologne, 1679), fol. 207r; Goulart, *Histoires admirables*, p. 238; Nynauld, *De la lycanthropie*, pp. 64-68. See also Summers, *The Werewolf*, pp. 44-45, and Otten, *A Lycanthropy Reader*, p. 47, for some examples of the few cases treated by physicians.

46. In the fourteenth century Bernard Gordonius said that some called lycanthropy "daemonium lupinum," *Lilium medicinae* (Lyon, 1573), vol. 2, pp. 19, 211; and Giovanni Arcolano da Verona distinguished two types of this mental affliction, one "lupine madness," and the other "demonic lupine madness," sufferers of which "no longer even look like human beings," he says, "but resemble wolves and demons," *Practica* (Venice, 1557), vol. 9, ch. 16, pp. 28-33; later, Jan van Hewin wrote that "often it is not without the demon that this calamity arises," *Opera omnia*, vol. 1, *De mania, de morbis capitis* (Lyon, 1658), p. 377; all three passages cited by Summers, *The Werewolf*, pp. 23, 42-43, 45. See also Jean Céard, "Folie et démonologie au XVIème siècle," in *Folie et déraison à la Renaissance*, ed. A. Gerlo (Brussels, 1976), pp. 129-47, esp. pp. 140-41, for some sixteenth-century physicians' opinions about demonic intervention in melancholy; also N. Jacques-Chaquin, "La représentation du corps sorcier à l'âge classique," in *La folie et le corps*, études réunies par J. Céard (Paris, 1985), pp. 201-22, and Sydney Anglo, "Melancholia and Witchcraft: The Debate Between Wier, Bodin and Scot," in *Folie et déraison*, pp. 209-27.

47. Boguet, *Examen of Witches*, pp. 143-45.

48. *Ibid.*, p. 146.

49. De Lancre, *Tableau de l'inconstance*, vol. 4.4, p. 227.

50. Boguet, *Examen of Witches*, p. 155.

51. *Ibid.*, pp. 146-47.

52. *Ibid.*, pp. 149-51. The observation that the children's clothes had been unbuttoned or untied is not simply evidence of human involvement in the crime – it is a sign of the extraordinary character of the attack, and evidence that the criminal was neither an ordinary wolf, nor a common murderer, but a werewolf.

53. H.C. Erik Midelfort, "Heartland of the Witchcraze," *History Today* 31 (February 1981), pp. 27-31, at p. 30; on the *Carolina*, see Midelfort, *Witch Hunting in Southwestern Germany, 1562-1684: The Social and Intellectual Foundations* (Stanford, Cal., 1972), p. 22. On the effects of the *Carolina* in Franche-Comté, see Brigitte Rochelandet, *Le "Fonds infernalia": Historique, inventaire, essai analytique,* Mémoire de D.E.A, Université de Franche-Comté (1985), p. 87.

54. Bavoux, *La sorcellerie en Franche-Comté (Pays de Quingey)* (Monaco, 1954), pp. 47-48; Monter, *Witchcraft*, p. 73.

55. Bavoux, *Sorcellerie*, pp. 31-43.

56. Rochelandet, "*Fonds infernalia*," pp. 16, 59-60.

57. See Lucien Febvre, *Philippe II et la Franche-Comté* (Paris, 1911), pp. 582-89.

58. Duparchy "Justice criminelle," p. 241, and Bavoux, "Les Bourgeois de Luxeuil et de Saint-Claude," *Mémoires de la société pour l'histoire du droit et des institutions des anciens pays bourguignons, comtois et romands* (1954), pp. 123-137.

59. Bavoux, *Sorcellerie*, p. 41; Boguet, *Examen of Witches*, chs. 1 and 4, pp. 3 and 7.

60. Boguet, "Instruction pour un Iuge en faict de sorcelerie," in *Examen of Witches*, pp. 211-38, arts. 7, 8, 11, 13.

61. *Ibid.*, arts. 27-42; Bavoux, *Sorcellerie*, pp. 42-44.

62. Bavoux, *Sorcellerie*, pp. 43-46; Rochelandet, "*Fonds infernalia*," pp. 15-16; Boguet, "Instruction," arts. 2, 39, 42-60; Bodin, *Démonomanie* (1580), vol. 4.2, fols. 175-186v.

63. Boguet, "Instruction," arts. 4, 14, 16, 37; *Examen of Witches*, ch. 2, pp. 43-44.

64. Boguet, "Instruction," arts. 17-19, 22-26, 43-49; Rochelandet, "*Fonds infernalia*," p. 16.

65. Bavoux, *Sorcellerie*, pp. 41-44.

66. Rochelandet, "*Fonds infernalia*," pp. 15-17; Aristide Dey, *Histoire de la sorcellerie au Comté de Bourgogne* (Vesoul, 1861), p. 69; Boguet, "Instruction," arts. 51-53, 57.

67. Of some thirty-five accused witches examined by Boguet, twenty-eight were condemned to death, four died in prison and two others were banished: Bavoux, "Boguet, grand juge de la terre de Saint-Claude," in *Académie des sciences, belles-lettres et arts de Besançon. Séances publiques* (1947-56), pp. 252-69, at p. 261.

68. Boguet, "Instruction," arts. 3, 8, 12-13, 17-19.

69. Rochelandet, "*Fonds infernalia*," p. 87.

70. Trials: Peter Stumpf, Bedburg, 1589 (figure 2); Michel Jacques, Val de Travers, Neuchâtel, 1590 (Monter, *Witchcraft*, p. 149n.); Jacques Roulet, Angers and Paris, 1598 (de Lancre, *Incrédulité*, pp. 785-90); three women of Vaud, 1602 (Monter, *Witchcraft*, p. 149n.); Jean Grenier, Bordeaux, 1603 (de Lancre, *Tableau de l'inconstance*, 4.2-4); one woman at Lucerne and five women at Cressi, Lausanne, 1604 (Nynauld, *De la lycanthropie*, pp. 52-53). Werewolves and lycanthropy discussed in: Nicolas Rémy, *Daemonolatriae Libri Tres* (Lyon, 1595), 2.5; Prieur, *Dialogue de la lycanthropie* (Louvain, 1596); King James I, *Daemonologie* (Edinburgh, 1597), pp. 60-62; *Arrest mémorable de la Cour de Parlement de Dole, du dixhuictiesme iour de Ianvier 1573, contre Gilles Garnier* (Sens: Jean Savine, 1574; reprint, Angers, 1598); Beauvois de Chauvincourt, *Discours de la lycanthropie* (Paris, 1599); Del Rio, *Disquisitionum magicarum* (Louvain, 1599), 2.18; Boguet, *Discours des sorciers* (Lyon, 1602, 1603, etc.); Jean Filesac, in his extensive ms. commentary of 1603 on Jean Grenier's trial, transcribed by Robert Mandrou, in *Possession et sorcellerie au XVIIème siècle* (Paris, 1979), pp. 35-109, at pp. 84-85, refers to trials in Rennes in 1598 and in Grenoble in 1603, and had clearly read Boguet's account of the trials in Saint-Claude.

71. De Lancre, *Incrédulité*, pp. 785-90.

72. Wier, *Histoires, disputes et discours*, vol. 2.6.13, pp. 262-76.

73. Daniel d'Auge, *Discours sur l'arrest donné au Parlement de Dole*, in *Arrest mémorable...contre Gilles Garnier*, p. 11.

74. Boguet, *Examen of Witches*, ch. 47, pp. 140 and 153.

75. See n.8 above concerning Roulet and Grenier.

76. On the magical practices of shepherds, see Alfred Soman, "La sorcellerie vue du Parlement de Paris au début du XVIIème siècle," in *Actes du 104ème Congrès national des Sociétés Savantes (Bordeaux, 1979), Section d'histoire moderne et contemporaine*, 2 vols. (Paris, 1981), vol. 2, pp. 393-405, at p. 403.

77. Febvre, *Philippe II*, pp. 3-4n.

78. ADD 2B 2000, fols. 220r-221v.

79. Bibliothèque nationale, Coll. Moreau, MS 903, fol. 267r, transcription by Bavoux, at ADD F "Fonds Bavoux," t. 27a.

80. Bavoux, "Loups-garous de Franche-Comté: Identification du refuge et observations sur le cas de Gilles Garnier," *Nouvelle revue Franc-Comtoise* 1 (1954), pp. 43-50, at p. 48.

81. Transcription by Bavoux from a register of the Parlement formerly numbered ADD B 52 (now lost) at ADD F "Fonds Bavoux," t. 27a.

82. *Arrest mémorable...contre Gilles Garnier*; also published in 1574 at Orléans by Eloy Gibier and

in Paris by Pierre des Hayes. For 1573, read 1574, as in Franche-Comté the year was still numbered as beginning at Easter.

83. Transcription by Bavoux at ADD F "Fonds Bavoux," t. 28a.

84. Bavoux, "Loups-garous" (1954), pp. 47-48.

85. Febvre, *Philippe II*, pp. 617-51. The Parlement's increased activity and attempts to speed up court business are attested by the fact that decrees in criminal cases ran to two volumes that year instead of the customary single annual volume. Unfortunately, the second volume is the register B 52 now missing from the series.

86. ADD 2B 3149, *Arrest 32*.

87. Jean Petremand, *Recueil des ordonnances et édicts de la Franche-Comté* (Lyon, 1664), p. 223.

88. See A. Molinier and N. Molinier-Meyer, "Environnement et histoire: Les loups et l'homme en France," *Revue d'histoire moderne et contemporaine* 38.2 (1981), pp. 225-45, esp. pp. 226-27.

89. In January 1600, Henri IV of France ordered the organization of three monthly wolfhunts; see Molinier and Molinier-Meyer, "Environnement et histoire," p. 238.

90. Records of witchcraft trials in Franche-Comté show three notable periods of crisis: 1598-1610, 1628-32, and 1658-61; see Rochelandet, *"Fonds infernalia,"* p. 86. To a certain extent, trials of were-wolves reflect the same increases in frequency. During the thirty-one years from 1598 to 1611, from 1626 to 1634 and from 1657 to 1664 at least twenty-five people were tried, and one lynched, for crimes including that of transformation into wolves. Outside these periods, from 1521 to 1597, from 1612 to 1625 and from 1635 to 1656 (112 years), only seven or eight other individuals are known to have been tried on similar charges.

91. Boguet, *Examen of Witches*, esp. ch. 47, pp. 136-63, Duparchy, "Justice criminelle," pp. 296-99.

92. Numbers in square brackets indicate relevant chapters in the second edition of Boguet's *Discours* (1606), trans. by E.A. Ashwin, *An Examen of Witches*, London, 1929.

93. Boguet, *Examen of Witches*, pp. 1-3, 99.

94. *Ibid.*, pp. 1-8, 11, 16, 29-31, 40-41, 44, 55, 62, 64, 66-67, 77, 85, 119-20, 122-23, 125-28.

95. *Ibid.*, pp. 47, 67-68, 129, 136, 155.

96. *Ibid.*, pp. 96, 169, 171-79, 193-98.

97. *Ibid.*, pp. 136-7, 140, 153.

98. *Ibid.*, p. 158.

99. *Ibid.*, pp. 21, 29, 31-33, 134.

100. *Ibid.*, pp. 25, 56, 58, 60, 150.

101. Duparchy, "Justice criminelle," p. 299; and ADD F "Fonds Bavoux," t. 6; Boguet, *Examen*

of Witches, pp. 130, 133.

102. Duparchy, "Justice criminelle," pp. 296-99.

103. Boguet, *Examen of Witches*, pp. 131-32, 138, 157, 196-97.

104. *Ibid.*, pp. 75, 98-99, 149, 165-66.

105. *Ibid.*, pp. 157-58, 165-66.

106. *Ibid.*, pp. 150-51. In 1610, Jean Grenier took part in a similar experiment at Pierre de Lancre's request, and demonstrated his remarkable speed and agility on all fours (de Lancre, *Tableau*, p. 229).

107. Boguet, "Instruction," art. 6 and *Examen of Witches*, pp. 116, 213. There was a long tradition of immunity to metamorphosis among saints, heroes and other superior mortals (Ulysses, for example, escapes the fate of his companions, transformed into pigs by Circe: *Odyssey* 10.229-43); immunity to demonic illusions among officers of the law might easily have been understood as an indication of their moral superiority.

108. Boguet, *Examen of Witches*, esp. ch. 47, pp. 136-55; Duparchy, "Justice criminelle," pp. 300-04; Bibliothèque Municipale de Besançon, MS 390, fols. 1-8; ADD F "Fonds Bavoux," t. 6, 27a.

109. Boguet, *Examen of Witches*, p. 149.

110. Duparchy, "Justice criminelle," pp. 303-04, and BMB MS 390, fols. 1-8.

111. Boguet, *Examen of Witches*, pp. 21, 29-30, 45; Duparchy, "Justice criminelle," p. 303.

112. Boguet, *Examen of Witches*, pp. 143, 150-51; Duparchy, "Justice criminelle," p. 304.

113. Duparchy, "Justice criminelle," pp. 300-02; Boguet, *Examen of Witches*, pp. 21, 129, 138.

114. Boguet, *Examen of Witches*, pp. 47-48.

115. ADD 2B 3160, fols. 104r-107r; ADD F "Fonds Bavoux," t. 17.

116. Maurice Garçon, *Les loups garous* (*Les Oeuvres Libres*, no. 229) (Paris, 1945), pp. 155-56.

117. Transcripts at ADD F "Fonds Bavoux," t. 28a.

118. Duparchy, "Justice criminelle," pp. 408-12; ADD F "Fonds Bavoux," t. 6, 7.

119. Gabriele Chiari, "Il lupo mannaro," in *Mal di luna*, ed. G. Lützenkirchen et al. (Rome, 1981), pp. 57-81, esp. pp. 59-60; Summers, *The Werewolf*, pp. 113-14, 116, 201, 204.

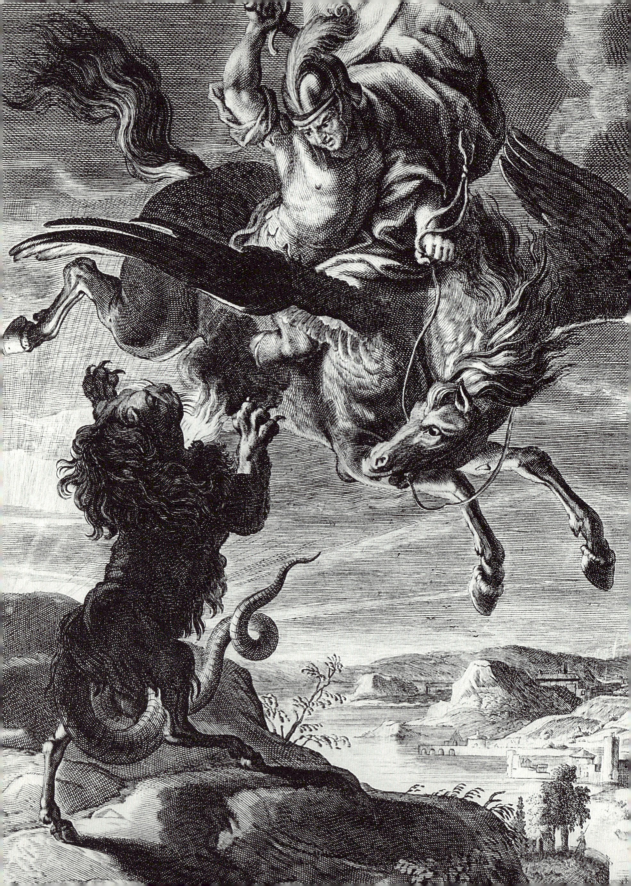

The Chimera Herself

Ginevra Bompiani

The Animal Sign

The Family of Chimera

> And Sea begat Nereus...who is true and lies not.... And yet again he got great Thaumas
> and proud Phorcys being mated with Earth and fair-cheeked Ceto.... And again, Ceto
> bare to Phorcys the fair-cheeked Graiae, sisters gray from their birth...and the Gorgons
> who dwell beyond glorious Ocean in the frontier land toward Night where are the clear-
> voiced Hesperides, Sthenno, and Euryale, and Medusa who suffered a woeful fate: she
> was mortal, but the two were undying and grew not old. With her lay the Dark-haired
> One in a soft meadow amid spring flowers. And when Perseus cut off her head, there
> sprang forth Chrysaor and the horse Pegasus.[1]

At the beginning of the world, living and imaginary, there is a double wedding:
Mother Earth weds her son Heaven and her son the Sea. The first marriage, which
is fruitful and harmonious, a love match, produces a line of gods and kings, but also
a line of envious fathers and rebellious sons: a problematically vertical line of descent,
because it is on the vertical axis that the struggles for the kingdom take place. The
other marriage – the union between Gaea and Pontus – which is a discordant one
(between the fruitful earth and the unfruitful sea), produces, instead, a line of monsters and prodigies, of brothers and sisters, along a horizontal axis dominated by two
factors: seriality and hybridization.

Even the incest in this line occurs on a different axis: vertical incest, between
mother and son, is replaced by horizontal incest, between brother and sister: the
lordly Phorcys and the lovely-cheeked Ceto.

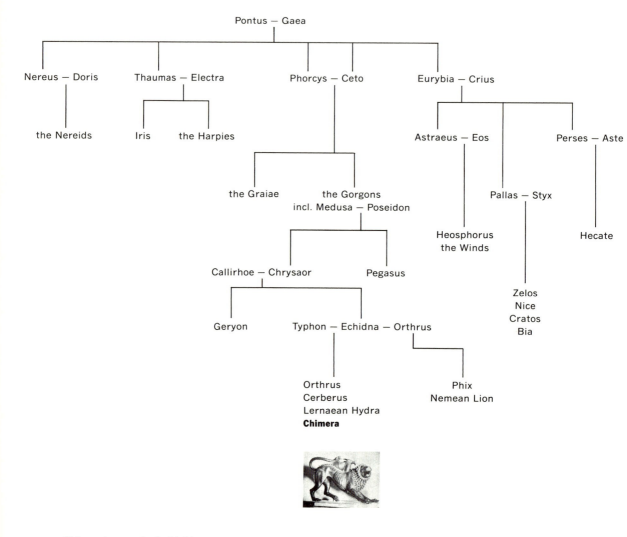

Pontus — Gaea

Nereus — Doris   Thaumas — Electra   Phorcys — Ceto   Eurybia — Crius

the Nereids   Iris   the Harpies   Astraeus — Eos   Perses — Aste

the Graiae   the Gorgons
incl. Medusa — Poseidon   Pallas — Styx   Hecate

Heosphorus
the Winds

Callirhoe — Chrysaor   Pegasus

Zelos
Nice
Cratos
Bia

Geryon   Typhon — Echidna — Orthrus

Orthrus
Cerberus
Lernaean Hydra
Chimera   Phix
Nemean Lion

Chimera's genealogical table.

The progeny of Phorcys and Ceto show the same pattern in all possible combinations: seriality (the Graiae, the Gorgons) is reproduced within the body – the three heads of Cerberus, and Hydra's innumerable necks. All the descendants of Phorcys and Ceto are hybrids combining human and animal features with exemplary fantasy (the Middle Ages, with a further proliferation of forms, will foster formlessness): Medusa with her snake-locks; winged Pegasus; Sphinx, part woman, part lion; Orthrus and Geryon, dog and master with two heads each; Typhon and Echidna, with a serpent's body beneath human head and shoulders. But there is none to equal Chimera, the triple animal, whose heads succeed one another in reverse order, so that the weakest will blow its steaming breath onto the neck of the strongest – an impossible union in an implausible order.

There are two main characteristics in this descending line. The first is the chthonic characteristic, marine and stygian. There is primitiveness, depth and uncertainty in these animals that come from the bowels of the earth, from the dark and the cold. They are true *grotesques*: searing blasts of fire and ice, damp breezes, rain-bearing sciroccos.[2] By divine will, their dwelling is on the edge of the world, far from men and gods; they are in the beyond, bounded by the river Styx:

> Such an oath, then, did the gods appoint the eternal and primeval water of Styx to be: and it spouts through a rugged place. And there, all in their order, are the sources and ends of the dark earth and misty Tartarus and the unfruitful sea and starry heaven, loathsome and dank, which even the gods abhor.[3]

> [T]he Gorgons belong to the line of Phorcys and Ceto, whose name evokes both a monstrous hugeness and, in the furthest depths of the sea or the earth, cavernous pits. In fact, all that the children of this couple have in common, besides monstrosity, is that they live "far from gods and men," in the subterranean regions, beyond the Ocean, at the edge of the Night, where they often perform the role of guardians, even scarecrows, barring the way to forbidden places.[4]

The second characteristic is an identity that wavers between the unique and the infinite. Either the monster is unique (like Cerberus or Chimera), or it has a tendency toward repetition (like the Harpies); and this oscillation is repeated within the body (thus, Cerberus has three, or five, or a hundred heads). Uncertainty is also

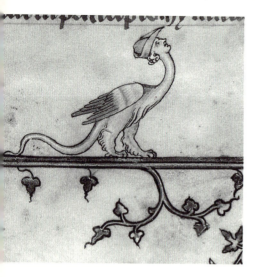

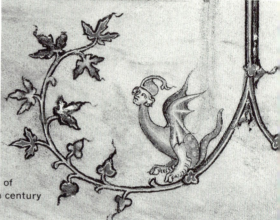

Figure 1: Fabulous Creatures. From the border of the pages of the *Heures de Savoie* manuscript, Jean Pucelle Atelier, 14th century (Paris, Musée Jacquemart-André).

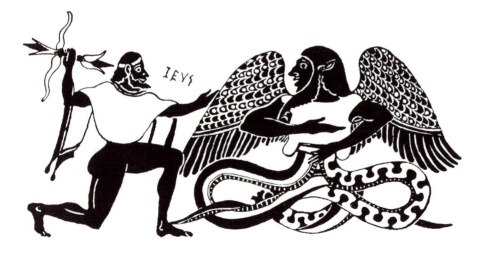

Figure 2: Zeus and Typhon. From J. Fontenrose, *Python, a Study of a Delphic Myth and Its Origins* (Berkeley, 1959).

zon

a chthonic and marine characteristic; it is in heaven that such beings assume their definitive, emblematic identity. Hence the monsters killed by heroes (such as the Nemean Lion) are taken into heaven to assume the form of a constellation or the position of messenger to the gods. Their identity then becomes permanently settled. But those whose destination is hell, as in the case of Chimera, never acquire a definite shape or identity. And Chimera will lose her uniqueness in the medieval chimeras whose infinite variety of forms protrude from cathedrals (figure 1).

TYPHOEUS

> And from Typhoeus come boisterous winds which blow damply except Notus and Boreas and clear Zephyr. These are a god-sent kind, and a great blessing to men; but the others blow fitfully upon the sea. Some rush upon the misty sea and work great havoc among men with their evil, raging blasts; for varying with the season they blow, scattering ships and destroying sailors. And the men who meet these upon the sea have no help against the mischief. Others again over the boundless, flowering earth spoil the fair fields of men who dwell below, filling them with dust and cruel uproar. But when the blessed gods had finished their toil, and settled by force their struggle for honor with the Titans, they pressed far-seeing Olympian Zeus to reign and to rule over them, by Earth's prompting. So he divided their dignities amongst them.[5]

A damp and violent north wind, blowing darkness, frost and mist from afar, an inhospitable wind, sonorous and infertile, that brings men thoughts of death and drives them from their lairs, pursues them and brings out their animal fear. In its icy blast, his ears assailed by a thousand voices, man forgets to remember that he is human, the gods forget they are gods. Or the violent mouth of an erupting volcano, spewing forth flaming foam, which multiplies and stretches and howls, shrieking words intelligible only to the gods. This is the aspect of Typhon, or Typhoeus, the father of Chimera, half man and half serpent (his head collided with the stars, his arms extended from the dawn to the dusk; from his loins issued a hundred snake heads with blazing eyes and mouths uttering discordant sounds: ululations, hisses and bellows). He belongs to the ranks of the swift. Only Zeus's thunderbolts — more fiery, more electric and swifter than he — will arrest him and pin him down in Tartarus, where he belongs (figure 2):

After the Gods had defeated the Gigantes, Gaea in anger mated with Tartarus and bore Typhon, a huge monster of mixed form. He attacked heaven, hurling flaming stones and belching fire from his mouth. The gods fled before him to Egypt, where they took animal forms to escape his notice – all except Zeus, who stood against him.[6]

In spite of his stormy nature, there is something of Circe in Typhon. He shows humans and gods their animal nature – not the nature of quiet and lascivious animals, like the Enchantress's swine, but the nature of wild animals in desperate flight. Only Zeus (who, for love, will take animal shape a thousand times) stands firm and fights him with his spiritual nature. The war between Zeus and Typhon is a war of spirit against spirit, fire against fire. The vicissitudes of this war testify to the similarity of the two rivals:

> Zeus followed him thither and grappled with him, a move that gave Typhon a chance to entangle Zeus in his coils. Taking Zeus's sickle from him, Typhon severed his sinews and carried the god, thus rendered impotent, over the sea to Cilicia, where he laid him in the Corycian Cave. The sinews he hid in a bearskin and set the dragoness Delphyne to guard them. But Hermes and Aigipan (Goat Pan) recovered the sinews and restored them to Zeus, who renewed battle, mounting his chariot and once more hurling thunderbolts.[7]

The war between Zeus and Typhon, in Apollodorus's version, which differs from Hesiod's, does not immediately reveal the superiority of Zeus over the primitive monster. In its changing fortunes it shows a more subtle superiority, harder to recognize and impose: the superiority of a more highly evolved civilization, of a more abstract use of language. The spirit of Olympus vanquishes the spirit of the wind: two different ways of unleashing the force of breath on the world. From that moment on, from the time of Zeus's victory, the force of the tempest no longer is only the force of the elements but has also become metaphor: "The ground beneath it rumbled, as when Zeus the lord / of lightning bolts, in anger at Typhoeus, / lashes the earth around Einarimos, / where his tremendous couch is said to be."[8]

ECHIDNA

And in a hollow cave she [Ceto] bare another monster, irresistible, in no wise like either to mortal men or to the undying gods, even the goddess fierce Echidna who is half a nymph with glancing eyes and fair cheeks, and half again a huge snake, great and awful, with speckled skin, eating raw flesh beneath the secret parts of the holy earth. And there she has a cave deep down under a hollow rock far from the deathless gods and mortal men. There, then, did the gods appoint her a glorious house to dwell in: and she keeps guard in Arima beneath the earth, grim* Echidna, a nymph who dies not nor grows old all her days. Men say that Typhon the terrible, outrageous and lawless, was joined in love to her, the maid with glancing eyes. So she conceived and brought forth fierce offspring.[9]

Similar only in appearance, but different in nature is Typhon's spouse, Echidna. Her name means "viper" and, like her husband, she has the head and shoulders of a human and the extremities of a serpent, but there is no movement in her, apart from the sluggish, murky motions of the cave dweller. Echidna is a subterranean monster, who by divine will was born and lived in a cave — astute, cruel and mournful. Tears and astuteness come both from her serpent's nature and from her subterranean quarters (from which she emerges only to devour young men). If Typhon has the vehemence of a hurricane, Echidna has the cruel and stagnant motions of the marshes, the seductive wiles of one who waits in the shadows. She belongs to the slow, immobile species, who dart at their prey. Young and immortal, she is known to have two killers: Argos and Heracles. Perhaps, confused by the shadows, they fancied that they had killed her (figure 3):

Hesiod doesn't make clear whether Echidna's parents were Phorcys and Ceto or Chrysaor and Callirhoe; but it is fairly certain that he means the former. Apollodoros agrees with Olympiodoros that she was the daughter of Tartaros and Gaea; therefore she was Typhon's sister.... Echidna...killed all men who came her way, as Apollodoros tells us; though it was Argos Panoptes who killed her in an Argive legend in which Argos has the heroic role of Zeus, Apollo or Heracles.[10]

The Siblings

[F]irst she bare Orthrus the hound of Geryon, and then again she bare a second, a monster not to be overcome and that may not be described, Cerberus who eats raw flesh,

---

*Translator's note: The Italian uses the word *lacrimevole*, meaning "tearful, mournful."

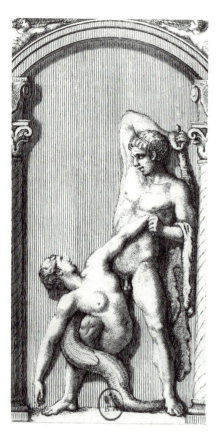

Figure 3: Hercules and Echidna
(Paris, Bibliothèque nationale).

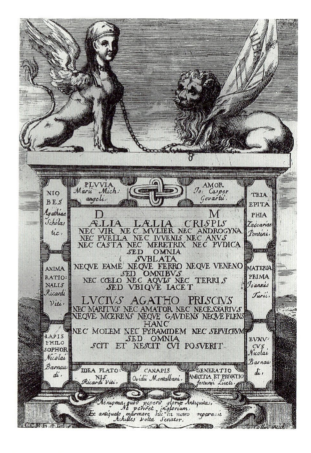

Figure 4: Frontispiece from *Aelia Laelia Crispis non Nata
Resurgens in Expositione Legali Caroli Caesaris Malvasiae*,
1683 (Paris, Bibliothèque nationale).

z o n e

the brazen-voiced hound of Hades, fifty-headed, relentless and strong. And again she bore a third, the evil-minded Hydra of Lerna, whom the goddess, white-armed Hera nourished, being angry beyond measure with the mighty Heracles....

She was the mother of Chimera who breathed raging fire, a creature fearful, great, swift-footed and strong, who had three heads, one of a grim-eyed lion, another of a goat, and another of a snake, a fierce dragon; in her forepart she was a lion; in her hinderpart a dragon; and in her middle, a goat, breathing forth a fearful blast of blazing fire. Her did Pegasus and noble Bellerophon slay; but Echidna was subject in love to Orthrus and brought forth the deadly Sphinx which destroyed the Cadmeans, and the Nemean Lion, which Hera, the good wife of Zeus, brought up...yet the strength of stout Heracles overcame him.[11]

Two of Chimera's siblings are dogs, the three-headed Cerberus and the two-headed Orthrus. (According to Robert Graves, Orthrus is none other than Sirius, the Dog Star that ushers in the Athenian new year. He has two heads, like Janus, and his two children, Sphinx and the Nemean Lion, are each the emblem of a half year.) Each was assigned to a master, Cerberus to Hades and Orthrus to Geryon, the son of Chrysaor, son of Medusa. Both are vanquished by Heracles, the hero par excellence, the conqueror of monsters. The Hydra of Lerna will also be killed by Heracles (since it is the fate of monsters to be slain by heroes, as it is the fate of heroes to regret their deed): her countless snake heads grew back with each hack of the sword, a feat that will win her a place of honor in the book of emblems, where whatever cannot be felled by a sword-blow or a reasonable word will be represented by her image. But the true siblings of Chimera, albeit by a different father, are Sphinx and the Lion. She will be constantly compared to one and often confused with the other. She and they are related by their common leonine nature. Like Sphinx and Hydra, Chimera is a hybrid. In fact, as we shall see, she is the supreme hybrid. Like Orthrus and Cerberus she is tame, though wild.

Of all these, only the Sphinx is still part human, having a woman's head on the body of a lioness. Chimera, even though she acquires, over the course of time, an ephemeral woman's face, is a purely animal composite, of female sex (figure 4).

Animality predominates among the children of Echidna. Only Sphinx has the power of speech, and she uses it as her siblings use brutal weapons: to kill, deceive

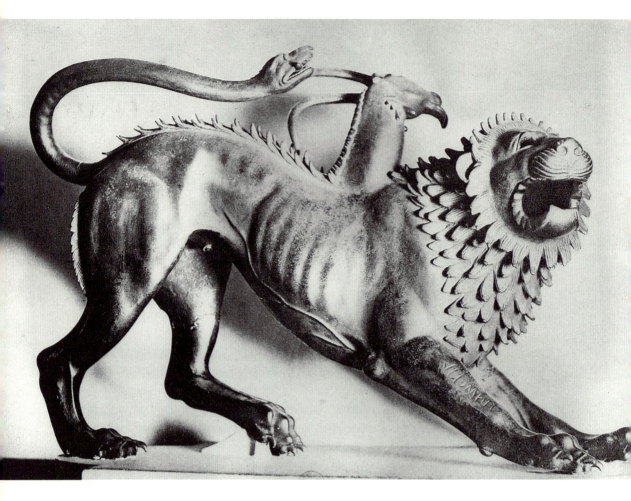

Figure 5: Chimera of Arezzo, 1558 (Florence, Galleria dei Uffizi).

and invent riddles. Sphinx and Chimera are killed not by the common enemy, Heracles, but by two renegades, two deluded, tragic heroes who, after killing them, both become blind, melancholy wanderers: Oedipus and Bellerophon.

All Echidna's children bear the stygian, tartarean stamp of Typhon, and foremost among them Cerberus, the watchdog of Hades. Aeneas will find them all at the gates of hell:[12]

> In the courtyard a shadowy giant elm
> Spreads ancient boughs, her ancient arms where dreams,
> False dreams, the old tale goes, beneath each leaf

Cling and are numberless. There, too,
About the doorway forms of monsters crowd —
Centaurs, triformed Scyllas, hundred-armed
Briareus, and the hernaean hydra
Hissing horribly, and the Chimera
Breathing dangerous flames, and Gorgons, Harpies,
Huge Geryon, triple-bodied ghost.[13]

Only some of the children have the subterranean nature of their mother: the Nemean Lion, whom Heracles drives from his den and kills in the depths of a cave, and Cerberus, the custodian of Hades. But Sphinx and Chimera are animals of the surface, even of high places — Sphinx keeps watch in the desert, Chimera in the mountains. Between them they share two other hereditary traits: Sphinx has immobility (but the immobility of the desert, not of the pond), Chimera has the speed, the lightness and the impetus of Typhon. This hallmark, lightness, will characterize her future history — her own, that of her slayer and that of the hundred figures sprouting from his seed.

The Chimera Herself

His guest should fight
and quell a foaming monster, the Khimaira,
of ghastly and inhuman origin,
her forepart lionish, her tail a snake's,
a she-goat in between [figure 5]. This thing exhaled
in jets a rolling fire.[14]

[I]t had the fore part of a lion, the tail of a dragon, and its third head, the middle one, was that of a goat, through which it belched fire. And it devastated the country and harried the cattle; for it was a single creature with the power of three beasts. It is said, too, that this Chimera was bred by Amisodares, as Homer also affirms (*Iliad* 16.328ff.) and that it was begotten by Typhon on Echidna, as Hesiod relates.[15]

[T]he ridge where dwelt Chimera, that fire-breathing monster with lion's head and neck and serpent's tail.[16]

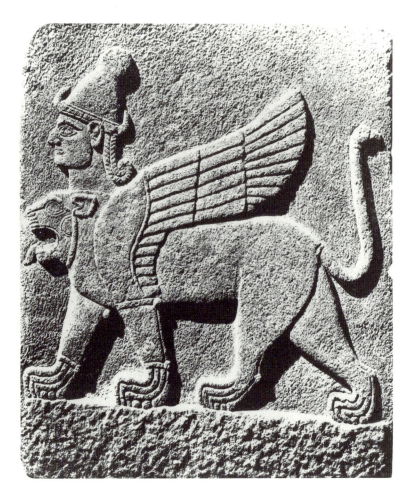

Figure 6: Chimera, Hittite Bas-relief. From M. Riemschneider,
Die Welt der Hethiter (Gustav Kilpper Verlag, 1954).

When classical authors mention Chimera it is to tell of her death or to deny the possibility of her existence (see, for example, Lucretius).[17] When Renaissance and modern authors speak of Chimera, they discuss her meaning, immediately transforming her impossibility into the sign of the possibility of other beings. Although she was unique, her proper name has always been preceded in translations (as is Sphinx's) by the definite article, making it a common noun, a multipliable entity. Her destiny is embodied in that article: the single character in a single story has become the prototype of every possible composite, every hybrid (including the contemporary hybrids of genetic engineering). The creature slain by Bellerophon in obedience to an order aimed, in reality, at killing him has become that which every-one has to kill within himself; the being that could not exist has become the supremely interpretable.

What we know about Chimera, before her death, is that she lived with King Amisodarus and – a contradictory piece of information – devastated the country (what country, the country of Amisodarus? Did he let her?): an animal both wild and tame, loved by one king and hated by another (Iobates), she was of the female sex, the sex of a sensuous she-goat. The goat predominated in her body because it was from her goat's head that she belched flames, and She-goat (Ximaira) was her name. Yet it was the lion that eventually predominated in iconology, to such an extent that she can be mistaken for an ordinary lioness, and can be identified only by the presence of Bellerophon. Other ancient variants of the chimera form are a woman's head, in a Hittite bas-relief, placed over a lion's head (figure 6) and the presence of wings. The goat's head sometimes faces the lion's head, sometimes the snake's head. The latter head is depicted sometimes turned toward the body, some-times fluttering backward.

Because of this uncertainty of form, she becomes more of a verbal than a picto-rial symbol. She who, in myths, was purely a fiery apparition, without a voice or a history, was to become, in the early days of modern philosophy, the *ens rationis*, the creature of language, the metaphor of metaphor.

The Chimera's Slayer

Bellerophon, son of Glaucus, son of Sisyphus, having accidentally killed his brother Deliades or, as some say, Piren, or, as others will have it, Alcimenes, came to Proetus and was purified. And Sthenoboea fell in love with him, and sent him proposals for a meet-ing; and when he rejected them, she told Proetus that Bellerophon had sent her a vicious proposal. Proetus believed her, and gave him a letter to take to Iobates, in which it was written that he was to kill Bellerophon. Having read the letter, Iobates ordered him to kill the Chimera, believing that he would be destroyed by the beast, for it was more than a match for many, let alone one; it had the fore part of a lion, the tail of a dragon, and its third head, the middle one, was that of a goat, through which it belched fire. And it devastated the country and harried the cattle; for it was a single creature with the power of three beasts.... So Bellerophon mounted his winged steed Pegasus, offspring of Medusa and Poseidon, and soaring on high shot down the Chimera from the height (figure 7). After that contest Iobates ordered him to fight the Solymi, and when he had finished that task also, he commanded him to combat the Amazons. And when he had killed them also, he picked out the reputed bravest of the Lycians and bade them lay an ambush and slay him. But when Bellerophon had killed them also to a man, Iobates, in admiration of his prowess, showed him the letter and begged him to stay with him; moreover he gave him his daughter Philonoe, and dying bequeathed to him the kingdom.[18]

> The King's daughter bore
> three children to Bellerophontes: Isandros,
> Hippólokhos, and Laodámeia.
> Zeus the Profound lay with Laodámeia,
> who bore Sarpedon, one of our great soldiers.
> But now one day Bellerophontes too
> incurred the Gods' wrath — and alone he moped
> on Aleion Plain, eating his heart out,
> shunning the beaten track of men. His son
> Isandros in a skirmish with Solymi
> met his death at insatiable Ares' hands,
> and angry Artemis killed Laodámeia.[19]

While we know little about the life of Chimera (in fact we hardly know anything about her except her death, and her two residences, before and after death), we do know a good deal about the life of Bellerophon. His existence begins with the involuntary homicide of his brother (indeed, it is said that he derived his name from this first misdeed). In him we see, reemerging, the hallmark of his father's father, Sisyphus, who keeps repeating the same useless effort again and again. Bellerophon's life is also to be full of fruitless labors. He goes to Proetus for purification, only to find himself involved in another involuntary crime: he wins the love of Proetus's wife, just as Hippolytus, son of Theseus, captivated Phaedra with his wildness. Like Hippolytus, Bellerophon is a chaste hero, afraid of women. What convinced Iobates of his innocence, apparently, was a stratagem on the part of the women whom Bellerophon confronted with a stormy sea (thereby providing evidence of his mari-

Figure 7: P.P. Rubens, Mounted on Pegasus, Bellerophon Pierces Chimera (Bayonne, Bonnat Museum).

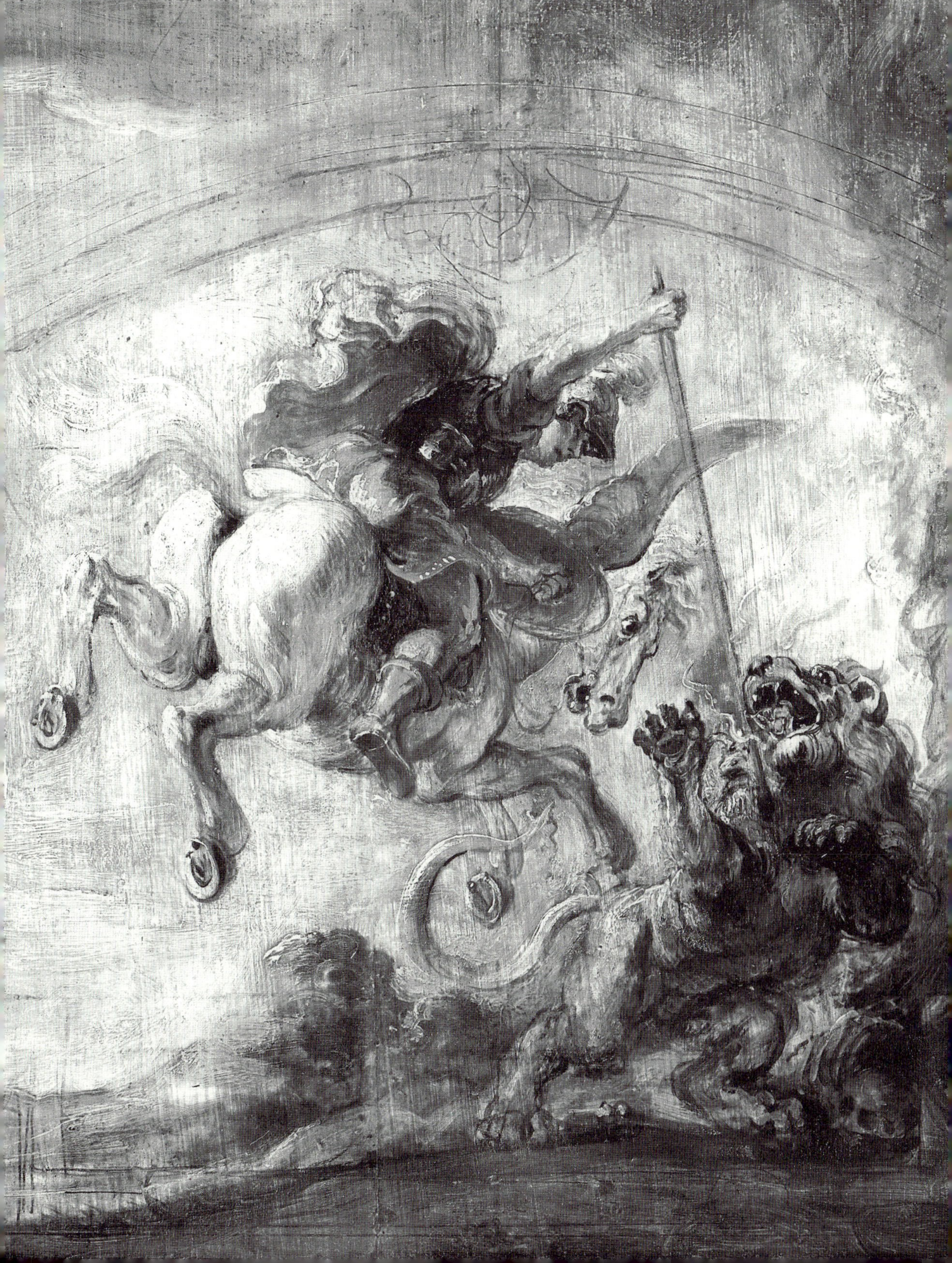

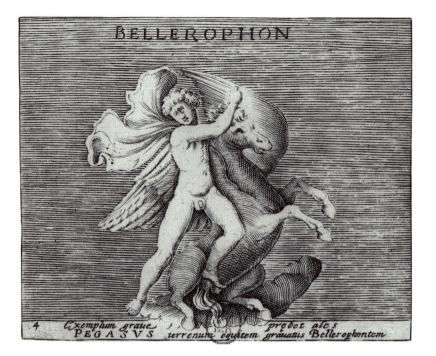

Figure 8: Anonymous, Bellerophon and Pegasus (Paris, Bibliothèque nationale).

time nature). The women lifted their skirts above their belts and Bellerophon fled in alarm, with the obedient sea following in his wake. Horace, therefore, calls him "chaste Bellerophon" (*Carmina* 3.7.14). To fight Chimera, on the orders of Iobates, Bellerophon captures the winged horse Pegasus, son of Medusa, and from above, hovering over Chimera's flaming jaws, he pours into them molten lead, which kills her when it cools. After many other adventures, when his life seemed becalmed in the quiet ranks of the kings, Bellerophon succumbs to a fatal folly: he mounts Pegasus and spurs him on to the celestial abodes, to the conquest of Olympus. Pegasus, inspired by Zeus, unseats his rider and sends him plummeting from the sky into the Lycian desert, where he loses his sight in the fall and is seized with a terrible melancholy. He is to end his days blind and solitary, having lost his sons and his kingdom, punished as heroes guilty of *hubris* always are (figure 8): "And thus, captive in his mind and blind in his soul, he went through life in solitude."[20]

Most striking about this fight between Bellerophon and the Chimera is the close link it establishes between these two characters. Like Saint George and the dragon, Bellerophon will be known primarily as "the slayer of the Chimera," so that his sad end will be attributed readily to this first enterprise, as to a necessary cause.

It is almost as if Bellerophon, in killing the Chimera, killed at the same time everything that the Chimera would become over the centuries: fantasy, poetic genius, dream, illusion.

In fact there is a deep-seated, secret solidarity between the two characters, and it is to be found in the word *hubris* – the sin that causes Bellerophon's downfall – and it is from *hubris* that the word "hybrid," which describes the Chimera, derives.

Hubris is the common characteristic of the characters engaged in the fight; the only one to escape it is Pegasus, whose claims (to flight, to form and to Olympus) are all honored. It is curious that the two fantastic creatures, goat and horse, later took on a very similar meaning, although with opposite connotations: poetic imagination. Almost as if Bellerophon were riding astride one form of poetic imagination to kill another. Or rather, the two animals shared between them the vocation for good and bad poetry. Of the three, the real master is Pegasus. He will dislodge his rider after helping him to slay the hybrid beast, and will fly to Olympus alone.

The combat unites the man and the animal, so that they share certain corporeal aspects between them:

1. Chimera is a being in whom lightness predominates. Even without wings, she has a tendency to go upward. Each of her heads clambers over the back of the next; flames rise from her body. Only the taller, the one higher up, can vanquish her. Swift and infinitely mobile, even the serpent part of her body rears imperiously. Although sensuous, she is not known to have had any loves. She is the epitome of seduction, not the marshy seduction of Echidna, nor the stony seduction of Sphinx, but the seduction of the nonexistent, of the contrived, the composite (Hopkins could be speaking of her when he thanks God "for dappled things"; and Flaubert in his *Temptation of Saint Anthony* quotes her as saying "I am light...").

2. Bellerophon, falling from Pegasus, reveals his heaviness, the heaviness of the melancholy, of one who is weighed down by a burdensome destiny. The fight between Bellerophon and Chimera is thus also the struggle between heaviness and lightness. But it is also the struggle between an incomprehensible destiny and a sign without a destiny, given to anyone who wishes to interpret it.

3. Chimera will lend herself to many interpretations, while the story of Bellerophon will remain mysterious. Why this sudden *hubris*? Chimera, like Sphinx, causes the downfall of her victims. But not in the same way as Sphinx; it is her

vanquisher who is toppled. She descends into the Underworld to bar the way to any interpretation.

4. There is another striking aspect to this duel: as in the fight between Perseus and Medusa, in order to vanquish Chimera one must avoid a head-on confrontation (all duels are fought face to face, except these[21]). Pegasus, springing from Medusa's neck, when her head is severed, will be Perseus's horse before belonging, temporarily, to Bellerophon. The body of Pegasus is interposed between the combatants in the duel, as the mirror-shield of Perseus was interposed. It is not simply a war between a man and an animal, it is a war waged by the human body on the animal body, a repetition of the war between Zeus and Typhon, between Apollo and Python, between Heracles and the Nemean Lion, and so many others. It shows that the human cannot be reduced to the animal. Hurled down to earth, blinded and maimed by the fall, a poor pathetic scrap of flesh, Bellerophon, wandering in the desert, is still a man — a melancholy man:

> Why is it that all those who have become eminent in philosophy or politics or poetry or the arts are clearly melancholics, and some of them to such an extent as to be affected by diseases caused by black bile? An example from heroic mythology is Heracles. For he apparently had this constitution, and therefore epileptic afflictions were called after him "the sacred disease" by the ancients. His mad fit in the incident with the children points to this, as well as the eruption of sores which happened before his disappearance on Mount Oeta; for this is with many people a symptom of black bile. Lysander the Lacedaemonian too suffered from such sores before his death. There are also the stories of Ajax and Bellerophon: the one went completely out of his mind, while the other sought out desert places for his habitation; wherefore Homer says: And since of all the Gods he was hated/Verily o'er the Aleian plain alone he would wander/Eating his own heart out, avoiding the pathway of mortals.[22]

> When the black bile, already present in preponderance, is inflamed, it causes deep depression and misanthropy; of this sort was Bellerophon's grief.[23]

> On his fate at the last I will keep silence. But to Pegasus were given on Olympus the lordly mangers of Zeus.[24]

The Interpretable Par Excellence

The Inhuman Body

The Renaissance was to change myths into signs. The Chimera's family could not escape this fate, but would offer its own set of enigmas for interpretation:

> The Hydra is "sophistic deceit." The Chimera is "wrath"; the Gorgons the charms of passion.[25]

> Morally, according to Fulgentius, Gorgon is interpreted as terror and fear. And the three Gorgons are perceived as the three aspects of terror. Sthenno is interpreted as "weakness"; Euryale is interpreted as "great profundity" and means madness. Medusa is interpreted as "oblivium," which not only disturbs the soul's vision but utterly confuses it.... The flying horse Pegasus signifies "fame, fanfare and renown, or eternal fountain." It also represents knowledge that flies all over the world, knows the nature of the universal, and furnishes poets with material for their song.[26]

But Chimera, most of all, will offer material for interpretation; and this is so because the ancients themselves never believed in her existence, or in her possibility — her image did not appear even in the most credulous bestiaries of the Middle Ages:

> It must not be supposed that atoms of every sort can be linked in every variety of combination. If that were so, you would see monsters coming into being everywhere. Hybrid growths of man and beast would arise. Lofty branches would sprout here and there from a living body. Limbs of land-beast and sea-beast would often be conjoined. Chimeras breathing flame from the hideous jaws would be reared by nature throughout the all-generating earth.... Since flame sears and burns the tawny frames of lions no less than any other form of flesh and blood that exists on earth, how could there be a Chimera with three bodies rolled into one, in front a lion, at the rear a serpent, in the middle the she-goat that her name implies, belching from her jaws a dire flame born of her body?[27]

Since she does not exist, the question arises as to what Chimera *is*. Since ancient times there has been a tendency to see in Chimera a landscape, a mountain or a volcano:

Alcimus in the state of Sicily and Nymphodorus of Syracuse say that the Chimera is a mountain in Lycia spewing fire, on whose summit there were many lions' dens and lairs.... Plutarch in the book of the virtuous deeds of women says that Chimera was a high mountain directly facing midday sun, which made large refractions and reverberations of the sun's rays, and consequently burning heat like fire on the mountain, which, overflowing and extending throughout the countryside, even dried and withered all the fruits of the earth.[28]

This explanation was repeated by Vincenzo Cartari:

I will not fail to mention Chimera, a monster utterly fabulous, and imagined by the poets, which, as described by Homer and later by Lucretius, had the head of a lion, the belly of a goat and the tail of a fierce dragon; and launched live flames from its mouth, as also related by Virgil, who places her in the first entrance to Hell, together with other terrible monsters. But the truth is that Chimera was not a beast but a mountain in Lycia, which, like Mount Etna, spouted live flames from its summit, and all around it were many lions; in the center of it there were trees and very pleasant pastures with various plants; and all around its foot, there were snakes, so that no one dared live there. This, however, was remedied by Bellerophon, whom Iobates sent there to be killed in revenge for the insult he had done (as Iobates believed) to Stheneboea, his daughter and wife of Proetus. Bellerophon ensured that from then on the mountain was safe for habitation. For which reason fables had it that Chimera was killed by Bellerophon.[29]

The concept of landscape gives unity to such disparate elements as mountain, sun, trees and animals. Frequently it is time, rather than space, that recomposes what interpretation decomposes:

[A]nd the Chimera is rhetorically transposed to allegory: indeed, the Chimera was a certain woman, the wife of Amisodarus, the King of Lycia. This woman had two brothers, Leo and Draco, who were destroying the conquerors on all the Lycian frontiers. The people thus called on these two brothers because of their unity and of the three-headed monster and also because of their skill in waging war, their swiftness and their fire-breathing. Bellerophon was skilled in waging war, and when he had conquered them, he placed them in servitude, thereby weighing down their lives.[30]

Chimera is no longer a composite being, but a multiple one, picked up from the battlefield: two brothers and one sister who fight against Bellerophon. Chimera is the name of the young woman who struggles behind Leo and in front of Draco — daughter or wife of Amisodarus: "In the third book of the history of Asia, Agatharcides of Cnidus says that Chimera was a wife of Amisodarus, king of Lycia, and she had three brothers."[31]

But the privileged mediator between myth and existence is climate, or rather that unity of space and time which climate produces:

> Nicander of Colophon claims that the main meaning of these fictions lies in the nature of rivers and torrents.... That monster was slain by Bellerophon riding on Pegasus, that is to say, by the heat of the sun — for Bellerophon and Pegasus are in fact the same thing, namely the power of the Sun.[32]

> The Chimera, or winter-goat...is a water that should be compared to the waters of winter, which in order to be fruitful must be channeled with skill.[33]

Besides these explanations, which replace an impossible story with a possible one, there are the allegorical interpretations, which transform an impossibility into a moral prohibition:

> Chimera, otherwise a Volcano in Lycia, an area made habitable by Bellerophon, is also "inordinate lust."[34]

> The Chimera, which has the head of a lion, the body of a goat, the tail of a serpent signifies love, which in adolescence assaults like a lion, then is realized in a disorderly way. This is represented by the body of a goat which is a very sensuous animal. For this reason, satyrs are so called because they are never sated with lustful activity and are depicted with goat's horns. The serpentine tail of the Chimera signifies remorse which ultimately pricks the conscience of the lustful. That Chimera signifies and represents love is clearly stated by Horace, who says to lovers: "Entangled, as thou art, in the triple-formed Chimera's toils, scare Pegasus shall set thee free" [Ode 1.27.22-23]. Ovid has the following to say: "the ridge where dwelt Chimera, that fire-breathing monster with lion's head and neck and serpent's tail" [*Metamorphoses*, 9.647-48].[35]

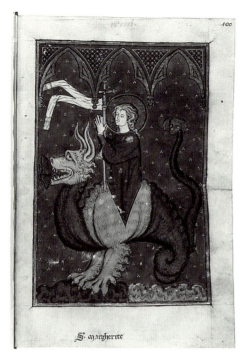

Figure 9: Saint Margaret, France, 13th century
(Paris, Bibliothèque nationale).

Allegorical interpretations do not neglect the other side of the struggle: the hero, his mandators and his allies. Both the physical and moral interpretations (figure 9) are considered:

> Those who interpret it in physical terms say that Bellerophon is nothing but the vapor raised by the intensity of the sun: because the air is stirred by the power of the sun, the heaviest part after being drawn up is sent back down, then grows heavy and accumulates in a pile which, falling down and coagulating, is called Pegasus. And since the lightest part rises to the region of the air, they say that the heaviest part was sent down below by Jupiter. Thus, since Pegasus rises out of the water by the movement which the sky makes during the day, Dawn breaks: it is said that Pegasus, not Bellerophon, brings daylight as sense judges it more clearly.[36]

Morally, Bellerophon is interpreted as "consultor sapientiae," the one who counsels knowledge. Proetus is interpreted as "sordidus," sordid or dirty. He is married to Anteia, interpreted as "contrarium," or contrary. Bellerophon, whose mission is the pursuit of knowledge, does not approve of the marriage between Anteia — lustfulness — and the sordid and dirty man. He is therefore sent to the Chimera, that is to say to temptation or inconstancy in love, for those who flee sexual love are among the ones she assails. But with the help of the horse Pegasus — courage and wisdom — he gains an easy victory. "She tells how a perfidious woman by false charges drove credulous Proetus to bring swift death on over-chaste Bellerophon" [*Odes* 3.7.13-16].[37]

This ambiguity of interpretation is found again in modern times. For Robert Graves, Chimera is a symbol of the calendar, tied to the tripartite year whose emblems were the lion, the goat and the serpent. On the other hand, Mount Chimera was a volcano, and this explains the fire it blew from its mouth. Paul Diel, in his *Symbolism in Greek Mythology*, dedicates a chapter to Bellerophon and Chimera. "The name," Diel confidently states, "leaves no doubt as to the meaning of this mythological figure." No image could better express the chimerical danger of imaginative exaltation. The myth externalizes the danger in the form of a monster encountered by chance. In truth the chimerical enemy is always present; every man carries secretly within himself the temptation of imaginative exaltation — that is, the devouring monster, Chimera. It is clear that "Chimera" and "perverse imagination" are synonymous.[38]

But, as the myth is gradually left behind, and Chimera, instead of being a character in a story, becomes an emblematic figure, an icon, the allegorical interpretation prevails. The final metamorphosis will be from the imaginary to the symbolic: "chimera becomes a figure of speech." And at this point the two symbolic sides of Chimera, the physical and the moral, will separate to their maximum distance: at the one end of the scale is an imaginary figure that bears no relation to anything real; at the other end is a reality which no longer contains any imaginary elements (figure 10).

Chimera is a composite but an unstable composite. In order to account for the disparity of her components (physical, geographical and pseudohistorical) and their antagonism, those who attempted an explanation always had to present the chimera in a particular situation (a mountain under the noonday sun, a river in winter, the evaporation of air, a combat, and so on). Even moral interpretations require something that can give unity to a figure which tends to decompose and recompose in a thousand different ways. The Chimera poses the same problem of identity that a

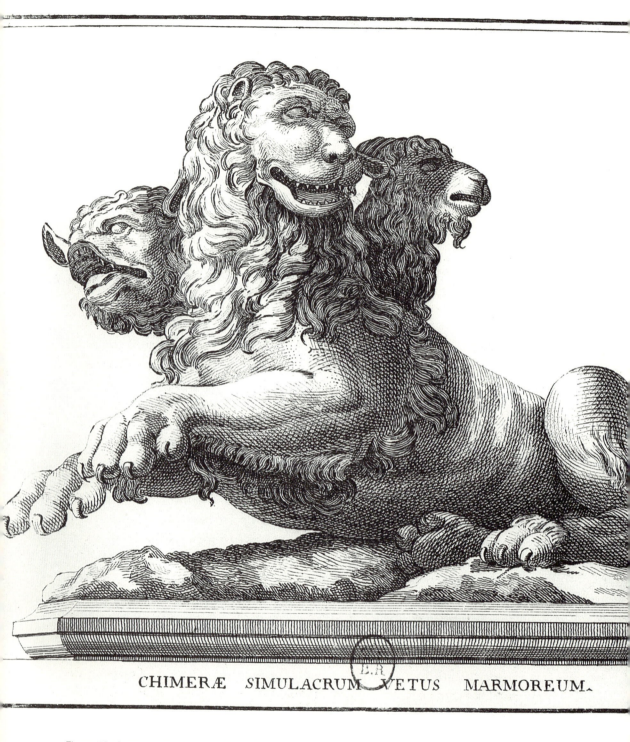

CHIMERÆ SIMULACRUM VETUS MARMOREUM.

Figure 10: Anonymous, Chimera (Paris, Bibliothèque nationale).

388

fairy tale poses: What makes the tale of Snow White recognizable in all the different versions? What makes a chimera into *the* Chimera?

In Renaissance emblems we find countless Hydras and Centaurs, Pegasuses and Sphinxes, but never Chimera by herself: she is either engaged in battle with Bellerophon or confronted face to face with her sister Sphinx. *Chimera is never alone.* She always exists in relation to something that negates her: Bellerophon who kills her or Sphinx who confronts her. This constant confrontation with another gives unity to this composite which is in danger of decomposing.

On the other hand, there is a determined effort to make Chimera a living creature: unique among all imaginary animals (so imaginary as to be excluded from the bestiaries), the Chimera exists today in three forms: animal (chimera monstruosa, a fish of the Holocephali family: figure 11), vegetable (chimera: a graft of parts of two individual plants of different species) and human ("a chimera is derived from two different zygotes, that is, from two different impregnations...that undergo a secondary fusion").[39]

Thus, the gap between the imaginary and the real has reached its maximum width. And it is precisely this rift that Chimera carries within herself, between myth, emblem and language.

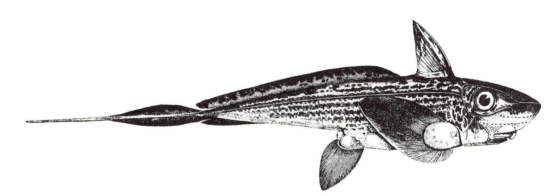

Figure 11: Monstrous Chimera. From *Dizionario Enciclopedico Italiano*, 1956.

The Metaphor

At the end of the seventeenth century, Chimera becomes part of the theory of poetic creation. In *An Apology for Poetry* by Sir Philip Sidney, Chimera is, together with other fantastic beings, the supreme example of creative freedom: man as poet is the creator of *another nature*:

> Only the poet, disdaining to be tied to any such subjection, lifted up with the vigour of his own invention, doth grow in effect into another nature, in making things either better than Nature bringeth forth, or, quite anew, forms such as never were in Nature, as the Heroes, Demigods, Cyclops, Chimeras, Furies, and such like: so as he goeth hand in hand with Nature, not enclosed within the narrow warrant of her gifts, but freely ranging only within the Zodiac of his own wit.[40]

But in subsequent discussions, from Hobbes to Coleridge, Chimera will become the figure of a form of imagination, if not perverse, certainly minor:

> Much memory, or memory of many things, is called *experience*. Again, imagination being only of those things which have been formerly perceived by sense, either all at once, or by parts at several times; the former (which is the imagining the whole object, as it was presented to the sense) is *simple* imagination; as when one imagineth a man, or horse, which he hath seen before. The other is *compounded*; as when from the sight of a man at one time, and of a horse at another, we conceive in our mind a centaur.[41]

Even if the Chimera is not mentioned here, she exemplifies, even better than the Centaur, the arbitrary union of many experiences: a spatial and temporal hybrid ("a man at one time, and...a horse at another"). In Coleridge Chimera becomes the very example of that *Fancy* which represents the model of mechanical and arbitrary, not fully creative, composition.

But an additional characteristic explains the fall of Chimera from her position as representative of poetic genius to that of a manneristic composition, namely, the irreality of Chimera, her impossibility:

> Some of my thoughts are, as it were, images of things; and to them alone strictly belongs the title "idea," e.g. when I represent to myself a man or a Chimera, or the sky, or an angel, or even God. Other thoughts have in addition other forms; for instance when I

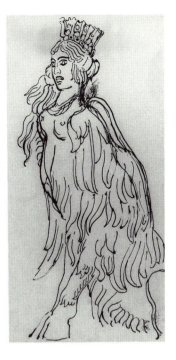

Figure 12: Gustave Moreau, Chimera (Paris, Musée Gustave Moreau).

will, fear, affirm, deny.... If ideas are considered only in themselves, and not as referred to some other thing, they cannot, strictly speaking, be false. For whether I imagine a goat or a Chimera, that I am imagining the latter is no less true than that I am imagining the former.[42]

Emanuele Tesauro, in his *Cannocchiale Aristotelico* (1654), would be the one to change Chimera from a mythological animal into a rhetorical figure of speech, the metaphor.[43] The function of the metaphor, in Tesauro's view, is that of connecting the most remote notions, of expressing "one concept by means of another very different one, of finding similarities in things that are dissimilar."[44] Like Chimera, the metaphor connects things distant from each other, and has its meaning outside itself. Like Chimera, the metaphor is, each time, the unique creature of its creator, the poet. As God makes something out of nothing, so the poet connects the most remote circumstances, and transforms one thing into its opposite (figure 12):

And this is the metaphor, mother of poetry, of symbols and emblems. And he is most ingenious, who can recognize and connect the most distant circumstances, as we shall relate...for just as God creates something out of nothing, so does inventive genius produce being from nonbeing; it causes a lion to become a man and an eagle a city. It grafts a woman onto a fish and produces a mermaid as the symbol of the seductress. It joins the bust of a goat to the rear of a snake and creates the Chimera as a hieroglyphic of insanity.[45]

Thus, what was hitherto a defect in Chimera (the heterogeneity of her components) becomes the sign of poetic invention. Chimera, taking up residence in the language (while still retaining her citizenship among proper nouns), acquires the meaning, apparently neutral, of invention. Soon, however, this will take on a negative connotation: "Here you see how, with so many ethereal chimeras, Nature ridicules the chimeras of men...I also include monsters among the jokes of Nature. But monsters are nothing but mysterious hieroglyphs and facetious images devised by Nature for the purpose of either deriding or educating mankind."[46]

But it is in the metaphor par excellence, which the heraldic figure is ("The Perfect Heraldic Figure is a Perfect Metaphor"),[47] that Chimera reveals her two faces of the impossible and of the symbol par excellence. With the specificity of her own being, Chimera foreshadows the heraldic figure:

Yet all these things have a real foundation. Add those that the intellect by merely imagining creates for itself, such as the *Fabulous Images of the Poetasters*, who, when taught by this symbolic Teacher, even when dreaming, teach; even when lying, tell the truth. Such were among the heraldic figures Argus, Icarus and Phaeton; and among the most famous heraldic figures, the Duke of Burgundy's Golden Fleece, Dolce's Pegasus, Sforza Pallavicino's Atlas, Duke Albert of Bavaria's Hercules wrestling with the Lions. So varied and mysterious are the images of the sky and of the Zodiac that all that huge arc seems an azure Shield decorated with symbolic figures and luminous emblems. For that reason many others placed on their coat of arms the Centaur, Aries, the constellation of Leo, the Boreal Dragon and a thousand other parts of Poetic Philosophy which reveal to the senses the secrets of the intellect.

Moreover the fecundity of this art is such that the monstrous monsters it spawns on marbles and shields were never procreated either by the desire of geniuses, or the lust of Africa in its hot sands. Such chimerical and monstrous bodies were the Onoandrous Man-Donkey on the Egyptian Pyramids; the Gorgonian Woman-Viper on the Shield of Pallas; the Sphinx Woman-Lion on the Shield of Polynices; the Chimera Dragon-Goat

Consilio et virtute Chimaeram superari
id est fortiores et deceptores

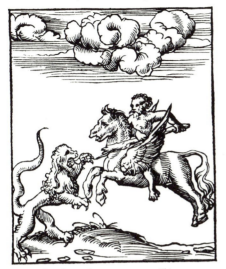

Bellerophon ut fortis eques superare Chimaeram
Et Licu potuit sternere monstra soli.
Sic tu Pegaseis vectus petis aethera pennis.
Consilioque animi monstra superba domas.

Figure 13: Andrea Alciati, Emblem.

on Turnus's Crest; the Capricorn Goat-Fish on Octavius Augustus's Medals and on Cosmo de Medici's coat of arms. All this indicates that this science, by combining substances which nature has studiously separated, turns nature upside down. Add to these the natural bodies chimerically paired, which are grotesque metaphors.[48] (Figure 13.)

Yet Chimera's unreality excludes her from the body of heraldry (in the same way, although for opposite reasons, as it excludes the human body). Chimerical and capricious bodies (such as the Man-Donkey or the Woman-Lion, or Chimera herself — the Dragon-Goat) must not appear on the heraldic device,

> not because they cannot suggest extremely witty and ingenious meanings, but because they would render the foundation more implausible and insignificant. Hence Virgil with deep wisdom shows us the Sun, a natural body, as the sign on King Latinus's Crest, on that of Turnus, a bizarre young man, he places a Chimera for which the chimerical bodies were named.[49]

Chimera and the human body are excluded from heraldry: one because it is too full of meaning to be real, the other because it is too real to be significant.

On the emblems, as well as in the myth, Chimera and the human body are paired in opposition.

There is, however, a characteristic of the emblem that places it at an equal distance from the human body and the chimerical body. The emblem is, in fact, an admirable composite, which has its soul outside the body:

> Therefore on the emblem, which is a painted Metaphor, the Figure with a Significant Feature constitutes the Body; the Person together with the Feature Signified, constitutes the Soul...therefore, the emblem is an admirable composite having its Soul outside its Body: having the Signifier perceptible on the Shield and the Signified intelligible in the mind.[50]

If the human body rejects this separation from the soul, at the cost of life, the chimerical body welcomes it in such a way that it is made into an emblem, but an emblem in reverse: the emblem of what is not and need not be.

The Soul of the Chimera

> The great horse, or Pegasus (whose master is Bellerophon), puffed up with honor,... chases Chimera through the highest stars. Jupiter throws the rider down headlong and brings the horse as witness to the impious crime to the stars. Thus, victory often destroys greedy leaders, who, when they have conquered most things, seek more.[51]

The emblem, states Emanuele Tesauro, is a composite of body and soul, which has its soul outside the body: its soul is in the concept (the signified) which accompanies the figure (the body, the signifier). If the signified is the soul of the emblem, what is the Chimera's soul? Perhaps we must look for it in one or in all of her meanings (why, in fact, should this multiplicity have only one soul?). It is here that one of Chimera's most mysterious characteristics emerges: the fact that she is never alone.

Just as the emblem degenerates, unless the figure is coupled with its concept in an indissoluble union, so *the* Chimera becomes any chimerical body; it becomes *a* chimera, unless another figure appears in the picture to give meaning to the image as a whole.

Either this second figure, as we have seen, is the fragile composite of horse and rider formed by Pegasus and Bellerophon, or, in pictures more remote from the myth, it is Sphinx, the antagonistic sister. Is it then in the antagonist, enemy or interlocutor that Chimera's meaning and soul are to be found?

One of the requirements of the heraldic emblem is that its body must be "True and Real." "For if you build a Metaphorical Signified over a Chimerical Signifier, you build the plausible over the implausible...since the true limits the forces of the intellect, and the imaginary is an unlimited and infinite thing."

Thus, if the heraldic emblem is a chimerical form, Chimera is not its body. The body, in fact, is necessarily limited, and Chimera is "unlimited and infinite." Chimera is an infinite Signifier, a "hieroglyphic of Insanity." In other words, she is a signifier that has the qualities of the signified, a body which has the properties of the soul, an *imaginary* thing which, instead of pointing toward the real, points toward the language.

If the emblem is an admirable composite, with its soul outside its body, Chimera is that hybrid in which the soul eternally nullifies the body and the body inexhaustibly dissipates the soul around it or, leaving aside the metaphor (if it is possible, when speaking of Chimera, to leave aside the metaphor), a hybrid in which the imaginary and the linguistic nullify each other.

*　*　*

In Flaubert's *Temptation of Saint Anthony*, inspired, as we know, by Callot's engraving, Sphinx and Chimera meet and attempt an impossible embrace (figure 14):

> *Chimera*: How is it that you constantly call me and reject me?
> *Sphinx*: It's you, untamable caprice, tearing and eddying past!
> *Chimera*: Is it my fault? How? Let me be!
> *Sphinx*: You're moving, you're out of reach!
> *Chimera*: Try again! — you're crushing me!
> *Sphinx*: No! impossible![52]

With the word "impossible" the encounter ends. In the dialogue, each of them had reflected the other, each has seen herself in the eyes of the other: Sphinx, mute, ponderous and immobile, traces alphabets in the desert sand; Chimera, swift, vociferous, fleeting, shouts and spouts flames. Sphinx calls Chimera "Fantasy." Chimera calls Sphinx "Unknown." Sphinx keeps her secret, dreams and calculates. Chimera,

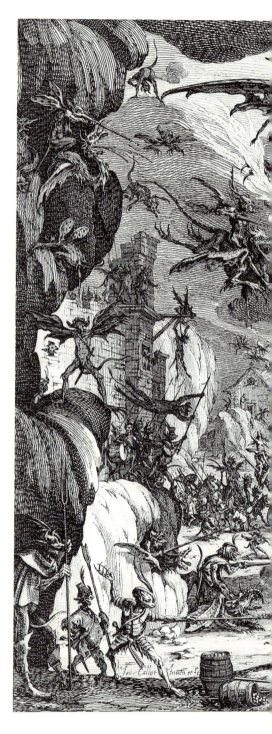

Figure 14: Jacques Callot, The Temptation of Saint Anthony, 1635 (Paris, Bibliothèque nationale).

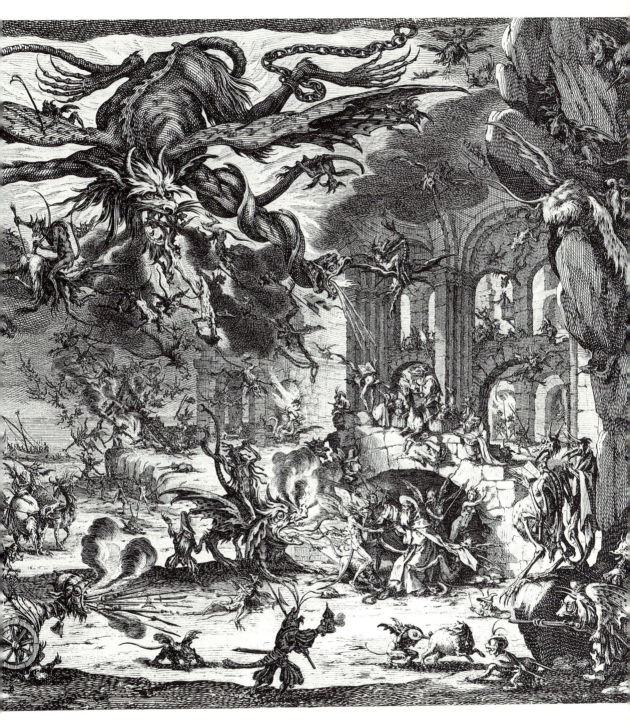

zone

light and playful, lascivious and seductive, seeks new perfumes, larger flowers, and pleasures never before experienced. She hates wisdom, just as Sphinx hates desire.

The impossible embrace culminates in the sinking of Sphinx into the desert, and in the disappearance of Chimera in spirals of smoke. We see again, as in the duel between Chimera and Bellerophon, the encounter of the light with the heavy, of the demonic with the melancholy; but if we take another look at the iconology of the battle (figure 15), we can hardly fail to note a certain erotic suggestion in the positioning of the winged horse above the lioness-goat, the prefigured impossible embrace.

Thus, in the modern dialogue between Sphinx and Chimera, an almost imperceptible secret, a cipher of the mythical duel reappears. The attempt at copenetration that ends with the explosion of the trio: Chimera ends up in hell, Pegasus on Olympus, Bellerophon, uprooted, in the desert. Similarly, although in opposite directions, Sphinx and Chimera, after having attempted a union, interpose between them as great a distance as separates the heavens from the abyss.

What makes this impossible, desired and hated embrace the fulcrum on which propinquity is changed into maximum distance? We recognize in the outcome of the encounter – the killing of Chimera or the sinking of Sphinx – a singular variant of the terrible dialectic of body and soul which so besets the allegory. In Flaubert's dialogue between Sphinx and Chimera, Yves Vadé sees the manifestation of a recurrent symbol of the romantic and post-romantic period (from Hugo to Nerval to Gustave Moreau, to Huysmans...): the confrontation between the enigma whose solution is the key to the universe ("The Sphinx is science enveloped in allegories," as Francis Bacon used to say) and the indecipherable whose cipher is illusory: "The Sphinx appears as the symbol of a hidden meaning whose reality, that is, her non-chimerical nature, is boldly stated; to recognize the Chimera as Chimera is tantamount to denying the Sphinx."

But what is the indecipherable? Is it not, perhaps, once again, a signifier that cannot coincide with anything signified, something signified which does not refer back to any signifier? If Sphinx contains within herself both the riddle and its answer (and dissolves as soon as one finds the other), Chimera contains both the riddle without an answer and an answer without a riddle. In other words, she contains the power to nullify any attempt at making sense, and to discourage any renunciation of it.

Body and Soul, Enigma and Indecipherable are figures of the same dialectic of the

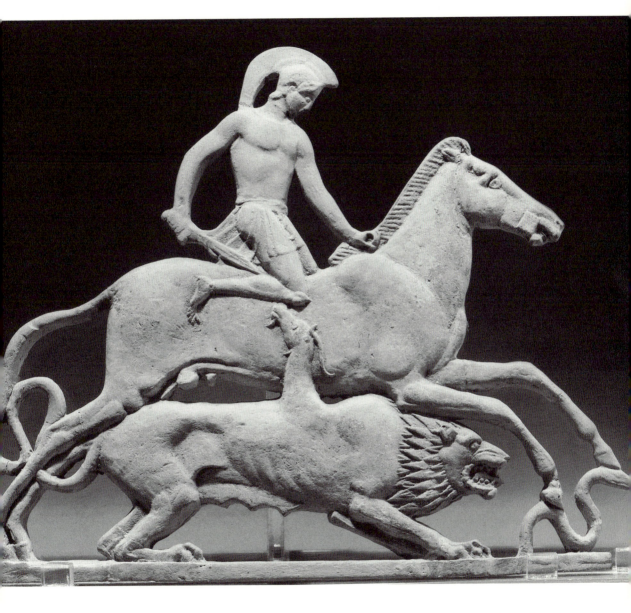

Figure 15: Bellerophon and Chimera (London, British Museum).

limited and the unlimited, which is at the root of any discussion of art. And just as the chimerical Body was excluded from the coat of arms, Chimera must be excluded from art. In the nineteenth century, as in the sixteenth, Chimera is once again the figure that, with its unlimited limitations, threatens art with meaninglessness.

In *Par les champs et par les grèves*, Flaubert posed the following question:

> If what we call monstrosities of nature have their own mutual anatomical, that is, plastic, relationships and their own physiological laws — laws necessary to their existence... why then should not all that also have its own beauty, its own ideal? Did the ancients not believe this? And is their mythology anything other than a monstrous and fantastic universe dressed up in forms alien to our nature and yet beautiful, since they are so right in themselves and in harmony with each other?... Who has not found the Chimera charming; who has not loved her lion's snout, her rustling eagle's wings, and her green-glinting rump?[53]

Later on in the text, he answers his own question:

> Art should not exceed the limits of the real.... There will never be any aesthetic value in inventing animals and plants which do not exist, in giving wings to a horse, fish tails to women's bodies, impossible existences, revelations that cannot be grasped.... The imagination in fact doesn't live on Chimeras; it has its own reality as you have yours.... It turns about and turns about again to beset it, and is happy only after having given it an existence that is real, palpable, durable, ponderable, indestructible.[54]

Like Tesauro's, Flaubert's Chimera is the representation of the unlimited, of that which has "no real, palpable, durable, ponderable, indestructible existence." Chimera's threat consists in her infinite impossibility (the infinite of impossible worlds) which nullifies the imaginary (figure 16). Chimera, in other words, is a bad Muse.[55] She leads one simultaneously into the temptation of omnipotence and of nihilism: everything is possible, everything is futile.

Facing her is Sphinx, a motionless monster of stone that counters the *hubris* of the indecipherable with its modest riddle, just as, in the myth, the couple Bellerophon and Pegasus, fragile harmony of the living, counters the unthinkable tangle of the three animal-bodies with its more agile and soluble composite. Even though Bellerophon poured molten lead into his cast (proceeding like a sculptor — the oppo-

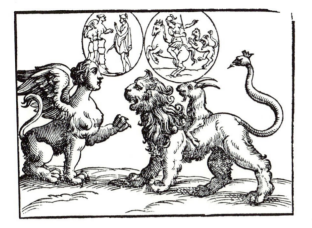

Figure 16: Vincenzo Cartari, *Seconda Novissima Editione della Imagini degli Dei Antichi*, 1626 (Paris, Bibliothèque nationale).

site of Pygmalion) and Sphinx crushes fiery Chimera with her massive weight, the weight falls always on the other side; the weight of the body (Bellerophon who plummets into the desert, Sphinx who sinks into the sand) and the weight of the soul (melancholy); as if the antagonist, in order to compose the unity of body and soul, deprived itself of the lightness of the spirit; as if Chimera's boundless body, breathing from its many souls, produced a sort of gas, a miasma, an evil exhalation. "When the black bile already present in preponderance, is inflamed, it causes deep depression and misanthropy; of this sort was Bellerophon's grief."

Hybrid, indecipherable, undetermined, hellish, interpretable, feminine, metaphorical, light, animal, fiery, raging, boundless, impossible, Chimera is the only monster which, when transformed from myth into language, brought along the same allurement, the same threat.

But not only into language. Daughter of a wind and a swamp, Chimera is that exhalation, that languor, which on hot evenings rises from a stagnant body of water and causes the soul to feel the grim heaviness of the body, and the body to feel the heaviness of the soul, and to desire (figure 17).

★   ★   ★

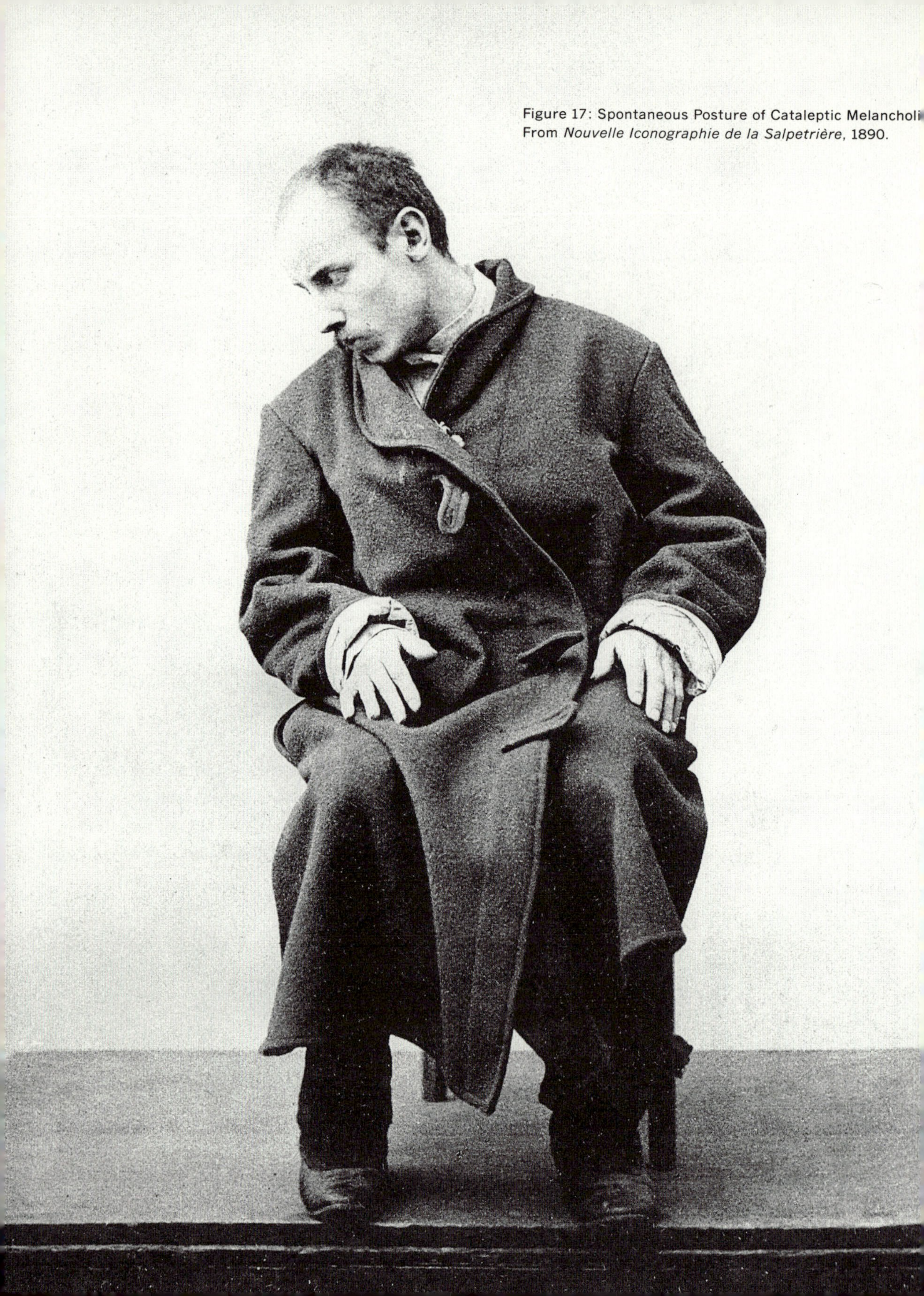

Figure 17: Spontaneous Posture of Cataleptic Melancholi
From *Nouvelle Iconographie de la Salpetrière*, 1890.

In an admirable text, only slightly later than Flaubert's *Temptation*, Baudelaire catches in a unique image the eternal dialogue between Chimera and her double: the dialogue between light and heavy, between desire and melancholy, between high and low, between the chimerical body and the human body. In an illustration, which was reproduced in the Florentine literary magazine *La Chimera*, a body appears, bent under the weight of its own chimera, in an apparent reversal which is no more than the last deciphering of a myth (and the transformation of a metaphor into a metonymy): Chimera has become heavy; like that which makes man aware of the weight of his body and of its mortal limitations, and encloses him in the aporia of hope and indifference (figure 18):

Under a vast gray sky, on a vast and dusty plain without paths, without grass, without a nettle or a thistle, I came upon several men bent double as they walked.

Each one carried on his back an enormous Chimera as heavy as a sack of flour, as a sack of coal, as the accoutrement of a Roman foot-soldier.

But the monstrous beast was no inanimate weight; on the contrary, it hugged and bore down heavily on the man with its elastic and powerful muscles; it clutched at the breast of its mount with enormous claws; and its fabulous head overhung the man's forehead like those horrible helmets with which ancient warriors tried to strike terror into their enemies.

I questioned one of these men and asked him where they were going like that. He replied that he did not know and that none of them knew; but that obviously they must be going somewhere since they were impelled by an irresistible urge to go on.

A curious thing to note: not one of these travelers seemed to resent the ferocious beast hanging around his neck and glued to his back; apparently they considered it a part of themselves. All those worn and serious faces showed not the least sign of despair; under the depressing dome of the sky, with their feet deep in the dust of the earth as desolate as the sky, they went along with the resigned look of men who are condemned to hope forever.

And the procession passed by me and disappeared in the haze of the horizon just where the rounded surface of the planet prevents man's gaze from following.

And for a few moments I persisted in trying to understand this mystery; but soon irresistible Indifference descended upon me, and I was more cruelly oppressed by its weight than those men had been by their crushing Chimeras.[56]

NOTES

1. Hesiod, *Theogony*, trans. Hugh G. Evelyn-White in *Hesiod, the Homeric Hymns and Homerica* (London and Cambridge, Mass.: Loeb Classical Library, 1982), 233-81.

2. "The name of Typhon also meant the burning Scirocco from the Southern Desert, a cause of havoc in Lybia and Greece," in Robert Graves, *The Greek Myths* (Baltimore: Penguin Books, 1955).

3. *Theogony* 805-10.

4. Jean-Pierre Vernant, *La mort dans les yeux* (Paris: Hachette, 1985), ch. 5.

5. *Theogony* 869-85.

6. Joseph Fontenrose, *Python: A Study of Delphic Myth and Its Origins* (Berkeley: University of California Press, 1959), p. 73.

7. *Ibid*.

8. Homer, *Iliad*, trans. Robert Fitzgerald (New York: Anchor Books, 1974), 2.781-85.

9. *Theogony* 295-308.

10. Fontenrose, *Python*, p. 95.

11. *Theogony* 309-332.

12. See Vincenzo Cartari, *Imagini degli dei delli antichi* (Venice, 1556): "As also related by Virgil who places the Chimera at the first entrance to hell with some other terrible monsters."

13. Virgil, *Aeneid*, trans. Robert Fitzgerald (New York: Random House, 1981), 6.282-89.

14. *Iliad* 6.179-82.

15. Apollodorus, *Biblioteca sive de Deorum origine* (Rome, 1555), 2.3. Translated by Sir James George Frazer as *The Library* (London, 1921), pp. 149-53.

16. Ovid, *Metamorphoses*, trans. F.J. Miller (London and Cambridge, Mass.: Loeb Classical Library, 1916), 9.647-48.

17. See also *The Oxford Classical Dictionary* (Oxford: Oxford University Press, 1949; repr. 1970), p. 186: "This is so oddly inorganic as to suggest an early misunderstanding of some kind, and there is much to be said for the theory...that originally (in Oriental art) it had wings ending in a goat-like head, a type known to exist...."

18. Apollodorus, *Biblioteca* 2.3.

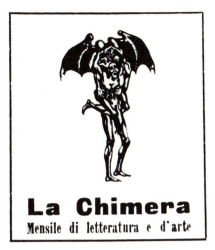

Figure 18: From *La Chimera* (Florence, 1954).

19. *Iliad* 6.197-207.

20. Joannes Tzetzes, *Lycophron* (Rome, 1803).

21. See also Jean Chevalier, *Dictionnaire des symboles* (Paris: R. Laffont, 1969): "The Chimera seduces and destroys those who surrender to her, she cannot be fought face to face, and must be hunted and caught by stealth in her lair."

22. Aristotle, *Problemata* 30, quoted in R. Klibansky, E. Panofsky and F. Saxl, *Saturn and Melancholy: Studies in the History of Natural Philosophy, Religion and Art* (London: Nelson, 1964), pp. 18-19.

23. Melanchthon, *De anima*, quoted in Klibansky, Panofsky and Saxl, *Saturn and Melancholy*, p. 90.

24. Pindar, *Olympia*, trans. Richmond Lattimore (Chicago: University of Chicago Press), 13.89-90.

25. See Christoforo Landino's commentary on the *Aeneid*, "Quaestiones Camaldolenses" (1480).

26. Jean Thenaud, *La lignée de Saturne*, (1511?) (Geneva, 1973).

27. Lucretius, *De rerum natura*, trans. R.E. Latham (New York: Penguin Books, 1951), 2.700-06, 5.901-05.

28. N. Conti, *Mythologie c'est-à-dire explication des fables* (Lyon: Paul Frelon, 1600), pp. 972-73.

29. Vincenzo Cartari, *Imagini degli dei*, p. 240.

30. J. Tzetzes, *Lycophron*.

31. N. Conti, *Mythologie*, p. 974.

32. *Ibid.*

33. *Encyclopédie des dieux et des héros* (Paris, 1773), vol. 2, p. 563.

34. Don Cameson Allen, *Mysteriously Meant: The Rediscovery of Pagan Symbolism and Allegorical Interpretation in the Renaissance* (Baltimore: Johns Hopkins Press, 1970), p. 189.

35. J. Thenaud, *La lignée*.

36. N. Conti, *Mythologie*, p. 978. The light–heavy dialectic of the duel between Chimera and Bellerophon is reproduced here in meteorological terms.

37. J. Thenaud, *La lignée*.

38. Paul Diel, *Symbolism in Greek Mythology*, trans. Vincent Stuart, Micheline Stuart and Rebecca Folkman (London, 1980). Diel's interpretation is striking for the absolute certainty with which it is presented. The fact that Chimera in Greek means "goat" and not "perverse imagination" does not diminish this certainty.

39. Jean de Grouchy, *Jumeaux, mosaïques, chimères* (Paris: Medsi, 1980).

40. Sir Philip Sidney, *An Apology for Poetry*, ed. Geoffrey Shepherd (Manchester: Manchester University Press, 1973), p. 100.

41. Thomas Hobbes, *Leviathan* (1651), pt.1, ch. 2.

42. René Descartes, *Meditations on First Philosophy*, in *Descartes' Philosophical Writings*, trans. Norman Kemp Smith (London: Macmillan, 1952).

43. See the discussion of the entire process in Helmut Papajewski's long article *Chimäre und Metaphor* (Anglia, 1964).

44. Emanuele Tesauro, *Il cannocchiale Aristotelico*, ed. Ezio Raimondi (Turin: Einaudi, 1987), p. 67.

45. *Ibid.*

46. *Ibid.*, pp. 22-24.

47. *Ibid.*, p. 395.

48. Tesauro, *Il cannocchiale Aristotelico* (Venice: P. Baglioni, 1663), p. 26.

49. *Ibid.*, p. 594.

50. *Ibid.*, p. 593.

51. *Ibid.*, p. 673.

52. Gustave Flaubert, *The Temptation of Saint Anthony*, trans. Kitty Mrosovsky (Ithaca, N.Y.: Cornell University Press, 1980), p. 222.

53. Gustave Flaubert, *Par les champs et par les grèves*, pp. 59-60.

54. *Ibid.*, p. 5.

55. As Ritter Santini Lea says in her book *Le immagini incrociate* (Bologna, 1986): "In the last decade of the nineteenth century, the image of the Chimera had become for poets and writers, as for painters, a metaphor for an enigmatic feminine principle which has the power to attract, conquer and annihilate the power of the artist." See also her analysis of D'Annunzio's Chimera.

56. Charles Baudelaire, "To Every Man His Chimera," *Paris Spleen* (1862), trans. Louise Varise (New York: New Directions, 1970), pp. 8-9.

BIBLIOGRAPHY

CLASSICAL PERIOD

Apollodorus, *Biblioteca sive de Deorum origine*. Rome, 1555. Translated by Sir James G. Frazer as *The Library*. London, 1921. 2.1-3.

Hesiod, *Theogony*. Translated by H.G. Evelyn-White, *Hesiod, the Homeric Hymns and Homerica*. London and Cambridge, Mass.: Loeb Classical Library, 1982. *Passim*.

Lucretius, *De rerum natura*. Translated by R.E. Latham. New York: Penguin Books, 1951. 2.700-06 and 5.900-06.

Homer, *Iliad*. Translated by R. Fitzgerald. New York: Anchor Books, 1974. 6.152-230 and 16.326-29.

Ovid, *Metamorphoses*. Translated by F.J. Miller. London and Cambridge, Mass.: Loeb Classical Library, 1916. 9.646-50.

Pindar, *Olympia*. Translated by R. Lattimore. Chicago: University of Chicago Press. 13.89-90.

Virgil, *Aeneid*. Translated by R. Fitzgerald. New York: Random House, 1981. Book 6.

MODERN PERIOD

Alciati, Andrea, *Emblemata*. 1531.

Anonymous, *La Chimère ou le phantasme de la mendicité*. Paris, 1607.

———, *Les Chimères de M. Jurieu*. Paris, 1688.

Vincenzo Cartari, *Imagini degli dei delli antichi*. Illustrated by Lorenzo Pignoria Padovano. Venice, 1556.

René Descartes, *Méditations*, in *Oeuvres*. Paris: Garnier, 1967, p. 433. Translated by Norman Kemp Smith as *Meditations on First Philosophy*, in *Descartes' Philosophical Writings*. London: Macmillan, 1952.

Hobbes, Thomas, *Leviathan*, 1.2. London, 1651.

Ripa, Cesare, *Iconologia*. Rome, 1593 and Venice, 1645.

Ruscelli, Girolamo, *Le Imprese illustri*. Venice, 1566.

Sidney, Sir Philip, *Apologie for Poetrie*. London, 1595. Reprint, *An Apology for Poetry*. Edited by Geoffrey Shepherd. Manchester: Manchester University Press, 1973.

Tesauro, Emanuele, *Il cannocchiale Aristotelico*. Venice, 1663. Reprint, Turin: Einaudi, 1987.

Thenaud, Jean, *La lignée de Saturne*, c. 1511. Reprint, Geneva, 1973.

Tzetzes, Joannes, *Lycophron*. Rome, 1803.

CONTEMPORARY PERIOD

Allen, Don Cameron, *Mysteriously Meant: The Rediscovery of Pagan Symbolism and Allegorical Interpretation in the Renaissance*. Baltimore: Johns Hopkins University Press, 1970.

Baltrusaitis, Jurgis, *Le Moyen Age fantastique: Antiquités et exotismes dans l'art gothique*. Paris: A. Colin, 1955.

_____. *Réveils et prodiges: Le gothique fantastique*. Paris: A. Colin, 1960.

Barth, John, *Chimera*. New York: Random House, 1972.

Baudelaire, Charles, "Chacun sa Chimère," in *Petits Poèmes en prose*, 1862. Translated by Louise Varise in *Paris Spleen*. New York: New Directions, 1970.

Chastel, André, *Umanesimo e simbolismo*. Turin: Einaudi, 1958.

_____. *Art et humanisme à Florence au temps de Laurent le Magnifique: Etudes sur la Renaissance et l'humanisme platonicien*. Paris: Presses Universitaires de France, 1959.

_____. *Fables, formes, figures*. Paris: Flammarion, 1978.

Chevalier, Jean, *Dictionnaire des symboles*. Paris: R. Laffont, 1969.

D'Annunzio, Gabriele, *Il Fuoco*.

_____. "La chimera e l'altra bocca," in *Il secondo amante di Lucrezia Buti*. Milan, 1929.

Defrance, Jean-Philippe André, *La figuration animale au Moyen-Age, compromis entre le normal et le monstrueux*. Thèse de Doctorat Vétérinaire, 1968.

Diel, Paul, *Le symbolisme dans la mythologie grecque*. Paris: Payot, 1966. Translated by V. Stuart, M. Stuart and R. Folkman as *Symbolism in Greek Mythology*. London, 1980.

Flaubert, Gustave, *La tentation de Saint-Antoine*. Translated by K. Mrosovsky as *The Temptation of Saint Anthony*. Ithaca, N.Y.: Cornell University Press, 1980.

Fontenrose, Joseph, *Python: A Study of Delphic Myth and Its Origins*. Berkeley: University of California Press, 1959.

Graves, Robert, *The Greek Myths*. Baltimore: Penguin Books, 1955.

de Grouchy, Jean, *Jumeaux, mosaïques, chimères et autres aléas*. Paris: Medsi, 1980.

Kerenyi, Karl, *The Gods of the Greeks*. London and New York: Thames and Hudson, 1951.

Klibansky, R., E. Panofsky, F. Saxl, *Saturn and Melancholy: Studies in the History of Natural Philosophy, Religion and Art*. London: Nelson, 1964.

Lea, Ritter Santini, *Le immagini incrociate*. Bologna: Il Mulino, 1986.

MacCullough, Florence, *Mediaeval Latin and French Bestiaries*. Chapel Hill: University of North Carolina Press, 1962.

Mâle, Emile, *L'art religieux du XII au XVIII siècle: Extraits choisis par l'auteur*. Paris: A. Colin, 1945.

_____. *La Cathedrale d'Albi: Photographies de Pierre Devinoy*. Paris: P. Hartmann, 1950.

_____. *L'art religieux du XIIIème siècle en France: Etude sur l'iconographie du Moyen Age et sur ses sources d'inspiration*. Paris: A. Colin, 1902.

de Nerval, Gérard, *Les chimères*. Translated by Peter Jay as *The Chimeras*. Redding Ridge, Conn.: Black Swan Books, 1984.

Panofsky, Erwin, *Meaning in the Visual Arts*. Chicago: University of Chicago Press, 1983.

_____. *Studies in Iconology*: *Humanistic Themes in the Art of the Renaissance*. New York: Harper and Row, 1972.

_____. *Renaissance and Renascences in Western Art*. New York: Harper and Row, 1972.

Papajewski, Helmut, *Chimära und Metaphor*. Anglia, 1964.

Rose, H.J., "Chimaera," in *The Oxford Classical Dictionary*. Oxford: Oxford University Press, 1949.

Seznec, Jean, *Nouvelle Etude sur la Tentation de Saint-Antoine*. London: Warburg Institute, 1949.

_____. *La Survivance des Dieux Antiques*: *Essais sur le rôle de la tradition mythologique dans l'humanisme et dans l'art de la Renaissance*. Paris: Flammarion, 1980.

Vadé, Yves, "Le Sphinx et la Chimère," in *Romantisme* 15 and 16. Paris: Flammarion, 1977.

Vernant, Jean-Pierre, *La mort dans les yeux: Figures de l'autre en Grèce Ancienne*. Paris: Hachette, 1985.

Veyrat, Claude, *Les Animaux dans la Mythologie Grecque*. Lyon: Thèse de Doctorat Vétérinaire, 1967.

Translated by Margaret Roberts and Frank Treccase.

Italian eighteenth-century mechanical
marionette with internal strings.
Unclothed, headless representative of
a type of so-called "mechanical"
marionette in which the strings that
moved the legs were run invisibly through
the body to the control rod that lifted
the puppet by its head.

Bologna, Collection of Civica Galleria
Davia-Bargellini.

410

The Inanimate Incarnate

Roman Paska

For centuries, puppet theory has concentrated on the puppet's symbolic relationship with human models, the puppet being primarily cast in the role of a surrogate human. Reflections on puppet theater, from the *Ṛg-Veda* to Marcus Aurelius to the present, have perpetuated an image of the puppet as a symbol of man manipulated by higher forces or beings, a metaphor in which the puppet is structurally interchangeable with its own controller, man.

But East and West historically diverge in their respective emphases on the importance of the puppet's mimetic aspect. While Asian and African cultures maintain cognizance of the puppet's innate "otherness," granting it its own ontological status distinct from man, the European puppet theater, particularly the theater of marionettes (the term "marionette" referring in English exclusively to the string puppet), exceeds all other traditions in making the duplication of human characteristics its chief aesthetic concern.

While this tendency in puppet theater is closely allied with the general progression of Western theater toward realism, the resulting effect for the notion of the puppet is to regard it as a diminished, artificial human proxy, a "mere" puppet in that it functions as a substitute for something as accessible and familiar as the human organism, rather than something mysterious, immaterial and pure — like an idea, a spirit or god.

But even in the mimetic atmosphere of Western puppetry, the simulation of human movement and gesture takes precedence over the realistic representation of form. A fact commonly misunderstood by critics of puppet theater, this principle applies to puppets of every genre (hand, rod, shadow and marionette). The essential fascination of puppet theater, its ability to engage and hold an audience, is a

411

function of its nature as a theatrical activity consisting in the animation of lifeless objects (dead things) through the active intervention of a living human operator. The theatrical destination of the puppet also determines its distinction from the automaton, the mannequin and the doll, with their passive claims to formal autonomy as objects. In the puppet theater, the use(fulness) of the object is far more significant than the object in itself. And when the object does take human form, sometimes even reproducing anatomical features quite extraneous to its integrity as a puppet, it often does so self-consciously, as if the attempt to camouflage its otherness were in fact a subterfuge for displaying it.

Kleist's appreciation of the marionette theater of his day is clearly conditioned by the Romantic view of the puppet as a representational figure intent on acquiring mechanical autonomy. But his glimpses of the psychology and metaphysics of the medium have given his essay the allure of a sacred text for twentieth-century practitioners and theorists of the art. For these heirs to a tradition of puppet apologists descended from Kleist, the puppet's inherent resistance to realism, which previously obstructed its acceptance as a respectable artistic form in the West, has now become its principal raison d'être.

**Marionette Lilith by W.A. Dwiggins,
prominent American book and puppet
designer (1880-1956), with concealed
cords for joints.**

From Dorothy Abbe, *The Dwiggins Marionettes*
(Boston, 1970).

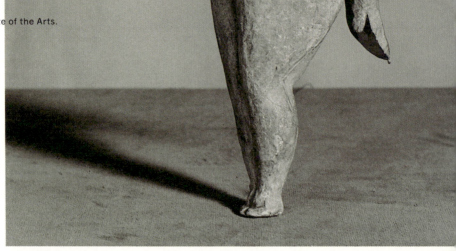

Nude marionette Queen designed by Michael Carr (active 1907-28) for experiments by Edward Gordon Craig. (Craig's controversial theory of the *übermarionette* was greatly influenced by Kleist's essay on the marionette theater.)

Detroit, Detroit Institute of the Arts.

On the Marionette Theater

Heinrich von Kleist

While I was passing the winter of 1801 in M——, one evening in a public garden there I met Herr C——, who had recently been engaged as the principal dancer at the opera in that city and was having an outstanding success with the public.

I told him I had been surprised to notice him several times at a puppet theater that had been set up in the marketplace and was entertaining the mob with little dramatic burlesques interspersed with song and dance.

He assured me that the pantomime of these puppets gave him great pleasure, and emphatically remarked that a dancer who wished to develop himself could learn a number of things from them.

As this comment seemed, by the way he expressed it, to be more than an idle fancy, I sat down beside him in order to listen in more detail to the arguments with which he could support such a curious statement.

He asked me if I had not, in fact, found some of the movements of the puppets, especially the smaller ones, very graceful in the dance.

This particular fact I could not deny. A group of four peasants, who danced a round in rapid time, could not have been more prettily depicted by Teniers.

I asked about the mechanism of these figures – how it was possible to control the individual limbs and their parts as the rhythm of the movements or the dance itself demanded, without having myriads of strings attached to one's fingers?

He answered that I mustn't imagine that every limb was pulled or positioned separately by the operator during the different moments of the dance.

Each movement, he said, had its center of gravity; it sufficed to control this point within the interior of the figure; the limbs, which were nothing but pendula, followed by themselves in a mechanical way without any further assistance.

He added that this movement was quite simple; that whenever the center of gravity was moved in a *straight line*, the limbs would still describe *curves*; and that the whole figure, shaken at random, often assumed a kind of rhythmical movement that was similar to dance.

The observation initially seemed to throw some light on the pleasure he pretended to find in the theater of marionettes. But I didn't even remotely suspect the conclusions he would later draw from it.

I asked him if he believed the mechanic who operated these puppets was himself a dancer, or at least must have some notion of the beautiful in dance.

He replied that even though the job was easy, from a mechanical point of view, that didn't mean that it could be done without feeling.

The line that the center of gravity had to describe was certainly simple and, he believed, in most cases straight. In cases where it was curved, its curvature seemed only of the first or at most the second degree; and in the latter case, it was only elliptical, a form of movement altogether natural to the human body (because of the joints), which therefore took the operator no great skill to indicate.

But from another point of view, this line was something very mysterious. For it was nothing other than the *path of the dancer's soul*; and he doubted if it could be found unless the operator imagines himself at the puppet's center of gravity — that is, in other words, dance.

I replied that this man's work had been represented to me as being rather spiritless — something like turning the crank that plays a hurdy-gurdy.

"Not at all," he answered. "In fact, the movements of his fingers are related to the movements of the puppets attached to them somewhat like numbers to their logarithms or the asymptote to the hyperbola."

But at the same time, he believed that even the last fragment of spirit of which he had spoken could be removed from the marionette, and that its dance could take place totally in the realm of mechanical forces — by means of a crank, as I imagined.

I expressed my surprise at seeing how attentively he evaluated this entertainment invented for the horde as if it were a fine art. Not only did he think it capable of higher development — he seemed to be involved in it himself.

He smiled and said he ventured to maintain that if a mechanic would build a marionette for him according to the requirements he gave him, he would perform a dance with it that neither he nor any capable dancer of his time, not excluding Vestris himself, was in a position to equal.

"Have you," he asked, as I cast my eyes silently to the ground, "have you heard of those mechanical legs that English artists fabricate for unfortunates who have lost their limbs?"

I said no, I had never set eyes on such things.

"That's too bad," he replied, "for if I tell you that those unfortunates dance with them, I'm almost afraid you won't believe me. What am I saying! Dance? Certainly the range of their movements is limited; but those at their disposal are accomplished with an ease, lightness and grace that astonish every sensitive mind."

I jokingly remarked that in that case, he had surely found his man. For the artist who was able to construct such a remarkable limb would no doubt also be able to assemble an entire marionette for him, according to his requirements.

"What," I asked, as he in turn was looking at the ground, a little embarrassed, "what then are the requirements you have in mind to achieve this artistic feat?"

"Nothing," he answered, "that isn't already found here as well — symmetry, mobility, lightness (but all to a higher degree), and especially a more natural arrangement of the centers of gravity."

"And the advantage this puppet would have over living dancers?"

"The advantage? First of all a negative one, my excellent friend; namely, that it would never be affected. For affectation appears, as you know, when the soul (*vis motrix*) is found at any point other than the movement's center of gravity. As the operator now has absolutely no other point in his control through the wire or string except this one, all of the other limbs are what they should be — dead, mere pendula, following the basic law of gravity — an admirable quality looked for in vain among the greater part of our dancers.

"Just look at P——," he continued, "when she plays Daphne and, pursued by Apollo, turns to look back at him; her soul is in the vertebrae of her lower back; she bends as if she were about to break, like a naiad from the school of Bernini. Or look at young F—— when, as Paris, he stands among the three goddesses and presents the apple to Venus; his soul is actually (it's frightful to see) in his elbow.

"Such mistakes," he added, stopping short, "are inevitable since we have eaten from the tree of knowledge. But paradise is barred and the cherub behind us; we must make the journey around the world to see if maybe there is still some opening from behind."

I laughed. "Of course," I thought, "the spirit cannot err where there is none."

417

But I noticed he still had more on his mind, and begged him to continue.

"In addition," he said, "these puppets have the advantage of being *antigravitational*. They know nothing of the inertia of matter, that property most inimical to dance, because the force that lifts them into the air is greater than the one that binds them to earth. What wouldn't our good G—— give if she could be sixty pounds lighter, or if a weight that size could assist her with her entrechats and pirouettes? The puppets only use the ground like elves, to *skim* it and reactivate the swinging of their limbs through an instantaneous pause; we use it to *rest* upon and recover from the effort of the dance — a moment that is obviously not dance itself, and allows for nothing better than to make it disappear as much as possible."

I said that no matter how deftly he presented the case for his paradoxes, he would never make me believe there could be more grace in a mechanical puppet than in the structure of the human body.

He responded that it was absolutely impossible for man even to equal the puppet in this. Only a god could compete with matter in this field; and here is the point where the two ends of the cyclical world connect.

I was more and more astonished, and didn't know what to say to such strange assertions.

It would seem, he responded, taking a pinch of snuff, that I had not read the third chapter of the first book of Moses attentively; and if someone wasn't familiar with that first period of human development, one couldn't very well speak with him about the following ones, much less the last.

I said I knew quite well what disorders consciousness could bring about in the natural grace of man. Through a mere remark, a young acquaintance of mine had lost his innocence before my very eyes, and despite all conceivable efforts, never regained that paradise afterward. "But what conclusions," I added, "can you draw from this?"

He asked me what sort of incident it was.

"About three years ago," I explained, "I went bathing with a young man whose constitution then displayed remarkable grace. He appeared to be about sixteen years old, and only from a distance were the initial traces of vanity, aroused by the attentions of women, perceptible. It happened that just a short time before, in Paris, we had seen the 'youth drawing a splinter from his foot'; the statue is well-known and copies are found in most German collections. A glance that he cast in a large mirror the moment he placed his foot on a stool to dry it off reminded him of it; he smiled and told me what a discovery he had made. In fact, I had made the same one at that same moment; but whether to test the certainty of the grace that possessed him, or to take a little salutary measure against his vanity, I laughed and replied that he was probably seeing ghosts! He blushed, and raised his foot a second time to show me; but, as could easily be foreseen, the experiment failed. Confused, he raised his foot a third and fourth, maybe even ten times. In vain! He was unable to produce the same movement again. What am I saying! The movements he made had such a comical aspect that I had trouble restraining my laughter.

"From that day, from that moment on, as it were, an incomprehensible change took place in this young man. He began to stand for days on end in front of the mirror, and one attractive quality after another deserted him. An invisible, incomprehensible force seemed to restrict the free play of his gestures like an iron net, and after a year had passed, there wasn't a trace left of the charm that had once delighted the eyes of those who surrounded him. Someone is still living who was a witness to that strange, unhappy incident, who could confirm it word for word as I have related it."

"At this juncture," said Herr C—— amicably, "I must tell you another story; you will easily understand how it belongs here.

"During my trip to Russia, I was on the country estate of Herr von G——, a Livonian nobleman whose sons were then intensively practicing fencing. The older one in particular, who had just come back from the university, acted the virtuoso, and one morning when I was in his room, he offered me a rapier. We fenced; but it turned out that I was superior to him; passion further increased his confusion; almost every thrust that I aimed struck home, and his rapier finally flew into the corner. Half joking, half hurt, he said, as he picked up the rapier, that he had met his master — but everything in the world has one, and he wanted to conduct me thenceforth to mine. The brothers burst out laughing and cried, 'Forward march! Down to the woodshed!' And with that they took me by the hand and led me to a bear which Herr von G——, their father, was having trained in the courtyard.

"As I stepped before him astonished, the bear stood on his hind feet, his back leaning up against the post to which he was fastened, his paw raised ready for battle, and looked me straight in the eye: that was his fencing pose. I thought I was

dreaming, faced with such an opponent; but 'Thrust! Thrust!' said Herr von G——,
'and see if you can hit him!' When I had recovered a little from my astonishment, I
lunged at him with the rapier; the bear made a slight movement with his paw and
parried the thrust. I tried to mislead him with feints; the bear didn't budge. I lunged
at him again with swift address; I would without fail have struck the breast of a man;
the bear made a slight movement of his paw and parried the thrust. Now I was almost
in the same situation as young Herr von G——. The seriousness of the bear served
to increase my discomfiture; thrusts and feints succeeded one another; I was drip-
ping with sweat — in vain! Not only did the bear parry all my thrusts like the best
fencer in the world, he never once followed a feint (which no fencer in the world
could imitate); eye to eye, as if he read my soul, he stood with his paw raised ready
for battle, and when my thrusts weren't meant in earnest, he didn't budge.

"Do you believe this story?"

"Completely!" I cried with hearty approval. "Coming from any stranger, it is so
probable; how much more then from you!"

"Now then, my excellent friend," said Herr C——, "you are in possession of
everything necessary to understand me. We see that in the organic world, to the
extent that reflection grows dimmer and weaker, the grace therein becomes more
brilliant and powerful. Yet, just as the intersection of two lines on one side of a point
suddenly appears again on the other side after passing through the infinite; or the
image in a concave mirror, after receding into the infinite, suddenly resurfaces close
before us — grace likewise reappears when knowledge has passed through the infinite, so that it appears purest simultaneously in the human body that has either none
at all or else infinite consciousness — that is, in the puppet or in the god."

"Consequently," I said, a little distraught, "we would have to eat again from the
tree of knowledge to fall back into the state of innocence?"

"Of course," he answered, "that is the last chapter of the history of the world."

Originally published as *Über das Marionettentheater*, in the *Berliner Abendblätter*,
December 12-14, 1810.
Translated by Roman Paska.

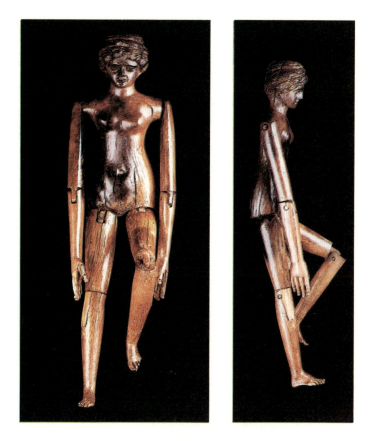

Roman doll with movable joints from the second century A.D. sarcophagus of Crepereia Tryphaena. Designed to produce anatomically accurate movements, this ivory doll (probably intended for votive use) is a fascinating indicator of late antique puppet technology.

Rome, Museo Capitolini.

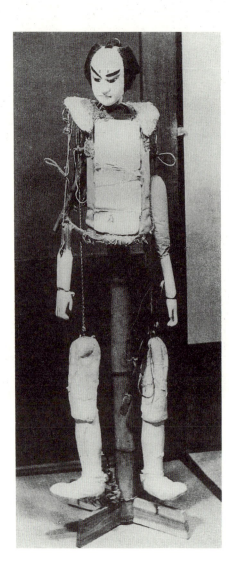

Naked Japanese Bunraku puppet, normally controlled by three manipulators, showing the basic structure of a male figure. Female puppets do not require legs.

From Saito Seijiro, Yamaguchi Hiroichi and Yoshinaga Takao, *Masterpieces of Japanese Puppetry* (Tokyo, 1958).

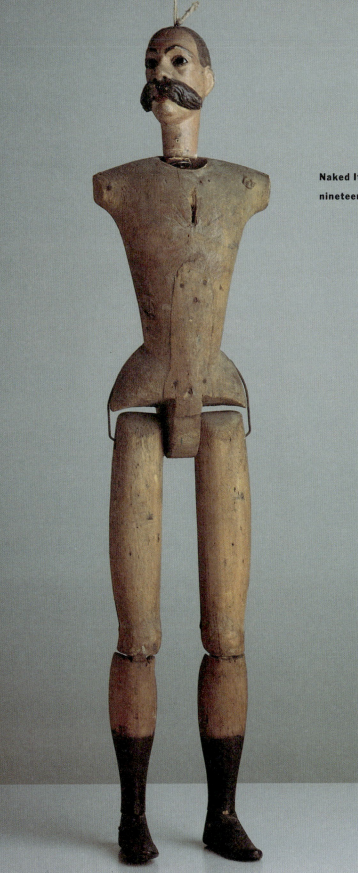

Naked Italian marionette, probably nineteenth-century (arms missing).

Orlando Pazzo (Crazy Orlando), nineteenth-century Sicilian marionette from the theater of Gaspare Canino (Alcamo). Intended for use in performance in this state of dress.

Palermo, Museo Internazionale della Marionetta.

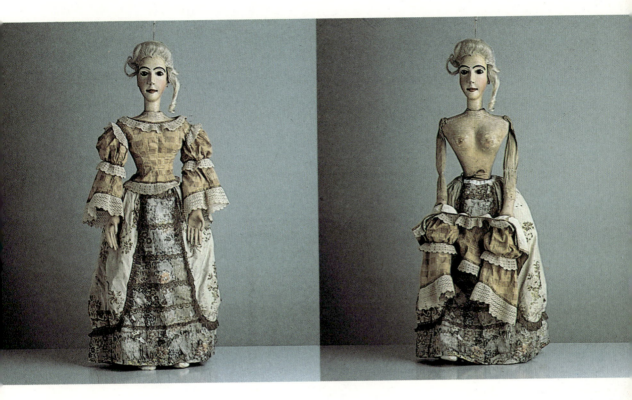

Young woman marionette with covered, unseen breasts entirely sculpted and painted. Probably late nineteenth-century Venetian, maybe a copy of an eighteenth-century figure. Controlled by a single rod to the head and strings to the hands only.

Milan, Private Collection of Roberto Leydi.

425

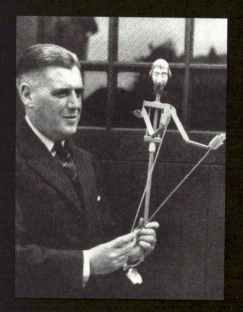

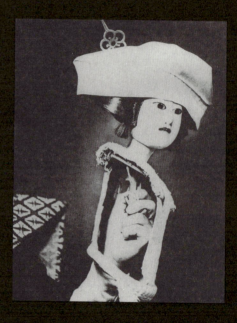

Undressed rod puppet. Mid-twentieth-century British example of figure worked from below with rigid rods attached to the hands instead of strings. In contemporary puppet theater, the rod puppet is often preferred to the marionette for its greater freedom from gravity.

From L.V. Wall et al., *The Puppet Book* (London, 1950).

Female Japanese Bunraku puppet, showing the position of the operator's hand inside the puppet. The puppeteer's fingers operate various levers on the internal rod to control such movable parts as eyeballs, eyebrows and mouth.

From Saito Seijiro et al., *Masterpieces of Japanese Puppetry* (Tokyo, 1958).

A hand puppet minus his costume, showing position of the operator's fingers
(British, ca. 1938). Devoid of rods,
strings or other mechanisms, the hand
puppet is usually considered the
essential puppet figure.

From David Frederick Milligan, *Fist Puppetry*
(New York, 1938).

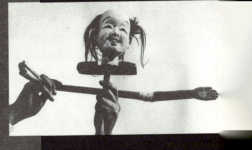

Japanese puppet operated by one man, who
manipulates internal armature by inserting
his hand in the back of the puppet's costume (Bunya theater, Sado Island).

From Donald Keene, *Bunraku: The Art of the
Japanese Puppet Theatre* (Tokyo, 1965).

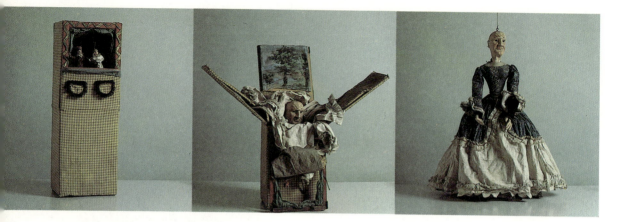

Early nineteenth-century Italian transformation puppet. A little hand puppet booth
with two puppets on stage (one of which is
Pulcinella), transformed into a woman
through a system of folding sections controlled by strings. A predecessor of later
so-called "specialty" marionettes on variety stages. From the 1820-30 "teatrino
Casa Borromeo."

Milan, Collezione Borromeo.

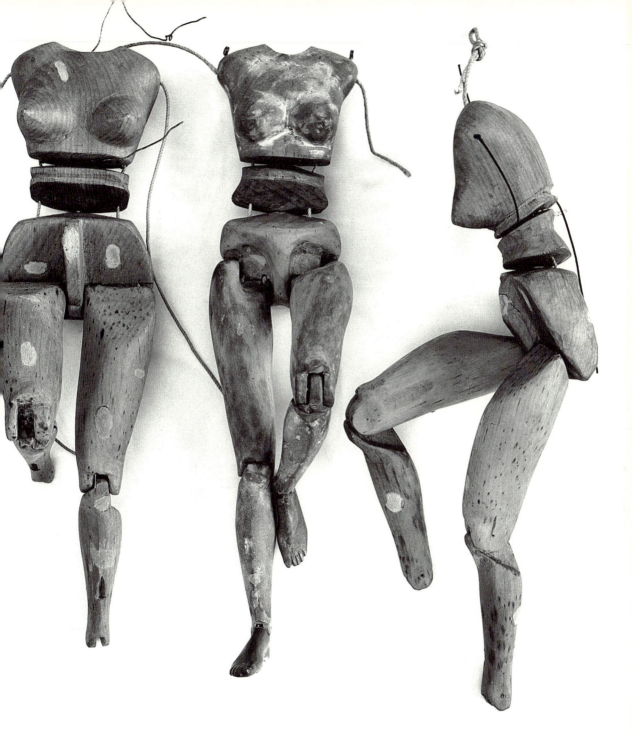

Unfinished marionettes by W.A. Dwiggins.

From Dorothy Abbe, *The Dwiggins Marionettes*
(Boston, 1970).

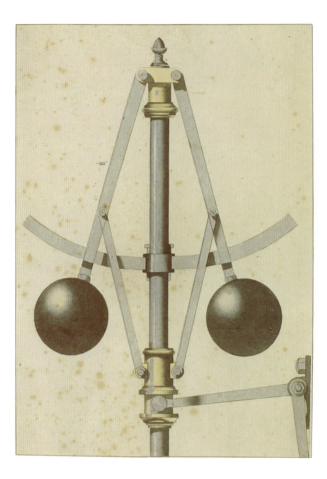

E. Gendreau, 1879. Private Collection.

The Classical Age of Automata:

An Impressionistic Survey from the Sixteenth

to the Nineteenth Century

Jean-Claude Beaune

An automaton is a machine that contains its own principle of motion. This Cartesian definition was advanced by Rabelais when, in *Gargantua* (1.24), he introduced the word "automate" into the French language: "and contrived a thousand little automatory engines, that is to say, moving of themselves." The English retained the Greek form "automaton" until its evocative power was supplanted by the new term "robot," coined in 1924 by the Czech writer, Karel Čapek. By then, however, the context had changed: the object itself was no longer the most important thing, at least from the technical point of view (although it continued to fascinate artists more than ever); rather, it was how the machines worked that mattered, their function, machines working en masse in industry and later in computing. The French adopted the term "automation," rather than keeping their own, more precise, "automatization," and today the word designates a whole technological world, governed by this principle. Even cybernetic or computer definitions of contemporary machines (like threshold automata, or semirecursive automata), which may be applied to mathematical entities far removed from the original machine, do not add anything to the main definition.

The Mechanical Myth. As a result of this, automata tend to be regarded as timeless. Ever since man has been capable of creating artifacts (which, in a sense, is the point at which he becomes fully human), he has dreamt of "autonomous" machines that could either imitate his own actions (thus providing a more reliable, more dependable automatic slave substitute) or could reproduce the course of the world as they function. Before it became a high-performance machine, an automaton was primarily a *techno-mythological idea* or, more precisely, the mythic distillation of technical processes and machines and, by extension, of tools or instruments. But this is

431

still basically the same idea; the "machines" that animated Egyptian temples operated on the same principle as the most sophisticated modern systems used in medicine, industry or art. Feedback from the so-called autonomous systems (the best example of which is Von Neumann's self-reproducing computer), far from exhausting the original fiction, has extended it and made it even more intense and disquieting. So, while each automaton is a separate machine, they all, within themselves and their image, have the capacity to preserve the profoundest essence of the whole technical domain.

Dissymmetry and Paradox. Two comments need to be made at this point. First, there is an obvious dissymmetry between machines and automata, in that machines are not always automatic, whereas automata seem invariably to be machines, whether real or imagined. In fact, the relationship between the two entities is far from simple: to put it briefly, we can say that automata represent the dream, the ideal form, the utopia of the machine, and that the gauge of their absolute perfection is their independence, which endows them from the first with an anthropomorphic or living quality. Machines, conversely, developed either according to their own norms or to norms determined by the scientific context. The "simple machines" of Galileo's treatise *Le meccaniche* are a direct expression of the force that should — according to contemporary theories — give man a purchase on the world. Television sets or motorcycles are not automatic insofar as they depend on an external energy source, and to the extent that their function seems to have lost that mythic dimension which gives the word "automaton" its primary sense.

This leads to the second of the two comments, a very different one, and one which should make us consider the real meaning of the culture and language of technology in a civilization that seems entirely bound up in the power of automata. At this point, we come up against what has to be called a curious paradox, and one which led Heidegger, among others, to ponder the way this sector of our activity has lost its meaning since ancient *poïesis* has been challenged and eventually subsumed by industrial civilization. It is a paradox which is all the more curious because this general absence of suitable language and of valorized education goes hand-in-hand with the proliferation of machines and an increase in their power, as well as an increase in their hold over man.

The Model Automaton. The combination of these two factors suggests that the idea of the automaton has lost none of its old evocative power, but, in fact, has taken on an exemplary function. On the one hand, it preserves the symbolic relationship between technology and man as something basic and metaphysical, involving the fundamental questions of life, the cosmos and culture; and, on the other, as contemporary artists have noticed, it plays the role of a "screen-image," of a sort of fatal necessity that allows man to escape from thinking about his contingency, individuality and, in the end, his freedom. Fate is thereby deliberately invested with the attributes of a factitious autonomy. There is no need for any reminder of the excesses of industrial and factory organization, which is rationalized into inhumanity, leaving almost no scope for the individual; in this respect automation has become a social — and, predominantly, an economic — idea, with the technical dimension constituting no more than a means, and man no more than a minor instrument. More concretely still, we can examine quickly some contemporary automatic machines designed to imitate, simulate or even replace human beings. Given the way not only philosophy, but aesthetics, literature and science in our culture are marked heavily by the duality of body and soul, of mind and matter, it is understandable that the earliest constructors of automata should have set themselves the task of simulating and replacing the body. Yet, as can be seen in Pascal, Leibniz and Babbage, as well as in the more recent concerns of Wiener and Turing, a desire to imitate and extend the calculating and intellectual faculties of the mind has gradually developed. And although the wilder fantasies of the 1950s have gone (nobody dreams of absolutes, like unbeatable automatic chess players, any more), this second enterprise has in fact been more successful than the first, since it is much easier to construct machines that are capable of high intellectual performance than it is to find an automaton capable of expressing in any real way ordinary, tangible sensations like hunger, sorrow or fear.

Chronology. The *mythical* automaton maintains a relationship with the cosmos, with the totality of things. This is the basis of the machine's primordial ambiguity and, at a more general level, of the whole realm of technology. The *mechanistic* automaton (from the Renaissance to the first machine-tools) is an attempt to dissect and copy the human body and the body of other living creatures (with a few notable *succès d'estime* rescued by collectors). The *mechanical* automaton (it is more useful in this context to talk about a general process of automation) groups together concentrations of machines, workshops and factories, in accordance with very inflexible rules. The *cybernetic* and *computing* automaton has been proliferating for the last forty years (in fact, since Ashby's homeostat, which was the first real modern autonomous machine), its definition sometimes becoming blurred by its links with neomechanisms endowed with at least semiautonomous intelligence or the ability to adapt, making it equivalent to a new kind of living creature. This sketchy typology ought also to make mention of the early calculating machines, a special group the benefits of which we are just beginning to receive; and the countless "bachelor machines" whose disconcerting, derisory ranks we owe to novelists, painters, sculptors, composers and directors. Finally, bringing the classification full circle, the living machine meets its mirror image, *live matter* (though the distance between them is small enough for some rational irrationality to revive their mutual rivalry), the atom of concentrated mechanicity inside the object, the golem, if you like – or, in a more profound way, the "eternal, unmoved, prime mover" that Aristotle puts at the center of both the universe and of his philosophy.

Technological Limit. So the automaton appears as a *sub-machine* which, depending on our fantasies and the logical way our reason works, connects up with the *super-machine*, often taking on its attributes, as if myth and technological utopia were conspiring in some osmosis of the "progressive image" and the "screen image." This nebula of dreams and visions is what provides the basis for technological development; it also enables us to understand how Heidegger's transmutation operates – how myth, under the pressure of social norms and relentless economic anxiety, becomes destiny and science, ideology or circumstantial discourse. A few more words about this "mutation": the conceptual displacement that turns myth into utopia, and what's more, gives rise to this seemingly inevitable positivistic doctrine, was not the result of underhand or malevolent wishes; it happened within what has to be called "active reason" – scientific, philosophical, cultural and historical reason (all victims of their own automatism, undermined by their systematic natures). The nineteenth-century experience of all the industrialized countries provides ample evidence of this transformation which was also the advent of a new age: the operation of the machine ethic, which is now the ethic of human beings, transformed desert islands of technicity into the social universe itself.

Automatic Language. As in the theory of general relativity, form and content cannot be treated separately; an automaton is not just a machine, it is also the language that makes it possible to explicate it. At a more general level, the automaton is the language that endows the people who are meant to know and communicate it with the privileges of totality which rational man thought he no longer had to confront. It is an experience devoid of rest, pity or distance; the limit of technology becomes the language of the techno-structure. The social and intellectual automaton nowadays makes up the "third type of world" we inhabit, a world in which the frontiers and the limits between body and mind, as well as those between nature and culture, and between life and death, have grown so thick, so enduring and so dense that when we look in the mirror each day we confront portraits of the living dead. These are the same ones that the simplest, most archaic automaton maintains at the heart of its myth, but which the anarchic yet rational development of technology has transformed into unfamiliar visions, rendered ghostly by their own presence.

The Classic Automaton. If we turn now to the "classic automaton," as it existed between the Renaissance and the latter part of the nineteenth century — when the industrial norm really established its hold over people — we find something apparently quite unassuming. Nonetheless, this automaton not only retains within it the myths of origin, which it preserves like a latent life, but it also clearly anticipates the utopias of the future. There are several general characteristics that we can apply to this group.

First, this automaton is a *mechanistic being*, and in this connection the Cartesian definition takes on its fullest sense: it acts by figure and motion, it is motion itself, the prime problem of physics, concentrated into exemplary machines. Here, as components, we find the simple machines of Galileo or Mersenne: balance, lathe, wheel, pulley, wedge, screw and so on. It is well adapted to structures of alternating or rotating movements and prepares the ground for the crank and connecting rod. Its mechanical skeleton is a living "encyclopedia" of the different mechanical pieces and of the machine parts available at the time.

Second, the automaton is basically a *mechanical individual*. It is often possible to discern some temptation toward group activity, of course, but not yet to such an extent as to affect its insularity. The combinations of instruments it presents are still visible, and its "character" still has an identity of its own. Moreover, this mechanical or technological individuality relates to the broader concept of the individual as it develops in philosophy from the Cartesian cogito to the "responsible man" of the Enlightenment.

Third, the automaton has *close links with living creatures* in all its different manifestations, but especially in relation to the medicine and physiology of the period. It dissects the living and imitates them sufficiently well to generate a gratifying illusion about its own nature; it proposes experimental protocols that link up with the old topics of the body, animals and man (compare Le Mettrie) as machines. It crops up wherever the awareness of man's physical functions becomes a pretext for investigating them and providing surgical prostheses – a precursor of organ transplants.

Fourth, as well as being a scientific individual, the automaton is also an *aesthetic* or more precisely, a *ludic* object. It simultaneously demonstrates and conceals the cunning artifice that makes it the supreme toy, and it also shares in the mathematical formalization of play. When dissection is complete, outward appearance reigns supreme and the automaton can make play of the ambiguities of the inside and outside of the body. Polished and powdered, it conjures up an image of Don Juan or Mozart (music being one of its favorite poles of attraction). Whether as entertainment for the great or as an illusion for the masses, it plays at denying its own trickery for the pleasure and pride of the spectators. As they watch, they admire themselves for being "philosophical" enough to suspend willingly their disbelief in what they know is the object's real nature; yet they also pretend to forget this suspension in order to share the great mysteries of the world with it. There are some sumptuous pretexts for artifice, especially in the eighteenth century.

Finally, at this period of history, as the world is somewhere being mapped and cataloged, the automaton represents a kind of primal mythology – not in terms of the old cosmicism, which Newton had done away with, but in relation to other secrets. The automaton achieves this through a *grasp of time* in which there is still some memory of the great era of monumental timepieces and Jacks of the clock. The automaton, as clock of the universe, is no longer happy making symbolic figures appear and strike the hour; rather, it keeps as its own mysterious secret the rudiments of a history of man and nature which emerges in the shadow of the science of space. The question of *primum mobile* persists in the problem of the origin and medium of forces. Even Newton did not solve this completely and the cunning automaton leaves a second way open for an overly pure rationality, the road that will be taken later, for example, by Hegel. This relationship between the automaton and time is probably the most important part of its originality; it is what separates the automaton from the machine that it, in fact, is, though it can never fully accept it.

Automatic Impressions. To illustrate this technological progress, I have chosen to present a sequence of images, one after another, like the damned in Dante's *Inferno* or assembly line workers waiting their turn. The automaton needs these slightly monotonous cohorts to express its temporality. So in fifteen or so images, with texts and linking notes, the automaton can march past, as if on parade, as the most effective way of expressing its properties at any given time. The order thus expressed is not a strictly chronological one, however, as the time thus displayed is neither that of the automata's origins nor necessarily that of their inevitable benefits. The automaton can still smile.

These are *automatic impressions*, images and texts to be read as a continuum, according to the "rule of suggestion" characteristic of the automata themselves; the reader must let himself or herself be taken over by the sequence of images and opinions, so that, at the end, the overall effect will enable him or her genuinely to share in this succinct genealogy and typology. Its purpose is to place the reader, if only temporarily, within the paradoxical logic of the technological object which plays endlessly at not being itself in order to assert more effectively its own identity.

Sharing in the trickery of the automaton is merely another way to define ourselves as human, that is, as both being and nothingness, presence and absence: the automaton is, in a way, our mirror...or our evil eye.

The Religious Automaton

The ancient temples of Egypt and Syria were, it is said, equipped with automatic mechanisms that controlled the opening of the doors, the sounding of trumpets and other "mysteries," like the aeolipyle of Alexandria.

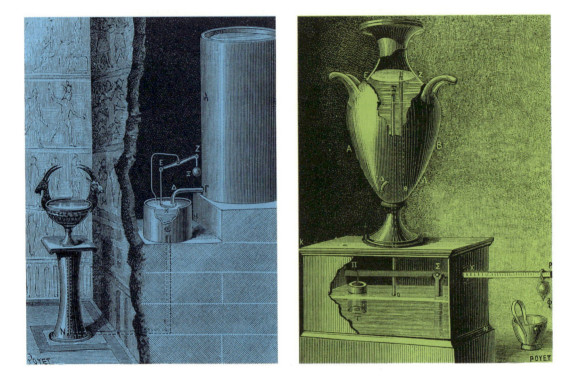

Figure 1: The amazing vase of Heron of Alexandria. No matter how much water is taken out of it, this vase always stays full.
Figure 2: Another amazing vase of Heron. Liquid flows according to the weight's movement.
From *La Nature*, 1883.

438

Sacred Time and Profane Time

There is a clear line from the music of the spheres to the sacred art of time. Medieval clocks with their Jacks (as at Strasbourg or Dijon) and clockmaking instruments mark a time when man had to know his place, including that of his death.

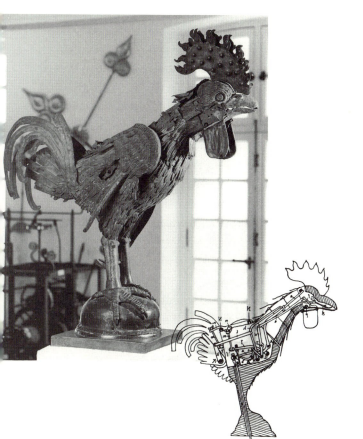

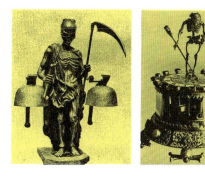

Figure 1: The cock from the astronomical clock in Strasbourg, 1354 (Strasbourg, Musée des Arts Décoratifs).
Figure 2: The mechanism of the Strasbourg cock. From A. Chapuis and E. Gélis, *Le monde des automates: Étude historique et technique* (Paris, 1928).
Figure 3: Death: one of the four stages of life as represented in the clock at the Cathedral of Strasbourg. From A. Chapuis and E. Gélis, *Le monde des automates: Étude historique et technique* (Paris, 1928).
Figure 4: A small clock from Augsburg, 1645. From A. Chapuis and E. Droz, *Les automates. Figures artificielles de l'homme et d'animaux* (Neuchâtel, 1949).

An Icarus myth for a less glorious reality?

It seems impossible to speak of Leonardo as a technician without at least mentioning the flying machine, which is at least equal to the *Mona Lisa*'s smile as a source of its author's fame. The fundamental idea of the engineer was that human flight is possible by a mechanical imitation of nature. It is exactly the same principle that Leonardo applied to the construction of textile machines: he had observed the workman at his task and had tried to reproduce mechanically movements into which the mind does not enter. Leonardo's first observations on the flight of birds led him to some important conclusions. Thus he notes that the kite "beats his wings moderately" and tries particularly to use air currents to keep him airborne. When he cannot find this support he replaces it by moving his wings more rapidly. When his wings are tired he can rest them by planning. We may say at the outset that the form of human flight envisaged by Leonardo was, in great part, what today we would call gliding. Observations then follow on wing positions, on the functions of feathers, whether they should be more or less open, on direction of flight which must be into the wind in order to rise. There is no doubt that the whole of this study is most remarkable.

The design for the machine itself certainly cannot be taken quite so seriously. For the wings he drew his inspiration from those of the bat, since these appeared to him to be the most logical and, no doubt, easier to create artificially than feathered wings. He then calculates the aerofoil required for given weights. It is easy to make similar calculations for birds: the wing of the pelican represents the square root of its weight. This analogy then led him to determine the shape of the wing, that is to say the ratios between length and width. The wing of the bat, which he took as a model, is not a rigid mechanism but is articulated....

The man must be placed vertically and move the wings with either his arms or his legs. The calculation of the force required was a much more difficult matter. Leonardo had come to the conclusion that a bird was a machine possessing superabundant power and that the availability of this power enabled it to attack and defend itself, which his flying man did not need to do.

There is no need to dwell upon a machine which has been abundantly reproduced and of which detailed studies have been made. Certainly there was some element of amazement in all these specifications which he gives on the materials to be used, on the probabilities of falling and on the means of escaping without injury. The idea was certainly not new and although mechanical reproduction of nature, which is the property of automata, had already been attempted, it is nevertheless true that Leonardo's observation was extraordinarily penetrating. (From B. Gille, *The Renaissance Engineers*, London: Lund Humphries, 1966, pp. 167-68.)

The baroque encyclopedist Father Athanasius Kircher made at least one invention, as recalled by Leibniz and Lully, which must rank as one of the most "cosmic" automata of all the strange machines ever dreamt.

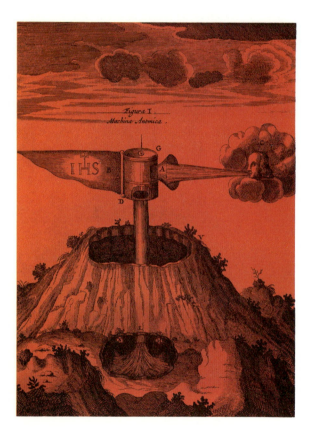

From *Mundus subterraneus*, 1664 (Paris, Bibliothèque nationale).

The First Prostheses

The idea itself was not new, but Ambroise Paré was the first to put it into practice. The "animal-machine" is born.

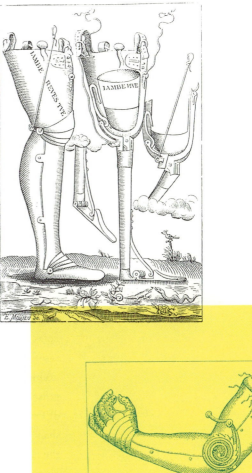

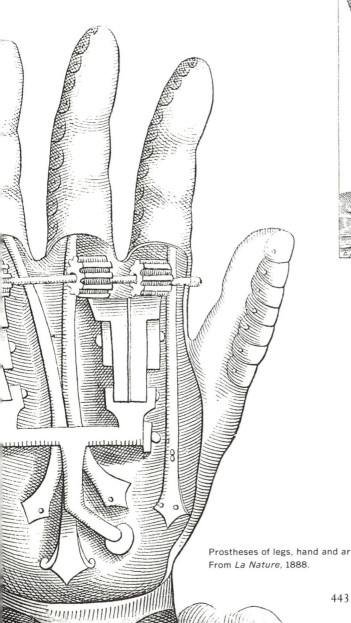

Prostheses of legs, hand and arm from the time of Ambroise Paré. From *La Nature*, 1888.

The opening words of Descartes's *Treatise of Man* are well-known: "I assume their body to be but a statue, an earthen machine formed intentionally by God to be as much as possible like us...." The following text, a letter from Descartes to Reneri for Pollot (April 1638), attempts to define the issue in more detail, without in any way simplifying it.

> Most of the actions of animals resemble ours, and throughout our lives this has given us many occasions to judge that they act by an interior principle like the one within ourselves, that is to say, by means of a soul which has feelings and passions like ours. All of us are deeply imbued with this opinion by nature. Whatever reasons there may be for denying it, it is hard to say publicly how the case stands without exposing oneself to the ridicule of children and feeble minds. But those who want to discover truth must distrust opinions rashly acquired in childhood. To make the right judgment about this, it seems to me, we must consider the following. Suppose that a man had been brought up all his life in some place where he had never seen any animals except men; and suppose that he was very devoted to the study of mechanics, and had made, or helped to make, various automata shaped like a man, a horse, a dog, a bird and so on, which walked, and ate, and breathed, and so far as possible imitated all the other actions of the animals they resembled, including the signs we use to express our passions, like crying when struck and running away when subjected to a loud noise. Suppose that sometimes he found it impossible to tell the difference between the real men and those which had only the shape of men, and had learned by experience that there were only the two ways of telling them apart which I explained [in] my *Discourse on Method*: first, that these automata never answered in word or sign, except by chance, to questions put to them; and second, that though their movements were often more regular and certain than those of the wisest men, yet in many things which they would have to do to imitate us, they failed more disastrously than the greatest fools. Now, I say, you must consider what would be the judgment of such a man when he saw the animals we have; especially if he was gifted with the knowledge of God, or at least had noticed how inferior is the best skill shown by men in their

artifacts when compared with that shown by nature in the composition of plants. Nature has packed plants with an infinity of tiny invisible ducts to convey certain liquids in such a way as to form leaves and flowers and fruits. Let us suppose that our man had noticed this, and so believed firmly that if there were automata made by God or nature to imitate our actions, they would imitate them more perfectly, and be incomparably more skillfully constructed than any which could be invented by men. Now suppose that this man were to see the animals we have, and noticed in their actions the same two things which make them differ from us, and which he had already been accustomed to notice in his automata. There is no doubt that he would not come to the conclusion that there was any real feeling or emotion in them, but would think they were automata, which, being made by nature, were incomparably more accomplished than any of those he had previously made himself. It only remains to consider whether the verdict he would give, with knowledge of the facts and unprejudiced by any false opinion, would be less credible than the one we made when we were children and have kept only through habit. We base our judgment solely on the resemblance between some exterior actions of animals and our own; but this is not at all a sufficient basis to prove that there is any resemblance between the corresponding interior actions.

Medicalized Man

Whether as machine-man or as human-machine, man does not emerge from surgery unscathed, as this plate from Diderot's *Encyclopedia* testifies.

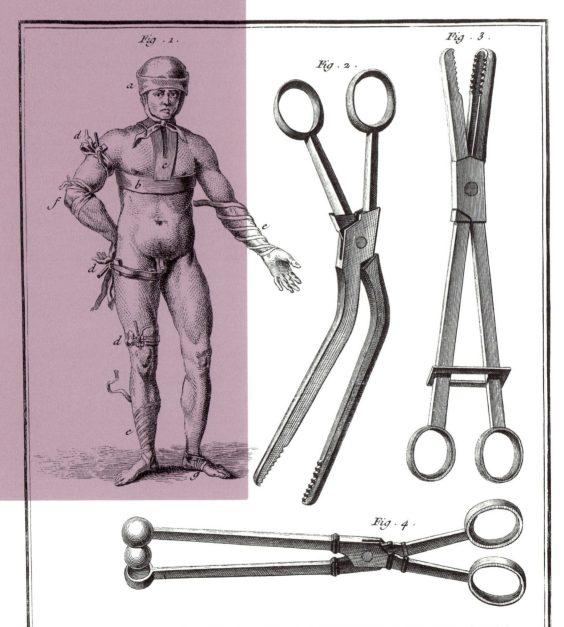

From Diderot and D'Alembert, *L'Encyclopédie ou Dictionnaire raisonné des sciences, des arts et des métiers*, 1763.

The *Encyclopedia*: An Automaton at Home

As a cultural automaton, the *Encyclopedia* can be seen as a total and systematic machine, characterized by an optimism as yet untainted by Borgesian anxieties. At this point, the imagined model is a house devoted to the pleasure of the lover of knowledge. Is this a laughable automaton, or is it, in a sense, an early sort of personal computer?

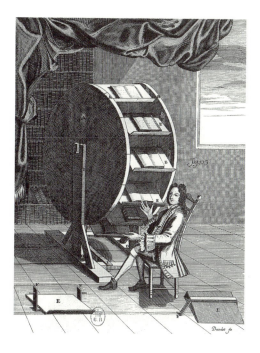

A peculiar and practical desk for scholars.
From Nicolas Grollier de Servière, *Recueil d'ouvrages curieux de mathématique et de mécanique* (Lyon, 1719).

How far can the Cartesian argument be taken? That is the question D'Alembert poses in this extract from the *Encyclopedia*. It is not just a philosophical question, for it encompasses a much broader problem which includes the language of beasts and that of human beings (as Condillac and Rousseau also understood).

Descartes is, therefore, the leading chief in this doctrine; conducted by his profound meditations to deny the beasts having a soul; to which paradox he gave an extraordinary vogue in the world. He probably would never have given into this opinion, if not impelled thereto by the unquestionable truth of a distinction between soul and body; to which distinction he first gave its greatest lustre, and by means of the then generally prevailing prejudice against beasts having a soul.

The doctrine of machines defeated two great objections; one, against the immortality of their souls; and the other, against the goodness of God: but from the moment that we adopt the system of automata, these two difficulties vanish; yet the abettors of it were not aware, that several others took their rise from it. Let it however be observed, that the philosophy of Descartes, notwithstanding all his enemies have uttered against it, tended always to the advantage of religion; and his hypothesis of the brute creation being no more than machinery, is a proof.

The Cartesian system hath always triumphed, whilst it had only to combat with the material souls of Aristotle, those incomplete substances deduced from the power of matter, to constitute therewith a knowing and thinking substance in beasts. But these chimerical entities of the schools have been so effectually defeated, that it is believed nobody will be in a hurry to revive them; because such phantoms could never stand the enquiry of an enlightened age like ours: for if there were not a medium between them and the automata of Descartes, we should be obliged to admit the latter.

Since the time of Descartes, a third party has luckily started into existence; by which all the ridicule of the automatic system has been displayed; and for which discovery we are obliged to the more accurate ideas that have been conceived about the intellectual world: whence it was established, that the system of the universe is more extensive than commonly believed, and contains several other sorts of inhabitants, besides angels and human souls; an ample resource for philosophers to fiddle off to, wherever the mechanical explanations stop short, and particularly where the actions of brutes are to be accounted for....

No inference can give a juster idea of Descartes's doctrine of automata, than Mr. Regis's comparison of some hydraulic machines, to be seen in certain grottos and fountains, that serve as ornaments to the splendid mansions of the great; where the water exerts itself by the disposition of the pipes, and some exterior pressure, by which means the machinery is put into motion. He compares the pipes of these fountains to the nerves, and the tendons, muscles, etc. to the other springs of motion that belong to the machinery; as, for instance, the animal spirits to the water, that communicates the first impulse of motion; the heart, to its source; and the cavities of the brain, to its reservoirs. The exterior objects, that by their presence act upon the organs of sense in animals, he compares to the strangers entering into a grotto, and who, according to the different prepared parts of the flooring, put certain figures, that have a correspondence therewith, into action: if they move towards Diana, she runs away, and plunges into a fountain; but if they proceed farther, Neptune advances with a menacing look, and a trident in his hand.

We may also, according to this system, compare animals to those organs that play several tunes by the movements given to them by water only. There may, add the Cartesians, be a particular organization in animals, agreeable to the supreme and creative will, and diversifiable in each different species, but always proportioned to the objects, having ever in view the great end of preserving the individual, and the species: and nothing could be more easy than such a disposition of things to the Omnipotent, that both intimately and perfectly knows the nature and tendency of all created beings. The establishment of such a correspondence and harmony could not oppose the least difficulty or trouble to his wisdom and power. The very idea of such an harmonizing plan is great, and worthy of the Deity; which alone, say the Cartesians, ought to gain over, accustom, and familiarise a philosophic mind to these paradoxes, at which vulgar prejudice takes so much offence, and gives so great an air of ridicule to the doctrine of Descartes on the present subject....

It is then in vain, Cartesians, that ye so often advance the vague idea of mechanism's possibilities that are unknown, and which neither ye can express, nor we conceive; yet that ye assert to be the primordial source, and the original cause, of all the phaenomena observable in animals. But we have a clear idea of quite another cause, which is, the idea of a sensitive principle, and that we perceive to have very distinct relations with all the phaenomena in question; satisfactorily explaining, and universally combining, all the different phaenomena.

Every one of us perceives, that our soul, in quality of this sensitive principle, produces a thousand different actions, and moves our bodies in a thousand different ways; and not unlike to those with which we see animals are actuated in similar circumstances. When we have allowed such a principle to reside in animals, we see the reason in the cause of all the movements which they make for the preservation of their machine: we know why a dog withdraws his foot from the fire when it burns him; why a dog yells when he is smitten; etc. But were this principle to be taken away, we can no longer perceive any reason, or any simple and only cause of all these actions. Wherefore we conclude, that in animals there is a sensitive principle; because the Deity is not a deceiver, and that he would be such, in case animals were mere machines; because he would exhibit to us a multitude of phaenomena, whence necessarily must result, in my mind, the idea of a cause, that at the same time cannot be: therefore the very same reasons, which directly show us an intelligent soul in every man, assure us also, that there is something more than matter, an intellectual principle, in animals.

But, to push this argument still farther, in order to comprehend its force the better, let us suppose, just for argument sake, an innate disposition in the machine, whence all these surprising operations arise: nay, let us even say, we believe it to be congruous with divine wisdom, to produce a machine that may be sufficient for its own preservation, because it inwardly possesses, through

450

virtue of its admirable organization, the principles of all the movements that concur to its being preserved. We now ask, What good purpose can be answered by such a machine? Wherefore was this wonderful apparatus of springs contrived? Wherefore are they endowed with organs so like to those of ourselves? Wherefore have they eyes, ears, nostrils, and a brain? It may be answered, that they may regulate the movements of the automata, by the different impressions which they receive from the exterior objects. But to what purpose all this? Why, to preserve the machine. But again, suppose this question were put: To what useful end, in this world, could machines be contributing, which can preserve themselves? The immediate answer given is, It is not our business to penetrate into the secret views of the Creator; or to scrutinise the ends which he assigns to himself in each of his works. But if he should manifestly discover his views to us, and by speaking signs, is it not consonant to reason, that we should gratefully acknowledge them? Have we not reason to say, that the ears are made to hear, and the eyes to see? that the fruits of the earth are destined for the nourishment of man? that air is necessary for the enjoyment of life, because the circulation of the blood could not be carried on without its pressure and influence? Can it be supposed, that the different parts of an animal's body were meant by the Creator for any other use, besides that which general experience hath indicated to us?

But to insist a little longer on this subject. The organs of our senses, which have been modelled by so wise an artificer, can be formed for no other purpose, comformable to the Creator's design, but to be capable of those sensations that are exerted in the soul through their mediation. Can it be doubted, that the body is made for the soul, to serve it as a principle of sensation, and be the instrument of its action? If this notion be true in regard to man, why is it not so in regard to animals? In the machinery of animals we discover a wise purpose, very worthy of the Deity, and verified by experience in all similar cases; which is to be united to a spiritual principle, and to serve it as a source of perception and an instrument of action. Therein appears an unity of end, to which is referred that prodigious combination of multiform springs, that compose an organised body. Take away this end; object to this intellectual principle, that feels through the machine, acts upon the machine and tends incessantly, through a motive of self-interest, to its preservation; I cannot see any purpose for which so admirable a work should have been contrived.

A machine like this ought to have been made for some end distinct from itself; because it is no more made for itself, than the wheels of a clock are made for it. Let it not be replied here, that a clock being made to mark the hours, its principal end is to furnish a just measure of time to mankind; and that the same may be said of animals, that they are machines constructed by the creator for the use of human beings. There would be a great error in such a sentiment; because there should be a careful distinction made between the accessary, and, as we may say, foreign uses of things, and their principal, their primary ends.

Besides, what a number of animals are there among the brute creation, from which man derives no manner of advantage! such as the savage beasts, insects, all those animalcula living in the air, the water, and that prey in crowds upon the surfaces of other bodies. The animals that prove subservient to man, are so but through accident. It is he, indeed, who breaks, who tames, who trains them up, and renders them pliantly obedient to all his purposes. We make use of dogs and horses for the removing, or the supplying of our wants, just as we make use of the wind to impel our ships upon the sea, and on land to turn our mills. It would be a very erroneous conclusion to affirm, that the natural use of the wind, and the chief end proposed for it by the Deity, in creating this meteor, was either to turn mills, or facilitate navigation. How much juster would that opinion be, that should assert, the use of the wind is to purify and freshen the air!

Now let us apply this to our subject. A clock is made to shew the hours, and for no other intent: the many different pieces, of which it is formed, are necessary to this end; in which too they all concur. But is there any proportion of comparison to be made between it, and the delicacy, the variety, and the multiplicity of organs in animal bodies, and the uses to which they are converted to by us? and those too in not many different species, and even among them but of the smallest part.

A clock is made for an end distinct from itself. But if we apply ourselves to contemplate animals, inspect their actions, and reconnoitre them in their natural state, while they are uncontrouled by the usurped authority of man, and that they are not industriously reduced to administer to our wants, and our capriciousness, they are entirely occupied by no other care but that of their preservation. How! that of the machine? cry those on the other side of the question: this answer does not satisfy us; mere matter cannot be the sole end of its formation; much less then can it be asserted of a portion of organized matter.

Therefore, the arrangement of a material being is made for some other end besides itself, and the sole conservation of its machine: though even this principle should be inherent in the very machinery, it must be the means, but not the end; and the more exquisite would it prove, the more of art discovered therein; and the more should I feel myself, in consequence, obliged to have recourse to something extraneous to the machine; that is, to some simple essence, for whose use this arrangement of matter was made, and with whose machinality is interwoven a connexion of obedience, for their mutual utility. Thus the ideas which we have of the truth and wisdom of the Deity, lead us directly to this general conclusion, which we may henceforward look upon as certain: Beasts, or animals, have an intellectual principle united to their machines, made purposely for them, as ours is made for us, and receive from it a variety of sensations, that make them perform actions which surprise us, through the different directions impressed by it on the moving powers of the machine. (From Diderot and D'Alembert, *Select Essays from the Encyclopedy*, London, 1772, pp. 148-69.)

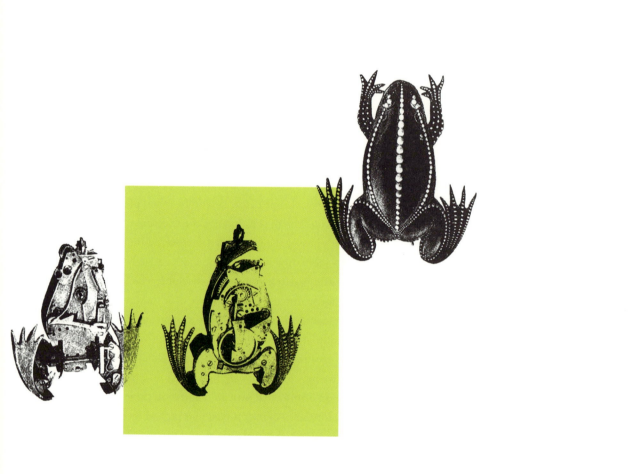
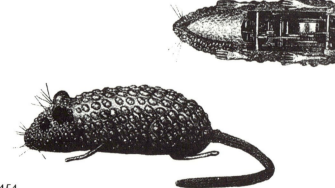

Some Mechanical Animals

Who can say whether these are experiments or toys? The automaton always occupies a relatively undefined position, as these clockwork animals — museum and collectors' pieces — clearly show. The mystery is more thinly spread, but it has not yet vanished altogether.

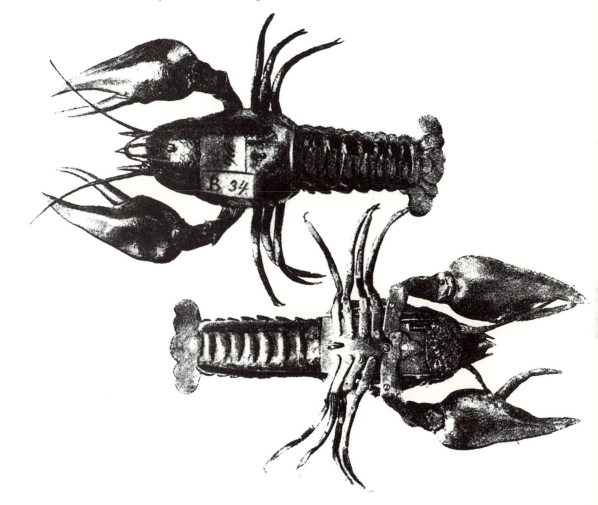

A mechanical mouse, frog and crawfish. From Chapuis and Gélis, *Le monde des automates.*

Vaucanson's Duck

Of all the contradictory fauna of mechanical animals, still unsystemized by a Buffon or a Linnaeus, the most outstanding was beyond doubt Vaucanson's Duck; Vaucanson intended to follow it with larger projects (such as an artificial man), but these never saw the light of day.

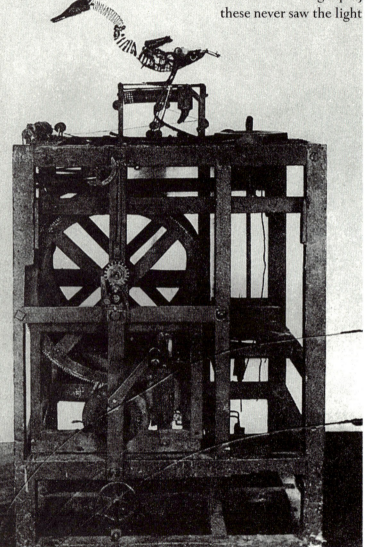

Figure 1: Device of the duck attributed to Vaucanson: the structure, weights, motor wheelwork.
Figure 2: Detail of the duck.
From Chapuis and Droz, *Les automates*.

Vaucanson: Engineer of Genius

Vaucanson was a doctor and later a factory owner, as well as an engineer. He applied his talents to textile machinery, and set up factories at Aubenas and Romans, but was not successful. It is perhaps more in keeping with the period to quote Voltaire's laudatory remarks.

> Monsieur Vaucanson is well-known for his various automatic machines, which have deservedly won for him the approbation of the Académie Royale des Sciences, and the applause of the Paris public; he has now come to this city, and Monsieur le Directeur has permitted him to be present at this session where he has shared with the Académie his plan to create an automatic figure whose motions will be an imitation of all animal operations, such as the circulation of the blood, respiration, digestion, the movement of muscles, tendons, nerves and so forth. He claims that by using this automaton we shall be able to carry out experiments on animal functions, and to draw conclusions from them which will allow us to recognize the different states of human health, in order to remedy his ills. This ingenious machine, by representing a human body, will be able to be used eventually for demonstration purposes in anatomy courses. (From *Registre contenant le Journal des Conférences de l'Académie de Lyon*, quoted in A. Doyon and L. Liaigre, *Jacques Vaucanson, mécanicien de génie*, Paris, 1966, p. 148.)

Mechanical Animals in the Salon

With the growth of illusionism, dollhouses, collections and exhibitions of surprising and graceful movement, from the salons of the eighteenth century to the soirées of the Second Empire, the automaton becomes a "character." Even more fascinating are the "animated tableaux," like this tableau of monkey-musicians, which certainly seems a far cry from mechanical tortoises.

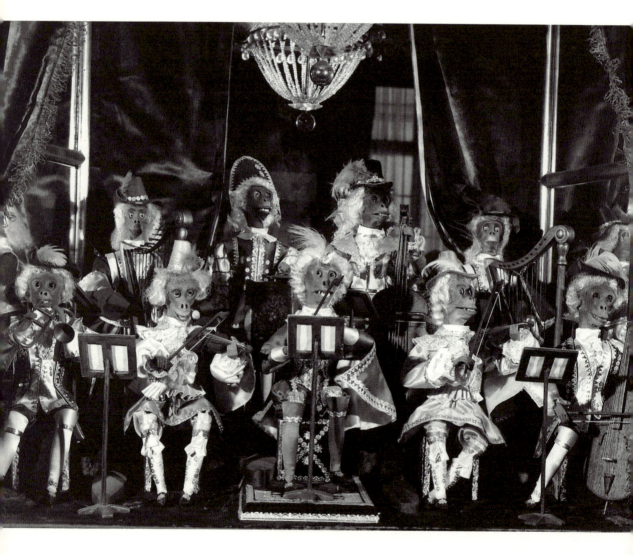

From Musée National de Monaco.

The Writing Automaton

Like clockmaking, with which it has many affinities, the tradition of constructing automata seems frequently to have found refuge in Switzerland. There are numerous minor masterpieces in the museum at Neuchâtel, prominent among them the *Harpsichord Player* and the *Writer of Jacquet-Droz*. The automaton is also a mirror of childhood.

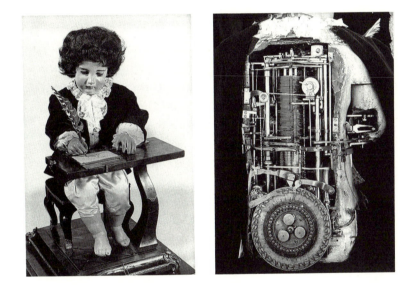

From Musée d'Art et d'Histoire, Neuchâtel.

Although copying bodies is fine, copying the mind is better. There is a degree of magic, perhaps even of satanism, in such projects: but, in any event, their history is edifying.

In the seventeenth century, Pascal and Leibniz designed machines to perform fixed operations (addition and multiplication). These machines had no memory, however, and were not, in modern parlance, programmable.

The first human to conceive of the immense computing potential of machinery was the Londoner Charles Babbage (1792-1871). A character who could almost have stepped out of the pages of the *Pickwick Papers*, Babbage was most famous during his lifetime for his vigorous campaign to rid London of "street nuisances" — organ grinders above all. These pests, loving to get his goat, would come and serenade him at any time of the day or night, and he would furiously chase them down the street. Today, we recognize in Babbage a man a hundred years ahead of his time: not only inventor of the basic principles of modern computers, he was also one of the first to battle noise pollution.

His first machine, the "Difference Engine," could generate mathematical tables of many kinds by the "method of differences." But before any model of the "D.E." had been built, Babbage became obsessed with a much more revolutionary idea: his "Analytical Engine." Rather immodestly, he wrote, "The course through which I arrived at it was the most entangled and perplexed which probably ever occupied the human mind." Unlike any previously designed machine, the "A.E." was to possess both a "store" (memory) and a "mill" (calculating and decision-making unit). These units were to be built of thousands of intricate geared cylinders interlocked in incredibly complex ways. Babbage had a vision of numbers swirling in and out of the mill under control of a *program* contained in punched cards — an idea inspired by the Jacquard loom, a card-controlled loom that wove amazingly complex patterns. Babbage's brilliant but ill-fated Countess friend, Lady Ada Lovelace (daughter of Lord Byron), poetically commented that "the Analytical Engine *weaves algebraic patterns* just as the Jacquard-loom weaves flowers and leaves." Unfortunately, her use of the present tense was misleading, for no "A.E." was ever built, and Babbage died a bitterly disappointed man.

Lady Lovelace, no less than Babbage, was profoundly aware that with the invention of the Analytical Engine, mankind was flirting with mechanized intelligence — particularly if the Engine were capable of "eating its own tail" (the way Babbage described the Strange Loop created when a machine reaches in and alters its own stored program). In an 1842 memoir, she wrote that the "A.E." "might act upon other things besides *number*." While Babbage dreamt of creating a chess or tic-tac-toe automaton, she suggested that his Engine, with pitches and harmonies coded into its spinning cylinders, "might compose elaborate and scientific pieces of music of any degree of complexity or extent." In nearly the same breath, however, she cautions that "The Analytical Engine has no pretensions whatever to *originate* anything. It can do whatever we *know how to order it* to perform." Though she well understood the power of artificial computations, Lady Lovelace was skeptical about the artificial creation of intelligence. However, could her keen insight allow her to dream of the potential that would be opened up with the taming of electricity?

In our century the time was ripe for computers — computers beyond the wildest dreams of Pascal, Leibniz, Babbage, or Lady Lovelace. In the 1930s and 1940s, the first "giant electronic brains" were designed and built. They catalyzed the convergence of three previously disparate areas: the theory of axiomatic reasoning, the study of mechanical computation, and the psychology of intelligence. (From D. Hofstadter, *Gödel, Escher, Bach: An Eternal Golden Braid*, New York: Basic, 1979, pp. 24-25.)

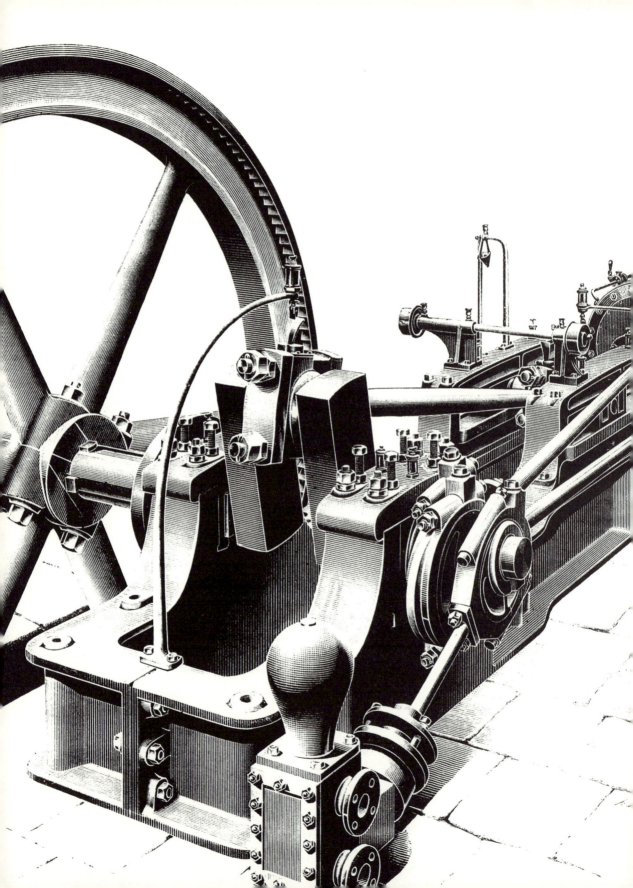

Weaving and the Beginnings of Industrial Automatism

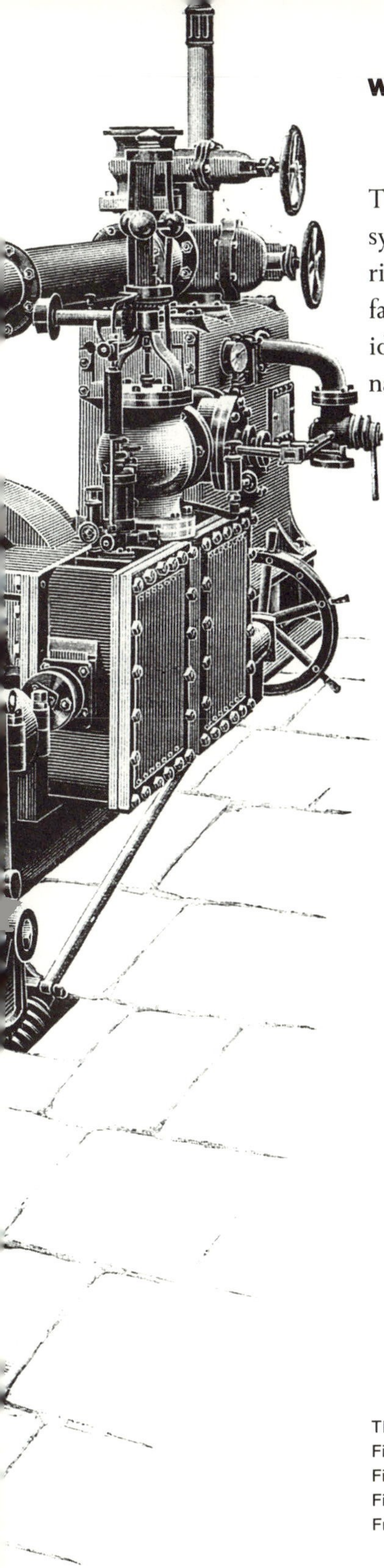

The threads are woven and rolled like language or mathematical symbols. Vaucanson, the inventor of a loom for brocaded material, tried to introduce automation into a small number of factories. When the Industrial Revolution got under way, the idea was taken up again and those looms or métiers gave their name to the first "real" machine-tools. The mutation had begun.

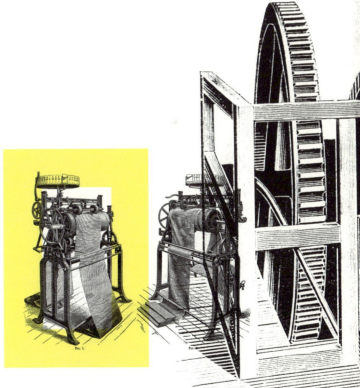

Three textile machines:
Figure 1: Horizontal engine for driving a rolling mill. From *Engineering*, 1892.
Figure 2: Cloth-measuring machine. From *Engineering*, 1893.
Figure 3: 100 horse-power main and tail rope electric haulage plant.
From *Engineering*, 1881.

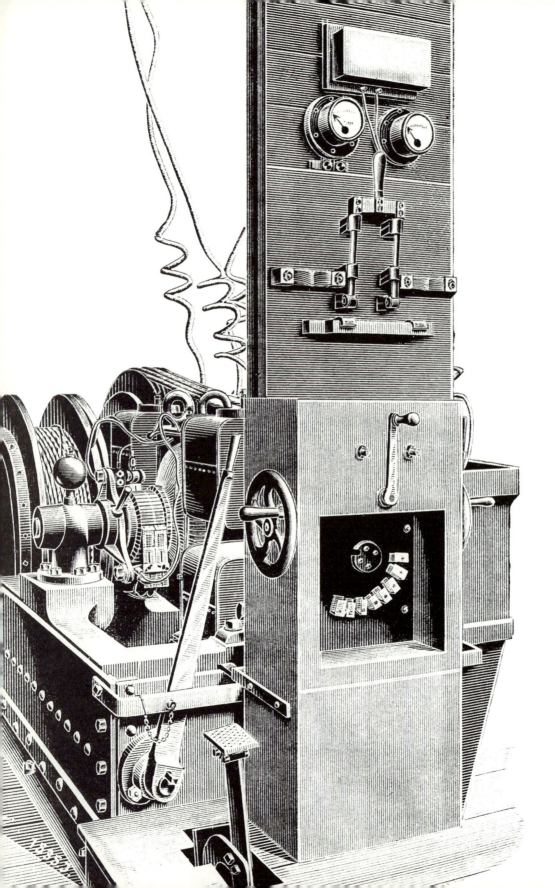

Factories did not spring up from nowhere: they developed from the need to coordinate actions, and from more or less explicit overall "automatization." This eighteenth-century factory has not yet reached its final form, but it's on the way there.

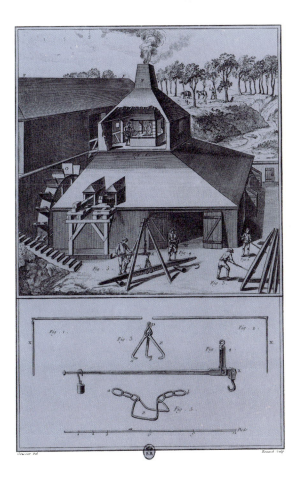

From Diderot and D'Alembert, *L'Encyclopédie*, 1763.

465

Automatism as a general efficient principle. Its consequences
for the world of labor are, of course, well known, but it also
affected human existence in a much more general way. Can this
all be attributed to the same automatism, and can we still talk
about "automata"?

Automation only became a new problem when it enabled the
integration of an autonomous operational cycle, involving definite
logical coherence, extended to all aspects of economic life as
manifested in any factory in all branches of industry.

In this perspective, therefore, it is not technology as such
which has direct social and psychological effects, so much as technology to the extent that it already finds expression in certain
social and economic relations – in a "context" to put it crudely.
The direct relationship between technology and individual psychology is almost always anecdotal, and cannot have any broad
social meaning. An isolated inventor can perfect a machine that
has particular effects on anybody working it, but to talk about
social effects, the machine must have come into general use,
imposed upon everybody by competition and progress and some
criterion of the society's general technological level. Vaucanson's
automaton had no social effects; the assembly line and the computer did, and on a very large scale.

What happened was that *automatism* ceased to be a *rare technological combination* and became a *general operational principle*. In
that sense, it plays a similar role to thermal energy, when its use
became widespread: the steam engine stopped being a novelty or a
curiosity and became the principle underlying the whole of industry; similarly, automation is not a rare and beneficial technical
process any longer, having become instead a generalized element
that defines the technical level of the whole of social production.
It is in this regard that we can speak of the social effects it brings
with it.

Descriptions of machinery, scientific laws and operating techniques provide direct knowledge about automation seen in this
way, but they do not provide a social explanation of it, as machinery,
even when it has been programmed to function automatically, it
is only used if its creators, its owners and its "managers" have

466

decided it should be. And they only decide that when there are pressing economic reasons, and the wherewithal to satisfy them, including disposable capital, trained personnel, the prospect of fairly long-term returns, a market to defend or new markets to capture, increased productivity, a decrease in the relative volume of wages or a need to maintain prestige.

Thus, the social and economic aspects of automation cannot be seen as direct consequences of the technological conditions for its introduction, any more than the social context for the expansion of thermal or electrical energy can be explained solely in terms of the scientific and technological nature of steam engines and electric motors. The development of automated production and management can only be explained in relation to preexisting social and economic structures. (From P. Naville, *Vers l'automatisme social?*, Paris, 1963, pp. 46-47.)

Today we are all aware of the importance of the agro-food sector, but the idea of automating it (in contrast with genetic planning) is not a recent one. The following machine is evidence of this and takes us to the edge of another kind of fantasy.

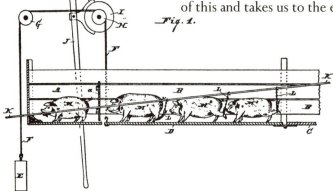

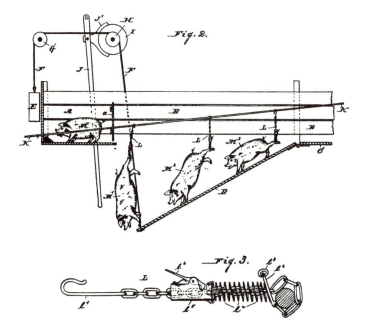

117. Apparatus for Catching and Suspending Hogs. 1882. *Here the living animal must be introduced into the 'disassembly' line. From the 1870's on when stunning was found too slow, devices were proposed to hoist the hog to the overhead rail without struggle:* 'The hog M acts as a decoy for the others, and much time and labor are thus saved. The brake is manipulated to allow the trap D to slowly descend until the hogs are completely suspended, when they slide off on the bar K to the place where they are to be killed.' (U. S. Patent 252,112, 10 January 1882)

From S. Geidion, *Mechanization Takes Command* (New York, 1948).

zone

How far can the imitation of human action and behavior be taken? Cohen's intriguing speculations require some thought:

It would seem that at least three things characteristically human are out of reach of contemporary automata. In the first place, they are incapable of laughter (or tears); secondly, they do not blush; thirdly, they do not commit suicide. It is conceivable that robots of the future may be capable of all three. However, until we have a better understanding of the nature of laughter it would be unwise to assume that we shall be able to teach robots how to laugh. The problem is rendered more complex by the fact that there seems to be a double relationship between the laughable and the automatic. We laugh when we see a human being behave like an automaton, if a speaker, for example, moves his head in a tic-like, stereotyped fashion. The appearance of mechanism where we expect life provokes laughter. And conversely we laugh when a true robot behaves like a man, and the closer the resemblance the more comical we find the situation. It is a little hard to imagine a true robot laughing because another true robot seems lifelike or, alternatively, because its designer appears to conduct himself like a fellow robot.

Blushing may not turn out to be much more manageable although both the anatomical and the psychological processes involved in blushing are fairly clear. The reader may wonder why blushing rather than other features of man is highlighted here. The answer is that blushing seems a singularly human phenomenon. It belongs to the expressive language of the human face. Its anatomical basis is an intricate system of capillaries which line the inner walls of the cheeks and which have a network of nerve fibres to serve them. This capillary action is the means of making our private feelings visible to an observer, for they make the blush possible. Monkeys flush in anger but they cannot be said to blush in shame. Perhaps the transition from flush to blush constitutes the dividing line between man and animal. Darwin called blushing "the most wondrous of all the wondrous powers of the mind . . . and the most human of all expressions." We blush when we feel exposed, physically or mentally, when we have been unmasked, when we have made what others see is a stupid mistake, when caught red-handed, when wrongly accused. We blush when we merely think about what someone else is thinking of what we are thinking. The common factor in these various situations is that we feel ourselves caught in an impasse. We cannot for the moment find a way out; so there is nothing to do but to blush. The blush is an outward manifestation of what subjectively is experienced as shame in the presence of others, and it takes place in the face because our experience of being in the presence of others is somehow localized in the face, which is that part of us offered for public display. But we do not only blush for shame. Darwin remarked that a pretty girl blushes when a boy gazes at her even though she knows perfectly well that his gaze is one of admiration. Her blush draws attention to herself while enhancing her charms.

As Buytendijk has remarked, with his customary shrewdness, girls blush more than boys because the significance of exposure is not the same for them as it is for boys. And this is due to the fact that a girl's relationship to her body differs from a boy's relationship to his, just as her relationships to other people are different from his. The adolescent girl, unlike her brother, feels her relationship to others mediated through her body, and particularly through her clothes, which serve the ambiguous purpose of covering and revealing at one and the same time. Adolescence, furthermore, is a phase when girls are more sensitive than ever to their appearance. The merest glance can provoke a blush, and the girl feels helpless, as if her protective covering had been torn aside.

In the light of this, we cannot now foresee how a future computer could be programmed to blush in suitable embarrassing circumstances, and we have to bear in mind that it is just as human not to blush when we should as to blush when we shouldn't.

Thirdly, suicide on the part of any future robot may have to be ruled out. A robot may be endowed with the capacity to bring about its own disorganization when conditions reach a given threshold of stress. But true suicide implies a foreknowledge of death and some idea of its significance, and this is a privilege of man.

In general, whatever refinements and novelties are introduced

470

into artefacts in the forseeable future, man is destined to remain for a very long time, the lightest, most reliable, most cheaply serviced and the most versatile general-purpose computing device made in large quantities by unskilled labour. (From J. Cohen, *Human Robots in Myth and Science*, London: George Allen and Unwin, 1966, pp. 137-39.)

A Famous Turk

zone

While it might well be objected that this reproduction is not famous, one cannot entirely avoid Maelzen's and Von Kempelen's chess-player, as analyzed by Edgar Allan Poe. And the reason why the analysis so effectively reveals the trickery is partly because Poe's reasoning is, in a sense, "machine-like," reminiscent of the kind of machines you find nowadays in every part of the office.

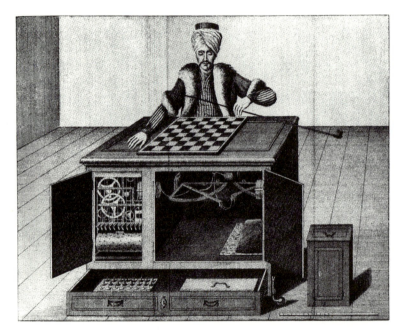

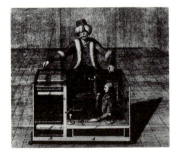

Figure 1: The chess player made by Von Kempelen showing its false machinery.
Figure 2: The accomplice hidden in the automaton.
From Chapuis and Droz, *Les automates*.

The Swimmer

This provides a somewhat more ironic note, before we conclude. Da Vinci, as we have seen, dreamed of a flying man. But
this curious mixture of swimmer and machine is, in its way,
almost moving. It could have been invented by Captain Nemo.
However, it would surely go faster if it had the webbed feet of
Vaucanson's duck.

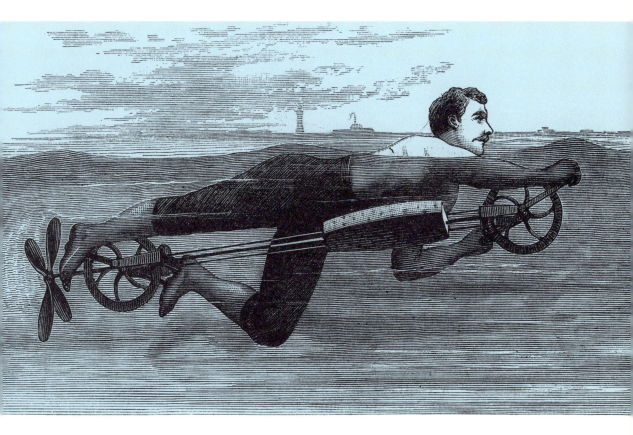

From *La Nature*, 1880.

The Pleasure of Ambiguity

By the mid-nineteenth century it is no longer Poe but his friend
Baudelaire who is addressing the question of the automaton, as
a being symbolizing the limits of the world, and André Pieyre
de Mandiargues draws a pleasing lesson from this:

> An automaton is an artificial representation of a human being, or
> an animal or a natural object, mechanically endowed with the
> power of movement. An android, which is a simulacrum of a man
> or a woman that has every appearance of being alive, ought – at
> least in theory – to be more accomplished than an automaton, and
> to deliver a more perfect imitation of its model. It is a question of
> language, of course, but androids belong more in the realm of
> magic, and automata in the realm of play and theater, where
> artifice rules. It is therefore quite right to be less concerned with
> the first, being more or less an ideal vision of the mind, than with
> the second. Yet there are a few questions which we ought to
> consider, nonetheless.

> As soon as we start talking about nature and artifice I find
> myself thinking of Baudelaire, whose entire work is divided between
> those two extremes. And there are a number of ways, it seems to
> me, in which automata relate to Baudelaire's world. That is what
> interests me most about them, that and the dandyism I perceive in
> collectors and enthusiasts. In fact, I think that what those people
> are looking for is not so much an accurate imitation of life as a
> kind of mask, a pretense which leans toward mockery, almost a
> brilliant joke produced at the expense of life, as the theater often
> is for theater-lovers. In Baudelaire's world the dandy loves the
> actress and the prostitute because they are both radically different
> from the natural woman, and not only in their costume and
> makeup. In *L'Eve future*, Villiers de l'Isle Adam describes a mechani-
> cal woman, an android, who has become the ideal woman for one
> extreme dandy, the only one he can tolerate. In fantasies of this
> sort, which are hard to imagine outside the context of "spleen,"
> luxury is extremely important. The automaton, likewise, has to be
> seen as a luxury plaything, quite as suitable to entertain fortune's
> favorites as to provide a moment's wonder for the underprivileged.
> The automaton is a thing of illusion, and its proper place should be
> a house of illusions. Baudelaire, who of course wrote a short *Morale*

du jouet, might easily have been inspired to write an essay on it.

Also, one of the main sources of pleasure in watching automata is the repetition of movement, something that man himself lacks, though one does find it in actors and soldiers on the parade ground. Yet the latter, men who have been turned into machines, are in fact as much the reverse of automata, which are machines in human form, as they are similar to them. And the word "automaton" contains a contradiction, because it applies both to spontaneity of movement and to the mechanization of it. Thus we come back to the idea of ambiguity and the light it casts on the strange spell automata exercise over us.

There is much more that could be said about the unsettling delight man takes in knowing full well that he is being deceived.... A fondness for automata is not such an innocent pleasure as it seems, even though there are no laws or religious prohibitions against it. If I carried on with this train of thought, it would not be long before I was back with Baudelaire again. (From André Pieyre de Mandiargues, *Les rouages de l'automate*, preface to Prasteau, *Les automates*, pp. 5-6.)

Electrified Madness

Doctors at the Salpetrière in the 1880s were just as much mechanists as they are today. But instead of scanners they used electric helmets to set vagabonds, "walking automata" and all kinds of neurotics back on the straight and narrow. Charcot seems to have given electrical treatment to 180 people per session. It is understandable that their descendants have "chosen health."

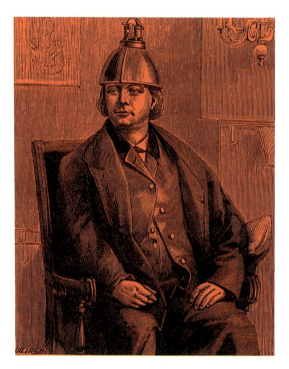

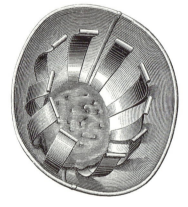

Figure 1: A vibrating helmet used for the curing of nervous disorders.
Figure 2: Inside view of the vibrating helmet.
From *La Nature*, 1892.

Waiting for the Sequel

Automatism also inspired military engineers, of course. Very early in the twentieth century armaments became vastly more rapid and more mobile. Like revolvers, they became automatic. We know the rest.

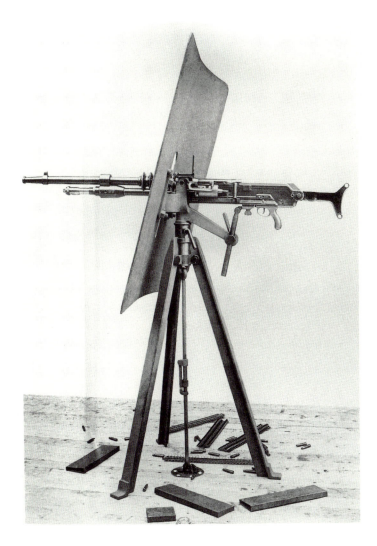

From *Catalogue du matériel de guerre*, Hotchkiss, 1900. Collection of the Institut J.-B. Dumay.

Parade's End. The procession has to come to an end. But the changes initiated by the all-powerful industrial era came about gradually, stage by stage. The classical automaton survives into the nineteenth century, although by then it has become a curiosity or a museum piece. But it is about to have to change, if not in its nature then at least in its aims and technical status; and this change can be viewed positively (as the final achievement by machines of the synthesis of labor and happiness on the basis of reason) or negatively, or even apocalyptically, if we share a common and more disturbing viewpoint. The fundamental point, as I have said, concerns the loss of technical knowledge and dignity which accompanies industrialization. Craftsmen had to serve a long apprenticeship before they were masters of their tools; they almost had to come to love them and, without getting bogged down in some convenient myth of tradeguild brotherhoods, they had to share their knowledge in order to secure it and their stake in it. Early forms of manufacture still implied a similar investment, for the most part. But as soon as you start from the principle that a worker's profitability depends on the degree of monotony and fragmentation of his job, and on his lack of understanding of the machine and the technological environment in which he moves (save for certain fixed and inflexible orders and rules), then these relationships are reversed. In the name of the great god profit, the machine symbolically takes back that share of knowledge which the worker is cheated of, and uses it – to employ an anthropomorphic image – to achieve a greater degree of independence, freedom and, in the long run, of automatism.

The Third Type of World. We can thus understand, though in no sense condone, the way in which technical culture and education have been profoundly affected by this delegation of competence. Such a tendency corresponds to "Heideggerian" angst about the hegemony of technology. Yet reality bears only the most approximate similarity to this schema. The industrial environment turns out, in actuality, to be extremely varied and diverse, up to the finest urban and manufacturing utopias. This is not inevitable, unless we pose the question at a deeper level where it has to do with the very being of the automaton, its perpetual oscillation between contingency and necessity, the haunting illusion it gives rise to of an artificial, material object which is capable, situated as it is at the limits of reason, of giving us access to this "third type of world" in which we wander.

The Automaton and Death. The automaton is both individual and totality, the extreme of artifice and an image of recreated, revitalized nature. During the period we have been examining it is the most singular and yet the most universal of beings. That is, it has a quality which embodies its power of mythical suggestiveness as much as its inexorable utopias; a quality of maintaining a special relationship with death — which is itself the most singular and most contingent moment of our lives, yet also the most universal, the one we know we cannot escape. It will return us, despite all the tricks and artifices of medicine or religion or anything else, to the cosmic clay from which we came. Universal and unique like death, both the one and the other: in this ambiguous finality lies the form of the automaton's own paradox, and the key to the general paradox of technology.

The Death Drive. The Renaissance Engineer, in Gille's sense, is the first who can properly be said to have conceived and constructed automata worthy of the name. But that complex and multifaceted individual — artist, architect, town-planner, utopian, physicist, mathematician and philosopher — was first and foremost a man of war. The machines he prepared for his prince were machines for killing; mobility, speed and camouflage belong with the arts of war that lie concentrated within the sequence of automata; later, while Don Juan counts the women and the moments of life still left to him, the powder factory of the salons merely shifted the grounds of the argument, while still resisting industrial progress. It is rather as the nineteenth century draws to a close that repetition finds a medical representation in the world of Charcot, Régis and Dubourdieu which is comparable to Zola's night: the vagabond is defined as an "ambulant automaton," social rejects, prostitutes and celibates as "degenerate dromomaniacs." Freud, who for a time was a pupil of Charcot, never forgot these shadowy figures. Although his whole conception of the unconscious was an attempt to replace these walking corpses with a symbolic force, they return with the "death drive," that ambiguous but disturbing diagnosis of our culture.

The Theater of Shadows. The moving figures were, of course, created as part of positive experiments: the human body, opened by Vesalius, finds a model in Cartesian mechanism and its extensions which medicine uses, sometimes to its advantage. When we come to Boerhaave, Borelli and particularly La Mettrie, the automaton rediscovers man and nature and slips between the two concepts as a recip-rocal reproach. Vaucanson creates a flute-player, a Provençal pipe-player and the duck, which earn him plentiful applause; the digestive mechanism in particular is copied schematically but effectively. And he doesn't stop there, but sets up facto-ries that anticipate the industrial automatism to come, the first real application of which will be to textile manufacture. In this rich, transitional period life and death are intertwined, as in tragedy: but Sophocles and Shakespeare are no longer pulling the strings, which have been taken over by engineer-inventors, scientists and automaticians, anxious about a nature that proffers them pitfalls and a life they know to be uncertain. The guillotine awaits its hour, as do massacres on a new and differ-ent scale. Today, man is still seeking to swim better, to run more quickly, to team up with a machine that, as de Sade shows, may embody more than a whiff of death. Yet people still take time out to dream of possessing perpetual motion, or of man flying, in Da Vinci's sense. Shadow and light. Automatism, in all its varied modes, is a demonstration that death is only the other side of life.

Translated by Ian Patterson.

Society Against the State
Essays in Political Anthropology by Pierre Clastres
$18.95 cloth, 218 pages

Foucault/Blanchot
Maurice Blanchot: The Thought From Outside by Michel Foucault
Michel Foucault as I Imagine Him by Maurice Blanchot
$16.95 cloth, 109 pages

Your Money or Your Life
Economy and Religion in the Middle Ages by Jacques Le Goff
$18.95 cloth, 116 pages

ZONE BOOKS

Matter and Memory by Henri Bergson
$21.95 cloth, 284 pages

Mitra-Varuna by Georges Dumézil
$21.95, 189 pages

Bergsonism by Gilles Deleuze
$19.95 cloth, 131 pages

The Accursed Share Volume I by Georges Bataille
$20.95 cloth, 197 pages

Theory of Religion by Georges Bataille
$17.95 cloth, 110 pages

Myth and Tragedy in Ancient Greece by Jean-Pierre Vernant and Pierre Vidal-Naquet
$28.95 cloth, 528 pages

Myth and Society in Ancient Greece by Jean-Pierre Vernant
$22.95 cloth, 280 pages

Zone 1/2: The Contemporary City
$20.00 paper, 480 pages

ZONE BOOKS
611 Broadway, Suite 838
New York, New York 10012

Zone 3: Fragments for a History of the Human Body, Part I
$19.95 paper, $37.95 cloth, 500 pages

Zone 4: Fragments for a History of the Human Body, Part II
$19.95 paper, $37.95 cloth, 576 pages

Zone 5: Fragments for a History of the Human Body, Part III
$19.95 paper, $37.95 cloth, 584 pages

Zone Books are distributed by The MIT Press, 55 Hayward Street, Cambridge, MA 02142

Subscribe today and engage in the latest critical discussion
of contemporary design culture.

assemblage

A Critical Journal of Architecture and Design Culture

K. Michael Hays, Editor
Alicia Kennedy, Executive Editor

Assemblage is an advanced journal of architectural theory and
criticism brought to bear on contemporary practice. Provocative,
polemical, and exploratory, *Assemblage* examines the
interrelationships between culture and design, between theory
and material reality.

Each extensively illustrated issue presents essays, projects,
and debates by leading and emerging scholars, theorists,
and practitioners. Work is drawn from a wide range of fields:
architectural and art history and theory, literary criticism,
philosophy, politics, and psychoanalysis.

Contributors to *Assemblage* include Micha Bandini, Eve Blau,
Yve-Alain Bois, Jean-Louis Cohen, Elizabeth Diller, Peter
Eisenman, Robin Evans, Mario Gandelsonas, Raphael Moneo,
Carlo Olmo, José Quetglas, Franco Rella, Alvaro Siza, Mark C.
Taylor, Georges Teyssot, and Anthony Vidler.

Published three times a year by the MIT Press, February, June,
and October. Founded 1986. ISSN 0889-3012.

MIT Press Journals
55 Hayward Street, Cambridge, MA 02142

Order Form

Yes! Please begin my one-year subscription (3 issues)
to *Assemblage.*

Year rates:

Individual $40.00
Institutional $65.00
Student $30.00
(photocopy of ID required)

Outside of U.S. and Canada add $9.00 surface mail or
$17.00 airmail postage.

Name

Address

City/State/Zip

____ Amount enclosed $ _____ or
____ Please charge my:
 ____ Visa or ____ MasterCard

Account # _____

Expiration date _____

Signature _____

Mail to:
MIT Press Journals
55 Hayward Street
Cambridge, MA 02142 USA
For credit card orders call
617-253-2889 M-F, 9–5

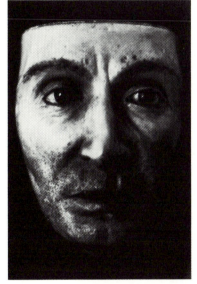
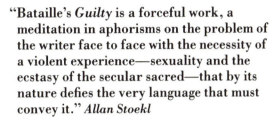

© COPYRIGHT

The journal of criticism encircled:
a tracing and exposing of networks of
knowledge, politics, gender, art, design,
and theory in contemporary culture.

FIN DE SIÈCLE 2000

Some of the artistic, political, and philosophical questions being raised as we
close out the second millennium.

Heidi Gilpin
Alice Jardine
Brian Massumi
R. E. Somol
Editors

Frances Bartkowski — Rosi Braidotti
Peter Canning — Thomas Hatch — Jeanne Hyvrard
Alice Jardine — Julia Kristeva — Richard Ledes
Rhonda Lieberman — Jean-François Lyotard
Brian Massumi — Chandra Talpade Mohanty
Toni Negri — R. E. Somol — Simon Watney

TECHNOBODY

Intersections of technology as political
technique and as *mēkhanē*: their combined effects on the body (as flesh)
and the polis (as ethics).

FUTURE ISSUES
COPYRIGHT 3
FEAR
COPYRIGHT 4
TOURISM

Single issues cost $7. Subscriptions (two issues) cost $13
for individuals (prepaid only) and $26 for institutions.

Outside the U.S. and Canada, add $2.00 (surface
mail) or $7.50 (air mail) per issue. Make checks or money
orders payable in U.S. funds to *COPYRIGHT*. Send your
name and complete address to:

Copyright, Center for Literary Studies, Harvard University,
61 Kirkland Street, Cambridge, Massachusetts 02138

Inquiries and submissions are welcome.

IMPULSE

MAGAZINE

THE ILLUSION OF CONTROL

16 SKEY LANE TORONTO, CANADA M6J 3S4 (416) 537-9551

Number 14: "Sexuality and the Social Body in the Nineteenth Century," edited by Catherine Gallagher and Thomas Laqueur, with contributions by Londa Schiebinger, Mary Poovey, D.A. Miller, Laura Engelstein, Christine Buci-Glucksmann, Alain Corbin, and the editors.

Number 17: "The Cultural Display of the Body," with contributions by Terry Castle, Glenn Harcourt, Luke Wilson, Peter Metcalf, Eve Kosofsky Sedgwick, and Harry Berger, Jr.

Number 20: "Misogyny, Misandry, and Misanthropy," edited by R. Howard Bloch and Frances Ferguson, with contributions by Joel Fineman, Jacqueline Lichtenstein, Naomi Schor, Gillian Brown, Charles Bernheimer, Carol J. Clover and the editors.

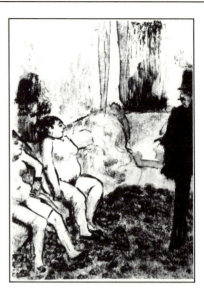

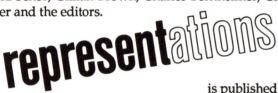

is published quarterly by the University of California Press. Special Issues: $8.00 each. Annual subscriptions: $22.00 individuals, $44.00 institutions. Send orders to: University of California Press, Journals Dept., 2120 Berkeley Way, Berkeley, California 94720 USA

Examine the central cultural issues of our times . . .

Art | *Theory* | *Criticism* | *Politics*

OCTOBER

Joan Copjec, Douglas Crimp, Rosalind Krauss and Annette Michelson, Editors   Published by the MIT Press

"OCTOBER is among the most advanced journals of the 1970s and 1980s in the fields of art theory, criticism, history and practice . . . . Few, if any, journals could receive a higher recommendation." – **Choice**

Recent special issues include the work of the late Belgian artist, Marcel Broodthaers, a cultural analysis of the AIDS epidemic, and German filmmaker Alexander Kluge. You'll find provocative and stimulating criticism – the most significant texts by and about leading contemporary artists, scholars, and critics – in each issue of OCTOBER.

Subscribe today and enrich your knowledge of the most important issues in the contemporary arts.

Yearly rates (4 issues):		Outside USA and	Mail to:
Individual	$25.00	Canada add:	**MIT Press Journals**
Institution	$55.00	$9.00 surface mail	55 Hayward Street
Student & Retired	$20.00	$17.00 airmail	Cambridge, MA 02142 USA
(photocopy of ID required)			For credit card orders call:
			617-253-2889 (M–F, 9–5)

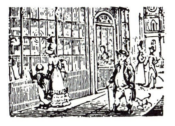
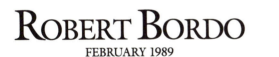
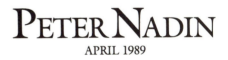
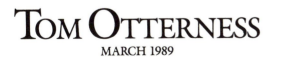
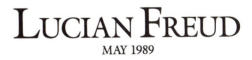

John Cage

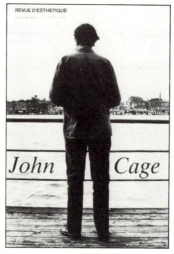

«Déconcertante» pour le grand public, la musique de John Cage est indissociable d'une **œuvre** : technique voire technologique, théorique, critique, graphique même. A tel point qu'un dialogue se perpétue à travers elle, depuis de nombreuses années, dans lequel sont impliquées les plus grandes voix de la philosophie, de la littérature, de l'esthétique et, bien évidemment, de la musique elle-même. La contribution de plusieurs artistes et penseurs japonais à ce numéro exceptionnel confirme le caractère «planétaire» de la démarche. John Cage, par ailleurs, donne ici plusieurs contributions inédites, textes, interviews, dessins et gravures.

REVUE D'ESTHETIQUE - Nouvelle série n° 13-14-15

1 vol., 580 pages dont 82 illustrations - 380 F

Le temps de la réflexion

Série dirigée par J.-B. Pontalis

IX

De la bêtise et des bêtes

SOMMAIRE

GALLIMARD nrf

Seminary Co-op Bookstore

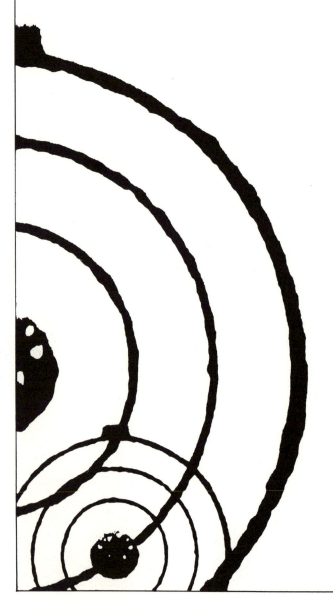

CRITICAL

HISTORICAL

PHILOSOPHICAL

5757 University
Chicago, Il 60637
(800) 777·1456

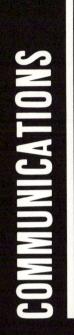

ISSN 0588-8018

COMMUNICATIONS

ÉCOLE DES HAUTES ÉTUDES EN SCIENCES SOCIALES · CENTRE D'ÉTUDES TRANSDISCIPLINAIRES
(SOCIOLOGIE. ANTHROPOLOGIE. POLITIQUE)

Variations
sur le thème

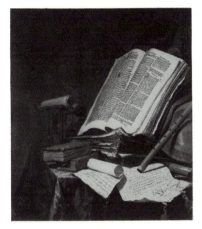

47

1988/Seuil

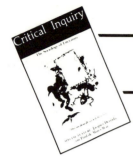

TELOS

A Quarterly Journal of Critical Thought

Since its first issue in May 1968, *Telos* has introduced into the English-speaking world the best trends in continental radical thought. Commited to the development of an *American* version of Critical Theory unencumbered by conformist communication theory or Freudianism, *Telos* continues to focus on international issues and, increasingly, on a critical analysis of American society.

ISSUE No. 76   SUMMER 1988

Subscriptions cost $24 per year (four issues) for individuals; $60 for institutions. Foreign orders add 10%. Checks must be in US funds. No Canadian checks will be accepted. Back issues are $7 each (institutions pay $15). Back issues available: 13, 17-76. For subscription, back issues or information, write:

Telos Press Ltd., 431 E. 12th Street, New York N.Y. 10009

Carl Andre
Jennifer Bartlett
Lynda Benglis
Jonathan Borofsky
Peter Campus
Robert Gober
Robert Grosvenor
Michael Hurson
Donald Judd
Robert Mangold
Elizabeth Murray
Joel Shapiro
Alan Shields
The Estate of Tony Smith
Robert Wilson
Jackie Winsor

Paula Cooper Gallery

155 Wooster Street New York 212 674.0766

CONTEMPORARY IMAGES

The Hidden Image
Photographs of the Male Nude in the Nineteenth and Twentieth Centuries
Peter Weiermair
translated by Claus Nielander
From the earliest daguerreotype of Hippolyte Bayard to the formalized fantasies of Robert Mapplethorpe, this is a stunning anthology of the changing iconography of the male nude and of the repression, the sublimation, and the taboos surrounding the depiction of the male body.
132 illustrations, 10 in color $45.00

Bestiarium
The Theatre Garden
Exhibition as Fiction
edited by Chris Dercon
Documents an extraordinary theatre garden created in 1988 by sixteen international artists. Distributed for the P.S. 1 Museum.
150 illustrations, color $25.00 paper

Blasted Allegories
An Anthology of Writings by Contemporary Artists
edited by Brian Wallis
The best writings (by such artists as Laurie Anderson, Richard Prince, and William Wegman) that record and interpret contemporary art and society over the last decade. Copublished with The New Museum of Contemporary Art, New York.
Illustrated $19.95

October
The First Decade
edited by Annette Michelson, Rosalind Krauss, Douglas Crimp, and Joan Copjec
A selection of some of the most important and representative texts, many from issues long out of print, that have appeared in OCTOBER, one of the foremost journals in art criticism and theory.
174 illustrations $24.95

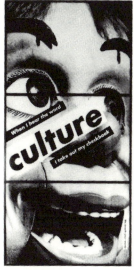

Barbara Kruger, Untitled, 1985 from *Modern Dreams: The Rise and Fall and Rise of Pop*

Modern Dreams
The Rise and Fall and Rise of Pop
edited by Brian Wallis, Tom Finkelpearl, Patricia Phillips, Glenn Weiss, and Thomas Lawson
Including essays by Reyner Banham, Kenneth Frampton, Leo Castelli, Claes Oldenburg, and Roy Lichtenstein, *Modern Dreams* explores the distinction between the pop art culture of London in the fifties and the conceptually related work of New York in the eighties. Distributed for the P.S. 1 Museum.
170 illustrations, 16 in color $25.00 paper

The Sphere and the Labyrinth
Avant-Gardes and Architecture from Piranesi to the 1970s
Manfredo Tafuri
translated by Pellegrino d'Acierno and Robert Connolly
Manfredo Tafuri presents his critique of traditional approaches to historical investigation and criticism, dismantling and reassembling the structure of the ideology of the avant-garde.
365 illustrations $39.95

Available at fine bookstores or directly from

The MIT Press

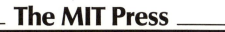

55 Hayward Street • Cambridge, MA 02142